Tetrahedrally Bonded Amorphous Semiconductors
(Carefree, Arizona, 1981)

AIP Conference Proceedings
Series Editor: Hugh C. Wolfe
Number 73

Tetrahedrally Bonded Amorphous Semiconductors

(Carefree, Arizona, 1981)

Editors
R.A. Street, D.K. Biegelsen, J.C. Knights
Xerox Palo Alto Research Center

American Institute of Physics
New York   1981

L.C. Catalog Card No. 81-67419
ISBN 0–88318–172–X
DOE CONF- 810331

PREFACE

A topical conference on Tetrahedrally Bonded Amorphous Semi-conductors was held at the Carefree Inn, Carefree, Arizona, from the 12th to the 14th of March, 1981. The conference was sponsored by the American Physical Society, with financial support from the Solar Energy Research Institute, Xerox Corporation and the National Science Foundation. The conference concentrated on the basic physics of hydrogenated amorphous silicon, and was organized in response to the rapidly growing interest in the technological applications of this material.

The Organizing Committee consisted of: D. K. Biegelesen (Xerox); M. H. Brodsky (IBM); D. Carlson (RCA); H. Fritzsche (University of Chicago); J. Joannopoulos (MIT); J. C. Knights (Xerox); G. Lucovsky (North Carolina State University); W. Paul (Harvard); B. Seraphin (University of Arizona); J. Stone (SERI); R. A. Street (Xerox), conference chairman; J. Tauc (Brown University); P. C. Taylor (NRL). The members of the International Advisory Committee were: I. Solomon (France); W. Spear (UK); J. Stuke (W. Germany); K. Tanaka (Japan). The Program Committee comprised D. Carlson (RCA); H. Fritzsche (University of Chicago); G. Lucovsky (North Carolina State University); R. A. Street (Xerox), chairman; P. C. Taylor (NRL).

These proceedings have been organized into chapters which reflect the range of interest of the submitted papers:

> Growth and Characterization of Films
> Atomic Structure and Bonding
> Electron States
> Electronic Transport
> Absorption and Recombination
> Surfaces and Interfaces

We are grateful to Violet Moffat, Erin Schreiner and Marilyn Tenney for their assistance in the organization of the conference and in the preparation of the proceedings. Our thanks also go to the projectionist, John Gill, and to the Carefree Inn and its staff for their contribution to the success of the conference.

> R. A. Street
> D. K. Biegelsen
> J. C. Knights
>
> Palo Alto, California
> April, 1981

TABLE OF CONTENTS

PREFACE

CHAPTER I: Growth and Characterization of Films

CHAPTER II: Atomic Structure and Bonding

CHAPTER III: Electronic Structure

CHAPTER V: Absorption and Recombination

OPTICAL EMISSION STUDIES OF
REACTIVE SPECIES IN PLASMA DEPOSITION*

F. J. Kampas and R. W. Griffith
Brookhaven National Laboratory
Upton, NY 11973

ABSTRACT

Optical emission studies of the glow-discharge deposition of
a-Si:H alloys reveal the presence of reactive species derived from
process gases and impurities. Studies of the dependences of emission
intensities upon deposition parameters elucidate the mechanisms of formation of these species. Effects of impurities detected by emission
spectroscopy upon a-Si:H film electronic properties are discussed. A
model of the chemical reactions involved in film growth is presented.

INTRODUCTION

Although the plasma deposition of a-Si:H is now common practice,
the chemical reactions involved in film growth are not well understood. The two techniques commonly used for studying the chemistry
of a-Si:H film deposition are optical emission spectroscopy and mass
spectrometry. In this paper we shall discuss the results of studies
of the optical emission from silane and disilane glow discharges and
also speculate about the nature of the chemical reactions responsible
for a-Si:H film growth.

RESULTS AND DISCUSSION

We have studied the silane glow discharge in great detail. In
this section we summarize results which are presented more completely
elsewhere.[1,2] The species observed in emission from the silane glow
discharge are Si, SiH, H, and H_2. The potentially important species
SiH_2 and SiH_3 have no known emission spectrum. In order to determine
the origin of the emitting species we studied the power dependences
of the emission intensities of the four species along with a small
amount of added N_2.[3] The emission intensities of Si, SiH, H, and H_2
varied as the 0.84, 0.78, 1.92, and 1.85 power of the N_2 emission intensity over a range of 10-100 W rf power. It was concluded that the
emitting excited states of Si and SiH are produced by one electron-
impact excitation, whereas the emitting excited states of H and H_2
require two electron-impact excitations. The following set of
energetically reasonable reactions is consistent with that conclusion:

$$e^- + SiH_4 \rightarrow SiH_4^* + e^- \tag{1}$$

*Work performed under the auspices of the U.S. Department of Energy
under Contract No. DE-AC02-76CH00016.

$$SiH_4^* \rightarrow Si^* + 2H_2 \qquad (2)$$

$$SiH_4^* \rightarrow SiH^* + H_2 + H \quad . \qquad (3)$$

The excited states Si^* and SiH^* emit the detected photons. However, the excited states H^* and H_2^* require another electron-impact excitation for their production. The anomalously high rotational and vibrational temperatures calculated from the SiH emission spectrum are explained by this mechanism.

A study of the photolysis of silane by 8.4 eV photons indicated that the primary products of silane photolysis are SiH_2 and SiH_3.[4] While these species were not detected directly, higher silanes produced by subsequent reactions were detected mass spectrometrically. That study is not inconsistent with our own work. The reactions given in Eqs. 2 and 3 may account for only a small part of the glow discharge decomposition of silane.

The emission spectrum of a <u>disilane</u> discharge also reveals the presence of Si, SiH, H, and H_2. The Si and SiH emission intensities are approximately one-tenth of their values for a monosilane discharge at the same pressure and rf power. The emission from H_2 and H are reduced by a similar factor compared to a monosilane discharge despite the fact that the deposition from disilane occurred at five times the rate as the deposition from monosilane. These facts imply that monosilane is a product of the disilane discharge. This supports the hypothesis of the IBM group[5] that the electron-impact dissociation of disilane proceeds in the following way:

$$e^- + Si_2H_6 \rightarrow SiH_2 + SiH_4 + e^- \quad . \qquad (4)$$

The fact that a-Si:H can be doped by the addition of PH_3 and B_2H_6 to the silane is central to photovoltaic applications. An understanding of the chemical reactions involved in doping would be useful for optimizing doping efficiency and reducing the number of defect states introduced in doping. We have found the species PH_2, PH, and P in the emission spectrum of a mixture of 1% PH_3 in SiH_4. See Figs. 1 and 2.

In studying the electronic properties of any material one must consider the unavoidable presence of impurities. We have described[2] at some length the synergistic doping effect of N_2 and O_2 in the plasma, as might be introduced by a small leak in the deposition system. Small air leaks can be detected quite easily by the emission from N_2. Sensitivities for N_2 of 100 ppm in the silane are easily obtainable. When oxygen concentrations ~0.1% are reached, emission from SiO appears in the spectrum.[1]

Another source of impurities is the process gas. A common impurity in silane is monochlorosilane (SiH_3Cl). We found that 1000 ppm SiH_3Cl in silane can result in a displacement of the Fermi level ~0.2 eV downward in the bandgap of the deposited film. This concentration of SiH_3Cl is easily detectable as emission from SiCl (281 nm) and results in 600 ppm incorporated Cl.

Outgassing of the deposition system is a third source of impurities. Emission from the species OH, CO, and N_2 is seen during an

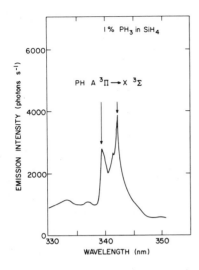

Fig. 1. Emission from PH in a 1% mixture of PH₃ in SiH₄.

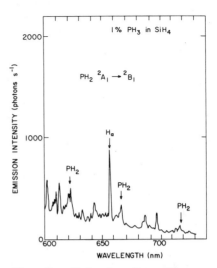

Fig. 2. Emission from PH₂. Bands not marked are due to H₂.

argon discharge used to clean the substrates. These species arise from H_2O, CO, and N_2 adsorbed onto the electrodes and chamber.

Metallic impurities are potentially very deleterious to the electronic properties of semiconductors. The argon cleaning discharge mentioned earlier shows emission from Mg and Zn when the substrate temperature is about 350 C. Emission from Zn is seen also in the silane discharge under these conditions. However, SIMS analysis of the deposited films show less than 0.2 ppm of Zn in the film bulk, 0.2 ppm being the sensitivity of the SIMS measurement. Thus emission spectroscopy of the discharge is more sensitive than SIMS for detecting Zn.

We turn now to the question of the chemical species involved in the growth of the a-Si:H film. Knights has stated that the species involved in film growth are probably SiH_2 and SiH_3.[6] As stated earlier, the reaction given in Eq. 4 has been advanced to explain the higher deposition rate in a disilane glow discharge. A rapid surface reaction was postulated to account for the fact that a-Si:H films have a smaller H to Si ratio than SiH_2, and the following reaction was proposed:[5]

$$SiH_2(g) \rightarrow SiH_x(s) + SiH_4(g) + H_2(g) \quad . \tag{5}$$

Lampe has proposed the following gas-phase reaction to explain results obtained in the photolysis of silane:[4]

$$SiH_2 + SiH_4 \rightarrow Si_2H_6^* \rightarrow Si_2H_6 \tag{6}$$

$$\rightarrow H_2 + SiH_3SiH \tag{7}$$

The species $Si_2H_6^*$ is a disilane molecule with an internal activation energy of 2.1 eV. We propose that hydrogen elimination during film deposition occurs through an analogous reaction:

$$SiH_2(g) + Si_xH_y(s) \xrightarrow{r_d} Si_{x+1}H^*_{y+2}(s) \xrightarrow{r_1} Si_{x+1}H_{y+2}(s) \qquad (8)$$

$$\xrightarrow{r_2} Si_{x+1}H_y(s) + H_2(g) \qquad (9)$$

The quantities r_d, r_1, and r_2 are the rates of the deposition, deactivation, and hydrogen elimination reactions, respectively. The ratio of the rates, r_2/r_1, can be calculated from the atomic hydrogen content of the film, c_H:

$$r_2/r_1 = 2c_H^{-1} - 3 \qquad (10)$$

This result follows from the fact that the film gains $r_1 + r_2$ silicon atoms per second but gains only $2r_1$ hydrogen atoms per second. An Arhennius plot of r_2/r_1 versus $1000/T_s$, where T_s is the substrate temperature, should give the difference in activation energy between the two rates. In Fig. 3 we have made such a plot using values of hydrogen concentration versus T_s taken from the literature.[7,8] The points fall close to straight lines for T_s less than 300 C. At 300 C, other mechanisms of hydrogen elimination, such as those that occur in the annealing of already deposited films, become important.

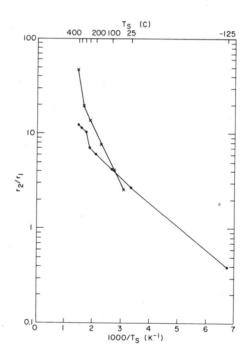

Fig. 3. Plot of log r_2/r_1 versus $1000/T_s$. o ref. 7; x ref. 8.

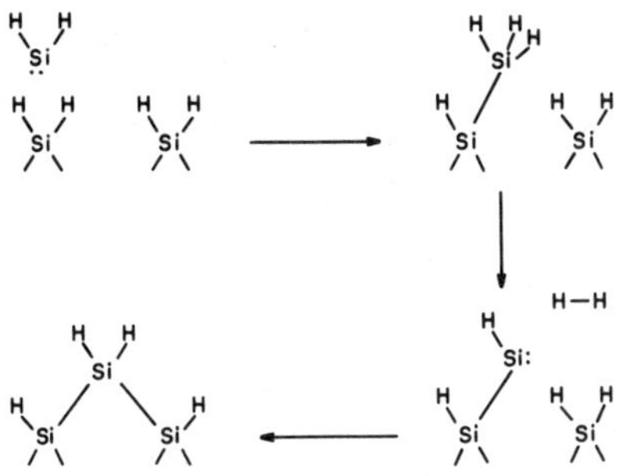

Fig. 4. Proposed mechanism of film growth, hydrogen elimination and cross-linking at film surface.

A model with SiH_4 elimination was also investigated using a set of equations analogous to Eqs. 8 and 9. In that case, straight lines were not obtained. The fact that straight lines were obtained from Eqs. 8 and 9 encouraged us sufficiently to consider the chemistry of the cross-linking step, which must follow hydrogen elimination. We propose that the divalent silicon atom resulting from hydrogen elimination inserts across a nearby Si-H bond, a well-known reaction.[9] The entire mechanism is shown in Fig. 4. The model we have presented is incomplete in that is does not explain the effect of electrode bias upon hydrogen content. Work on that problem is in progress.

REFERENCES

1. F. J. Kampas and R. W. Griffith, Solar Cells 2, 385 (1980).
2. R. W. Griffith, F. J. Kampas, P. E. Vanier, and M. D. Hirsch, J. Non-Cryst. Solids 35/36, 391 (1980).
3. F. J. Kampas and R. W. Griffith, J. Appl. Phys. in press.
4. G. G. A. Perkins, E. R. Austin, and F. W. Lampe, J. Am. Chem. Soc. 101, 1109 (1979).
5. B. A. Scott, M. H. Brodsky, D. C. Green, P. B. Kirby, R. M. Plecnik, and E. E. Simonyi, Appl. Phys. Lett. 37, 725 (1980).
6. J. C. Knights, J. Non-Cryst. Solids 35/36, 159 (1980).
7. J. C. Knights, G. Lucovsky, and R. J. Nemanich, J. Non-Cryst. Solids 32, 393 (1979).
8. M. Milleville, W. Fuhs, F. J. Demond, H. Mannsperger, G. Muller, and S. Kalbitzer, Appl. Phys. Lett. 34, 173 (1979).
9. I. M. T. Davidson, Quart. Rev. Chem. Soc. 25, 111 (1971).

DEPOSITION AND DOPING OF a-Si:H FROM Si$_2$H$_6$ PLASMAS

B. A. Scott, M. H. Brodsky, D. C. Green, R. M. Plecenik, E. E. Simonyi and R. Serino

IBM T. J. Watson Research Center, Yorktown Heights, NY 10598

ABSTRACT

Compared to SiH$_4$, the plasma deposition of amorphous hydrogenated silicon from Si$_2$H$_6$ results in compositionally similar films, deposited at rates at least an order of magnitude higher. The films also display larger dark and photoconductivities, a result related directly to higher E$_f$ in the intrinsic Si$_2$H$_6$-prepared material. The effect is structural, not impurity-dominated. Dopant incorporation is also found to be strongly influenced by the silicon source, as is the doping efficiency. For a given gas phase concentration of n-type dopant (PH$_3$), the distribution coefficient is C$_{eff}$<1 for Si$_2$H$_6$ plasmas, compared to C$_{eff}$>1 for depositions from SiH$_4$, yet film electrical properties are comparable. On the p-type side, much smaller differences are observed with B$_2$H$_6$ doping of the two sources. Finally, a-Si:H plasma deposition chemistry is examined within the context of a neutral radical model and hydrogen etching experiments.

INTRODUCTION

The use of higher silanes for various CVD silicon processes offers potential advantages over SiH$_4$, including higher deposition rates and/or lower temperature growth. This is related to the lower stability of the higher hydrides, due more to kinetic[1] than thermodynamic factors. We have been investigating the deposition of amorphous hydrogenated silicon (a-Si:H) by plasma decomposition of higher silanes to determine whether the resulting compositional, structural and transport properties differ from SiH$_4$-deposited material. In addition, studies using such source compounds can lead to insight concerning the important chemical mechanistic questions of a-Si:H film growth[2,3].

FILM PREPARATION

Disilane was synthesized by the reduction of hexachlorodisilane with LiAlH$_4$, using a modification of the method reported by Bethke and Wilson[4]. Small quantities of Si$_2$H$_6$ were also synthesized by the electric discharge technique for comparison purposes[5]. Since Si$_2$H$_6$ boils at 259 K, purification was performed in a series of low temperature distillation steps, followed by analysis using gas chromatography/mass spectroscopy[5]. Purities >99.9% were obtained exclusive of higher silanes, which are always present at ~ 1% levels. Depositions were carried out in an inductively-coupled plasma apparatus described elsewhere[6].

INTRINSIC a-Si:H

In earlier work[2] we found two major differences between disilane- and monosilane-prepared films. First, deposition from Si$_2$H$_6$ occurs at rates over an order of magnitude larger than those obtained with SiH$_4$ under comparable conditions. Secondly, we have consistently observed higher dark and AM1 photoconductivities in Si$_2$H$_6$-prepared films (substrate temperature T$_s$=300°C). In a subsequent section we examine possible mechanistic reasons for the deposition rates observed from SiH$_4$ and Si$_2$H$_6$. The difference in transport properties can be ascribed to the results shown in Fig. 1. Here the activation energies for intrinsic Si$_2$H$_6$-deposited films generally fall below those of SiH$_4$-prepared films deposited at the same T$_s$. This would make E$_c$-E$_F$ smaller and thus E$_F$ lies higher in

ISSN:0094-243X/81/730006-04$1.50 Copyright 1981 American Institute of Physics

the gap. Using the Anderson-Spear model[7], a higher E_F implies a lower number of positively-charged recombination centers.

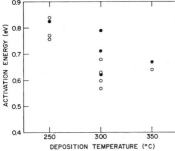

Fig. 1: Dark conductivity activation energy for SiH_4 (●) and Si_2H_6 (○) deposited films.

Although greater E_F could be due to n-type impurities, we have carried out extensive chemical analysis by electron microprobe on the film series shown in Table I. Impurities such a P and As were not observed. Their electrical effects on a-Si:H are known to occur at levels well within microprobe sensitivity limits. We find, in fact, that where non-neglible amounts of impurities are present, photoconductivity is lowest. Si_2H_6-prepared samples with the lowest inpurity levels show the greatest enhancements over SiH_4-deposited material. Hence, we conclude that there exist subtle but nevertheless real structural differences leading to the somewhat higher photoconductivities observed for Si_2H_6-prepared films.

Table I. COMPARISON OF DISILANE-PREPARED INTRINSIC a-Si(H) FILMS[†]

Sample	Log(ohm•cm)			ΔE_{dark} (eV)	ΔE_{pc} (eV)	Comments
	ρ_{pc}	ρ_{dark}	ρ_0			
507(2.0)	3.37	6.77	−3.97	0.63	0.15	Si_2H_6 from electric discharge
659(1.2)	3.65	6.33	−3.25	0.57	0.13	Oxygen <200 ppm Chlorine <60 ppm
509(2.0)	3.85	7.73	−3.73	0.68	0.16	Si_2H_6 from electric discharge
704(1.2)	4.35	7.78	−2.48	0.60	0.12	Oxygen 800 ppm; Chlorine 70 ppm

[†]Substrate temperature 300°C; r.f. power given in ( )

DOPED a-Si:H

A detailed series of experiments were carried out with n- and p-type dopants PH_3, AsH_3 and B_2H_6 mixed into the SiH_4 and Si_2H_6 source gases. The main results of this study are illustrated in Table II, where the room temperature conductivity is presented for a series of monosilane and disilane films prepared under identical plasma conditions at a gas phase doping ratio $(N_{dopant}/N_{Si})_{gas} = 1\%$. Also shown is the dopant/Si ratio in the solid and the distribution coefficient, C_{eff}[8]. For the n-type dopants we have the following significant results. Although there is little difference between the room temperature conductivities of SiH_4- and Si_2H_6-prepared films using PH_3, the actual amount of phosphorus incorporated in each case differs significantly. Over an order of magnitude more phosphorus must be incorporated in the SiH_4-prepared films to attain a comparable conductivity. The doping efficiency is therefore much less for n-doped SiH_4-deposited films. An even lower doping efficiency is observed for AsH_3/SiH_4. The conductivity is nearly two orders of magnitude poorer, yet films show the largest actual incorporation of n-type dopant. On the other hand, essentially the opposite result is observed for B_2H_6-doping: comparably high conductivities are achieved with somewhat less boron actually incorporated in SiH_4-deposited a-Si:H. Note that with neither source gas are dark conductivities above 10^{-2} $(\Omega\text{-cm})^{-1}$ attained on the n- or p-doped side.

Table II. Doping Parameters (1 at % gas phase level)

Gas	Dopant	$(N_{dopant}/N_{Si})_{solid}$	C_{eff}	$\log \sigma_{RT}$ $(\Omega\text{-cm})^{-1}$
SiH_4	AsH_3	0.055	5.5	-4.6
SiH_4	PH_3	0.034	3.4	-2.6
Si_2H_6	PH_3	0.0025	0.25	-2.6
SiH_4	B_2H_6*	0.0032	0.16	-3.6
Si_2H_6	B_2H_6	0.0054	0.54	-3.5

* Gas concentration 2 at %

The results of Table II can be very simply explained for the n-doped depositions if it is recalled that a-Si:H formation from Si_2H_6 occurs at more than an order of magnitude greater rate than that from SiH_4. Hence, phosphorus deposition from PH_3 occurs independently of silicon deposition from SiH_4 and Si_2H_6, because for phosphorus the ratio $C_{eff}(Si_2H_6)/C_{eff}(SiH_4) \approx 14$ reflects the ratio of deposition rates. On the p-doped side, however, C_{eff} does not scale in this way, and we surmise that appreciable interaction occurs in the gas phase between B_2H_6 and both SiH_4 and Si_2H_6.

DEPOSITION CHEMISTRY

In previous studies[2] we suggested that the plasma decomposition modes of both SiH_4 and Si_2H_6 might parallel their thermolysis chemistries, but with diminished kinetic barriers. The initial and rate determining step in the thermal decomposition chemistries can be written[1,9]:

$$SiH_4 \rightarrow SiH_2 + H_2 \qquad (1)$$

$$Si_2H_6 \rightarrow SiH_2 + SiH_4, \qquad (2)$$

where the rates are about two orders of magnitude higher for reaction (2) at 400°C, for example. Therefore, the a-Si:H deposition velocity enhancements observed from Si_2H_6 plasmas could be attributed to either the higher rate of SiH_2 formation and/or the presence of plasma-generated hydrogen, which might increase the velocity of back reaction (etching) in the SiH_4 case. To test the latter hypothesis, we carried out a series of SiH_4/H_2 depositions in an attempt to influence the rate. The results are shown in Table III along with those of experiments in which a hydrogen plasma was generated after film growth to determine the etch rate of a-Si:H in the absence of SiH_4. Table III indicates that film etching by H_2 (i.e., the reverse of eq. (1)) is not a significant factor in the lower deposition rate observed in SiH_4 plasmas at low r.f. power levels. We therefore conclude, assuming our analogy with silicon hydride thermolysis chemistry is correct, that the greater rate of homogeneous SiH_2 production could explain the higher a-Si:H deposition rates obtained with Si_2H_6.

ACKNOWLEDGMENT

We wish to thank J. Kuptsis and W. Reuter for carrying out film analysis by electron microprobe and SIMS. This work was partially supported by SERI subcontract ZZ-0-9319.

Table III. FILM DEPOSITION AND ETCHING EXPERIMENTS*

GAS COMP.	FLOW RATE scc/min	PRESSURE Torr	GROWTH RATE A/sec
SiH_4	3	0.1	0.35
$SiH_4 + H_2$	6	0.1	0.32
$SiH_4 + H_2$	6	0.2	0.31
H_2	3	0.1	0.0(etch)
(Film deposited, air exposed, followed by H_2-plasma treatment)			
H_2	3	0.1	0.0(etch)
(Film deposited for fixed period, followed by H_2-plasma treatment)			

*1.2 watts r.f. power; $T_s = 300°C$

REFERENCES

1. M. A. Ring, in *Homoatomic Rings, Chains and Macromolecules of Main Group Elements*, edited by A. Rheingold (Elsevier, New York, 1977).

2. B. A. Scott, M. H. Brodsky, D. C. Green, P. B. Kirby, R. M. Plecenik and E. E. Simonyi, Appl. Phys. Lett. **37**, 727 (1980).

3. B. A. Scott, R. M. Plecenik and E. E. Simonyi, submitted to Appl. Phys. Lett.

4. G. W. Bethke and M. K. Wilson, J. Chem. Phys. **26**, 1107 (1957).

5. B. A. Scott, M. H. Brodsky, D. C. Green, R. M. Plecenik, E. E. Simony and R. Serino, to be published.

6. M. H. Brodsky, Manuel Cardona, and J. J. Cuomo, Phys. Rev. B, **16**, 3556 (1977).

7. D. A. Anderson and W. E. Spear, Phil. Mag. **36**, 695 (1977).

8. $C_{eff} = (N_{dopant}/N_{Si})_{solid}/(N_{dopant}/N_{Si})_{gas}$

9. M. Bowrey and J. H. Purnell, Proc. R. Soc., A **341**, 371 (1971).

10. A. P. Webb and S. Veprek, Chem. Phys. Lett. **62**, 173 (1979).

NEW INSIGHTS ON GROWTH MECHANISM OF a-Si:H FROM OPTICAL EMISSION
SPECTROSCOPY

M. Hirose, T. Hamasaki, Y. Mishima, H. Kurata, and Y. Osaka
Department of Electrical Engineering, Hiroshima University, Hiroshima
730, Japan.

ABSTRACT

Optical emission spectra from the silane plasma have been measured as a function of silane flow rate. The relative concentrations
of the emissive species, SiH (414 nm), Si (288 nm), and H (656 nm),
have been determined. The growth rate and vibrational spectra of the
resulting films are interpreted in terms of the emission intensities
of the SiH and H radicals, and the diffusional mass transport of
these neutral radicals is suggested to be responsible for the deposition process of a-Si:H. From the optical emission spectroscopy of
doping gases, decomposition rate of diborane is found to be much less
than that of phosphine. Extremely high doping efficiencies of boron
and phosphorus atoms have been realized by lowering the emission intensity of the SiH band with respect to the H_2 line.

INTRODUCTION

Mass spectrometry[1-3] and optical emission spectroscopy[4-6] of the
silane plasma have revealed some features of the growth process of
a-Si:H. The majority of the glow discharges produce mostly neutral
fragments of silane and the diffusional mass transport of the neutral
radicals is assumed to be important for the growth of a-Si:H.[1,2]
The mean electron density of the order of 10^{10} cm^{-3} in the plasma
column appears to be insufficient to produce a high density of ionic
species, because the generation rate of neutral radicals is much
higher than the ionization rate.[1] On the other hand, Haller[3] suggested that ionic polymerization could be a significant pathway in the
mass transport of Si in the plasma from SiH_4 to a-Si:H, but he had to
assume further reaction steps to explain the hydrogen content of the
deposited film. In the mass spectrometry it is difficult to make
direct observation of neutral radicals. Optical emission spectroscopy (OES) has a great advantage in this sense, and the presence of the
neutral radicals, Si, SiH, H_2, and H has been demonstrated by OES.[4,5]
Furthermore, it is found that the emission intensities of the SiH
band and the H line exhibit a correlation with the concentration of
SiH_2 units in a-Si:H.[6] In this paper, we shall discuss the growth
mechanism and doping kinetics of a-Si:H in conjunction with results
of optical emission spectroscopy.

EXPERIMENTAL

A schematic of the experimental arrangement is shown in Fig. 1.
The reactor consists of a quartz tube (radius 30 mm) with two external ring electrodes for supplying rf power (13.56 MHz). A magnetic

ISSN:0094-243X/81/730010-05$1.50 Copyright 1981 American Institute of Physics

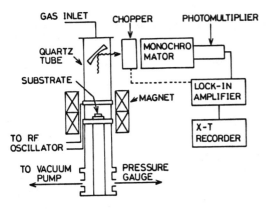

Fig. 1. Experimental setup for depositing a-Si:H and for optical emission spectroscopy.

field was applied perpendicular to the substrate surface. Optical emission spectra from the silane discharge were obtained as a calibrated photomultiplier output through a grating monochromator with a slit width of 50 μm. The measured intensities of the emission lines were corrected by taking into account the diffraction efficiency of the monochromator and the sensitivity of the photomultiplier. SiH_4, PH_3 and B_2H_6 gases were diluted with H_2 gas.

RESULTS

1. Growth process

For the quantitative discussion of results of OES, the relative concentrations of the emissive Si (288 nm), SiH (414 nm), and H (656 nm) have been determined by the optical transition probabilities for the corresponding species.[7-9] Using the measured intensities and the transition probabilities from the excited states of Si, SiH, and H being, respectively, 1.75×10^8, 1.43×10^6, and 6.4

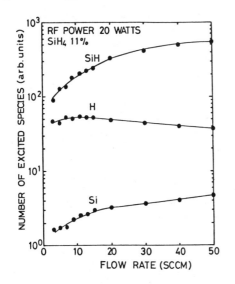

Fig. 2. Silane flow-rate dependence of the concentrations of reactive species in the plasma at a constant gas pressure of 0.64 Torr.

1×10^7 sec^{-1}, the silane flow-rate dependence of these concentrations was obtained as shown in Fig. 2. Figure 3 (a) shows the growth rate of a-Si:H and the product of the concentrations for the SiH and H radicals [SiH][H] as a function of silane flow rate. This result implies that the chemical reaction as $SiH + H \rightarrow Si + H_2$ might occur on the substrate and the mass transport of the SiH and H radicals plays an important role in the growth of a-Si:H. Further importance of the reactive SiH and H is shown by a correlation between the concentration ratio of SiH to H [SiH]/[H] and the content of SiH_2 units in the resulting films (Fig. 3 (b)). Incorporation of SiH_2 units is significant when the concentration ratio

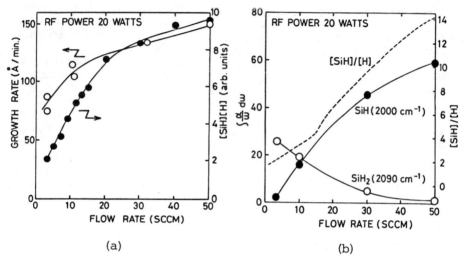

(a) (b)

Fig. 3. (a) Silane flow-rate dependence of the growth rate and the product of the reactive SiH and H [SiH][H]. (b) Integrated absorption of SiH and SiH$_2$ stretching modes as a function of silane flow rate. The dashed line refers to the concentration ratio of the reactive SiH to H [SiH]/[H].

is low, possibly because the reaction SiH + H → SiH$_2$ proceeds on the substrate in addition to the reaction SiH + H → Si + H$_2$.[6] At high concentration ratios, direct incorporation of the impinging SiH into the film becomes appreciable compared to the reaction SiH + H → SiH$_2$, leading to an increase in the content of SiH units in the film. From these results we propose that the reactive SiH and H are the dominant species for the mass transport to the wall, although other neutral radicals like SiH$_2$ and SiH$_3$ may exist in the plasma.[1]

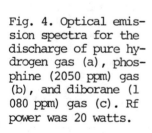

Fig. 4. Optical emission spectra for the discharge of pure hydrogen gas (a), phosphine (2050 ppm) gas (b), and diborane (1080 ppm) gas (c). Rf power was 20 watts.

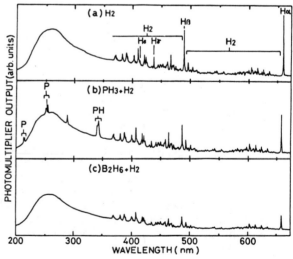

2. Doping kinetics

We have observed optical emission from the glow discharge of the PH_3 (1080 ppm)$-H_2$ and B_2H_6 (2050 ppm)$-H_2$ mixture gases for looking at the decomposition process of the doping gases. The optical emission from the PH band (342 nm)[10] and P lines (214, 215, 253, 254, and 255 nm)[7] were clearly detected, as shown in Fig. 4, while no BH (433 nm)[10] and B (250 nm)[7] lines appeared in the diborane plasma generated at the same discharge conditions as phosphine. Since the enthalpy change in the decomposition of PH_3 (231 kcal/mol) is appreciably small compared with that of B_2H_6 (652 kcal/mol) and since the optical transition probability of the BH radical (433 nm) is larger than that of PH (342 nm), the concentration of the excited BH molecules should be much less than that of the PH radicals. Therefore, a poor doping efficiency of boron in a-Si:H could be connected with a low decomposition rate of B_2H_6. Of course, we could not neglect the influence of the energy distribution of gap states on doping efficiency. From the above it is suggested that a relatively high rf power will be necessary to improve the doping efficiency, particularly in boron doping. Indeed dramatic increase in the doping efficiency (7.8 $\Omega^{-1}cm^{-1}$ for p-type Si:H and 27 $\Omega^{-1}cm^{-1}$ for n-type) has been achieved at an rf power of 30 watts for boron doping and 20 watts for phosphorus doping.[11,12] The optical emission spectra indicated that a high-doping efficiency could be achieved when the SiH band emission is weakened compared to the H_2 lines (Fig. 5). The concentration of SiH_4 should be lowered to obtain such a weak emission of the SiH band ; boron doping needed a lower concentration of silane than phosphorus. Very high doping efficiency mostly accompanies with microcrystallite formation in the a-Si:H network.[11,12] Precipitation of microcrystallites could be attributed to excited hydrogen atoms and molecules, because they attack the substrate surface and transfer the excess energy to the surface silicon atoms which causes partial crystallization of the network.

DISCUSSION

The surface reaction described as SiH_2(g) + Si(s) → 2Si-H* is a rate-limiting process of the thermal decomposition of SiH_4 at a temperature above 500°C, where g,s, and * denote the gas, solid, and adsorbed molecules, respectively.[13] In the case of the glow discharge, considerable amount of the SiH radicals are present in the plasma, and the sticking probability of the emissive SiH may be larger than that of neutral SiH_x (x = 2, 3) radicals, which are not emissive. The SiH radical ad-

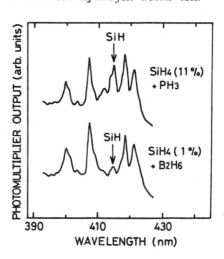

Fig. 5. Optical emission spectra during the deposition of a-Si:H with an extremely high doping efficiency.

sorbed on the substrate can give rise to the growth of a-Si:H even at a temperature much less than 500°C. The result of Fig. 3 strongly suggests the presence of the mass transport of the SiH and H radicals to the substrate. At present, we could not rule out the presence of further reaction steps of the radicals in the dark space around the substrate, but the primary deposition process appears to be understood in terms of the SiH and H radicals. The emissive Si is less important for the deposition since the concentration is two orders of magnitude less than the SiH radical. The doping kinetics is also assessed by the emission intensities of SiH and H_2; the emission intensity of the SiH band with respect to the H_2 lines is substantially important to achieve a high doping efficiency.

Turban et al.[1] studied the reaction mechanisms of the SiH_4 (5%)-He plasma and proposed that the neutral radicals SiH_x (x = 2, 3, 1) created by electron-molecule collisions are transported by diffusion and convection towards the wall. Recently Kampas and Griffith[5] measured the rf power dependence of the emission intensities for the species Si, SiH, H, H_2 and added N_2 in the silane plasma. They found that the emissive Si and SiH are primary products of the silane decomposition. This finding is consistent with our observation that the intensity of the SiH band emission exhibits a correlation with the deposition rate and composition of a-Si:H.

In conclusion, we would suggest that the growth of a-Si:H could primarily be attributed to the mass transport of the emissive SiH and H radicals.

REFERENCES

1. G. Turban, Y. Catherine, and B. Grolleau, Thin Solid Films, 60, 147 (1979).
2. B. Drevillon, J. Huc, A. Llret, J. Perrin, G. deRosny, and J. P. M. Schmitt, Appl. Phys. Lett. 37, 646 (1980).
3. I. Haller, Appl. Phys. Lett. 37, 282 (1980).
4. A. Matsuda, K. Nakagawa, K. Tanaka, M. Matsumura, S. Yamasaki, H. Okushi, and S. Iizima, J. Non-Cryst. Solids 35-36, 183 (1980).
5. F. J. Kampas and R. W. Griffith, J. Appl. Phys. in press.
6. M. Taniguchi, M. Hirose, T. Hamasaki, and Y. Osaka, Appl. Phys. Lett. 37, 787 (1980).
7. W. L. Wiese, M. W. Smith, and B. M. Miles, Atomic Transition Probabilities (National Standard Reference Data System, Washington, D. C. , 1969), Vol.1, p.25, Vol.2, p.71, 105.
8. W. H. Smith, J. Chem. Phys. 51, 520 (1969).
9. H. Bethe, Quantenmechanik der Ein- und Zwei- Elektronenprobleme (Springer-Verlag, Berlin, 1935), p.444.
10. K. P. Huber and G. Hertzberg, Molecular Spectra and Molecular Structure (Van Nonstrand Reinhold Company, N.Y.,1979), p.88,534.
11. T. Hamasaki, H. Kurata, M. Hirose, and Y. Osaka, Jpn. J. Appl. Phys. 20, 237 (1981).
12. T. Hamasaki, H. Kurata, M. Hirose, and Y. Osaka, Appl. Phys. Lett. 37, 1084 (1980).
13. Y. Ban, H. Tsuchikawa, and K. Maeda, Semiconductor Silicon (Electrochem. Soc., 1973), p.292.

"F-ETCHED a-SI FILMS"

Vikram L. Dalal, Charles M. Fortmann, and Erten Eser
Institute of Energy Conversion
University of Delaware
Newark, Delaware - 19711

ABSTRACT

A model which suggests that a-Si films deposited from $(SiF_4 + H_2)$ mixtures are subjected to strong ionic etching during growth is proposed. It is shown that many of the properties of these a-Si films, such as high conductivity in doped layers and growth, H incorporation, and bandgap data, can be explained by this model. High conductivities are achieved without any detectable F in the film.

INTRODUCTION

a-Si:F,H films grown from gases containing Si, F and H are of considerable technological importance[1,2,3]. It has been shown that under certain deposition conditions, the n-type doped a-Si:F,H films have very high conductivities, exceeding $\sigma = 1/\Omega$-cm. This high conductivity was originally attributed to low midgap density of states in a-Si:F,H[1,4]. These desirable properties of a-Si:F,H are attributed to the strong Si:F bonds, which satisfy dangling bonds in a-Si lattice [5]. However, this model fails to explain why, if F satisfies the dangling bonds, H is needed to achieve the desirable properties. The model also fails to account for some other properties of a-Si:F,H films, such as very slow growth rates, high stress levels, bandgap changes, strong influence of growth and properties on electrical bias on the sample during growth, and the occurance of microcrystallinity in doped films[6,7].

In this paper, we suggest a possible model for the growth of a-Si films from SiF_4 and H_2 which can explain most of these phenomena and describe some preliminary confirming experiments.

PROPOSED MODEL

We propose that a-Si films being grown from SiF_4 and H_2 mixtures are subjected to strong reactive ion etching[8-10], and ion bombardment, with the net growth rate being determined by a balance between deposition and etching, in a manner analogous to RF bias sputtering of thin films[11]. We consider this reactive-ion etching to be the major distinguishing feature between a-Si:H and a-Si:F,H, since a-Si:H are generally subjected to only very light etching during growth. Reactive ion etching using SiF_4 plasmas is, of course, a well known technology for crystalline Si[8-10].

Several consequences of this model are immediately apparent.
1. The model suggests that the growth rate will depend very strongly on electrical bias conditions on the sample, unlike the case of a-Si:H films.

ISSN:0094-243X/81/730015-05$1.50 Copyright 1981 American Institute of Physics

2. Under certain growth conditions, where the films may be subjected to strong ion bombardment, microcrystallinity could be promoted, along with high conductivity.
3. If the major role of F is to provide reactive ions to etch the films, then H would still be necessary to satisfy the dangling bonds.
4. It is possible that F will etch the weakly bonded Si atoms; i.e., atoms which are weakly bonded with at least one unsatisfied bond. If so, there will be fewer dangling bonds for H to satisfy. Then, the concentration of H in these films would be lower than in a-Si:H films deposited from SiH_4.
5. It is possible that, in addition to reducing number of atoms with one unsatisfied bond, F may also etch the weakest Si:Si bonds, namely the ones at the top of the valence band. Thus, F will promote an increase in bandgap.
6. If the doped films become microcrystalline, in analogy with O_2 in C-Si, O_2 in the plasma would have a minimal influence on conductivity, much less than the influence of O_2 on SiH_4-deposited a-Si films.

In the next section, we describe some of the preliminary experimental data that indicate that some of the above consequences are observed.

EXPERIMENTAL DATA

1. Influence of Bias. We have found that RF (cathodic) films deposited from $(SiF_4 + H_2)$ are much easier to dope to high σ than RF (anodic) films. At the same time, doped RF(C) films have higher band-gaps than RF(A) films. Figures 1 and 2 show our data. Both films were deposited from gas mixtures with identical relative concentrations of SiF_4, H_2 and AsH_3. These observations support the contention that strong etching and ion bombardment are necessary to produce microcrystallinity and attendant high doping, since cathodic films are subjected to strong negative self-induced bias, typically - 100V in our samples.
The achievement of high conductivity in RF(Ground) films only occurs when the power levels on RF target electrodes are very high ($\sim$ several W/cm^2) and plasma voltage is also large (+20V). The achievement of high σ state is aided by inclusion of Ar in the gas mixture, which can be expected to add to the bombardment of the film, leading to microcrystallinity.
2. Influence of Temperature on Bandgap. We have observed that increasing temperature decreases the growth rate and decreases the absorption constant. See Figure 3. Film 81/93 was grown at 350C and had a growth rate of 1.46Å/sec. Film 81/94 was grown at 450C and had a growth rate of 0.96Å/sec. All the other conditions were identical for the two samples. The increase in Eg with temperature is in sharp contrast to the case for a-Si:H films grown from SiH_4, where Eg decreases and growth rate increases, with temperature [12].
3. Auger Data. A study of our heavily doped films by Auger electron spectroscopy shows no evidence for F in the film, indicating that F is < 1%. This is contrary to the results of Madan et al [1], who found F > 2-4%. We still get the high σ supposedly ascribed to F.

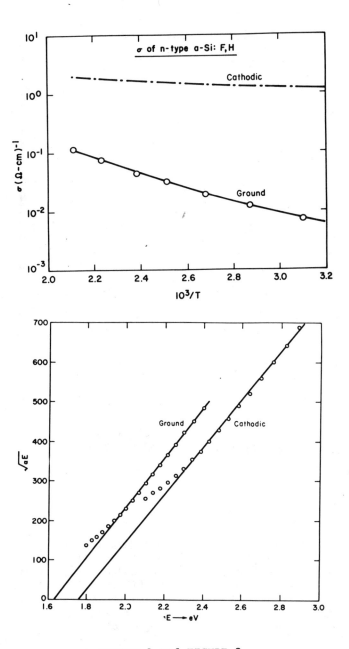

FIGURE 1 and FIGURE 2

Conductivity and optical absorption of As-doped a-Si films.
T=350C. SiF$_4$/H$_2$=3. AsH$_3$/SiF$_4$=1000 ppm.

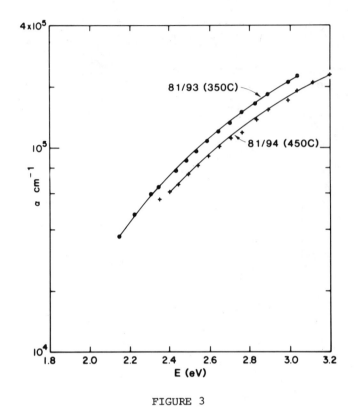

FIGURE 3

Optical absorption for two As-doped
RF(Ground) films prepared at 350 and 450C.

4. Influence of O_2. Preliminary experiments on addition of
O_2 (at $\sim$ 0.3 - 0.5% in the gas phase) to the plasma containing SiF_4,
AsH_3 and H_2 yield a film with higher bandgap, but retain the high
conductivity characteristic of these films ($\sim$ 1/Ω-cm). This suggests
that the films are microcrystalline and therefore, O_2 should not
reduce the conductivity significantly, unlike the case for a-Si:H
deposited for SiH_4. The increased O_2 clearly shows up in Auger scans
of the oxygenated films. The addition of O_2 thus may be used
advantageously to increase the bandgap while retaining high σ, a
consideration useful for transparent junction solar cells.

CONCLUSION

In conclusion, we propose that many of the properties of a-Si films prepared from (SiF$_4$ + H$_2$) mixtures can be understood if these films are subjected to strong reactive ion etching during growth. It is proposed that the electronic properties of these films are primarily due to H passivating the dangling bonds, with little electronic effect from F. The high conductivity in doped films may be primarily due to microcrystallinity, promoted by strong ionic etching during growth.

REFERENCES

1. A. Madan, S. Ovshinsky, and E. Benn, Phil. Mag. B40, 259 (1979).
2. A. Madan, et al. Appl. Phys. Lett. (1980).
3. P. Nielsen and V. L. Dalal, Appl. Phys. Lett. 37, 1090 (1980).
4. M. Shur, W. Czubatiyj, and A. Madan, J. Noncryst. Solids 35-36, 731 (1980).
5. S. R. Ovshinsky and A. Madan, U.S. Patent 4,226,898 (1980).
6. R. Tsu, M. Izu, S. R. Ovshinsky and F. H. Pollak, Bull. Am. Phys. Soc. 25, 295 (1980).
7. A Matsuda, et al. Japan. J. Appl. Phys. 19, L 305 (1980).
8. J. Hayes and T. Pandhumsoporn, Solid State Tech. 23, #11, 72 (1980).
9. Geraldine Schwartz and Paul Schaible, ibid, p. 85 (1980).
10. P. M. Scharble and G. C. Schwartz, J. Vac. Sci. Techn. 16, 377 (1979).
11. Leon Maissel, Physics of Thin Films 3, (1974).
12. P. Zanzuchi, C. Wronski and D. Carlson, J. Appl. Phys. 48, 5227 (1977).
13. V. L. Dalal, Solar Cells 2, 261 (1980).

EXPERIMENTAL EVIDENCE FOR A KINETIC MODEL OF HYDROGEN INCORPORATION INTO SPUTTERED a-Si*

T.D. Moustakas and T. Tiedje
Corporate Research Laboratory
Exxon Research and Engineering Company
Linden, N.J. 07036

W.A. Lanford
State University of N.Y.
Albany, N.Y. 12222

ABSTRACT

The dependence of hydrogen content, on the partial pressure of hydrogen, substrate bias, deposition rate, and deposition temperature was found to be consistent with a kinetic model of hydrogen incorporation into a-SiH$_x$ films, produced by reactive sputtering in an Ar+H plasma.

INTRODUCTION

Reactively sputtered hydrogenated amorphous Si films were found to have properties similar to those produced by glow discharge decomposition of silane[1,2]. However, the film growth process appears to be different in these two methods of film formation. For example, there is ample evidence[3] that during the glow discharge decomposition of silane the film is formed from Si$_x$H$_y$ species condensing on the top of the substrate. Spectroscopic studies of sputtering plasmas on the other hand give ambiguous information about the H incorporation mechanism. In one study[3] the results suggest that SiH$_x$ molecules are formed in the sputtering plasma. However, the results are not quantitative enough to suggest any correlation between these SiH$_x$ molecules and the film's H content. In the second study[4] the results suggest no silicon-hydrogen gas phase reactions.

In this paper we adopt the view that the reaction of Si with H occurs at the substrate surface. We also suggest that the Si and H reactions are kinetically controlled[5,6]. In support of this kinetic model of hydrogen incorporation we present hydrogen content data as a function of partial pressure of hydrogen, substrate biasing, deposition rate, and deposition temperature.

EXPERIMENTAL RESULTS-DISCUSSION

The relative amount of bonded hydrogen in the films discussed in this paper was inferred from the integrated intensity under the Si-H vibrational modes. We find no difference in the functional behavior if we plot the integrated intensity under the Si-H stretching or Si-H wagging vibration vs the different deposition parameters. Throughout this paper, therefore, we will use the integrated intensity under the stretching vibration to infer the relative amount of bonded hydrogen.

*Work supported partly by SERI (Contract No. XZ-0-9219).

The absolute amount of incorporated hydrogen in a few samples has also been measured by the nuclear reaction $^{15}N + ^{1}H \rightarrow ^{12}C + ^{4}He + \gamma$ [7].

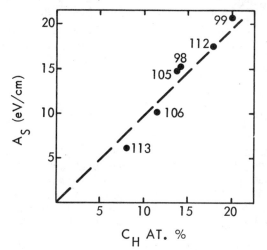

Fig. 1 shows that there is a one-to-one relation between the integrated intensity under the stretching vibration and the hydrogen content determined by the ^{15}N reaction. With this calibration we will present the rest of the hydrogen content data in terms of the integrated intensity under the Si-H stretching vibration.

Fig. 1. Correlation between infrared absorption and H content

Fig. 2 shows the relation between the hydrogen content and the partial pressure of hydrogen in the discharge for two series of films. Both series of films were produced at $T_s = 275°C$ a total pressure of 15 mTorr and power in the discharge of 1.6 watts/cm^2. The only difference is that during the deposition of one series (solid circles) the substrates were electrically grounded while in the second series (open circles) the substrates were biased to a positive potential.

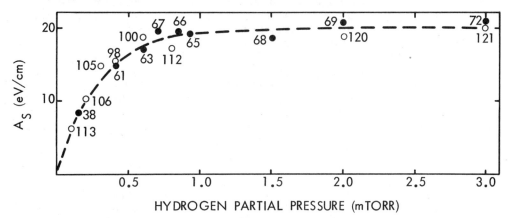

Fig. 2. Integrated infrared absorption as a function of hydrogen partial pressure.

The relationship shown in Fig. 2 between the H content of the film and the partial pressure of hydrogen in the sputtering plasma can be explained by a kinetic model of the H incorporation as follows[6]. We neglect any gas phase reactions between Si and H, and assume that the H incorporation arises from surface reactions. In the absence of any significant desorption of bonded H, the time dependence of the H coverage on the growing surface is given by,

$$\frac{dN}{dt} = F\theta\sigma \ (N_{Max}-N) \tag{1}$$

where N is the number of surface sites occupied by H, N_{Max} is the total number of available sites, F is the flux of hydrogen onto the surface, and θ and σ are respectively the sticking coefficient and capture crossection of the bonding sites for hydrogen. If the film deposition rate is R (in monolayers/s), then each surface layer has an average time 1/R available during which it can capture H atoms.

Taking into account this time limit, we conclude from Eq. (1) that the H content or integrated infrared osciallator strength As, obeys the relation,

$$A_s = A_{Max} \ (1-e^{-\frac{F\theta\sigma}{R}}). \tag{2}$$

Although it is not obvious which species of hydrogen (ion, molecule, atom) is most important in the incorporation process, we expect the flux of all of these species to be proportional to the partial pressure of H in the sputtering gas. To check whether these ideas are reasonable, we can fit the data in Fig. 2 with Eq. (2) and estimate a sticking coefficient θ. From the fit indicated by the dashed line in Fig. 2 we find θ =0.03 based on the measured deposition rate of 1.1 monolayers/s, the calculated flux F of neutral H_2 molecules onto the surface in a hypothetical neutral gas at the same temperature and pressure and an assumed capture cross-section of $10^{-16}cm^2$. This rather small value for the sticking coefficient (0.03) is reasonable, since only a fraction of the H_2 molecules are decomposed into atomic H in the plasma, and the molecular H is not likely to bond to dangling Si bonds. The close agreement in Fig. 2 between the biased and un-biased substrates demonstrates that the dominant H species in the in-corporation process is electrically neutral, probably atomic hydrogen.

According to the kinetic model of the H incorporation process, the hydrogen content should also depend on the film deposition rate. From Eq. (2) we expect the H content to depend on the ratio of the H flux F to the film deposition rate R and not on the two parameters separate-ly. In Fig. 3 we have plotted the integrated IR absorption as a func-tion of P_H/R for three different deposition rates from 1-4 A/sec. Note that the three sets of data fall on the same curve as expected in the kinetic model.

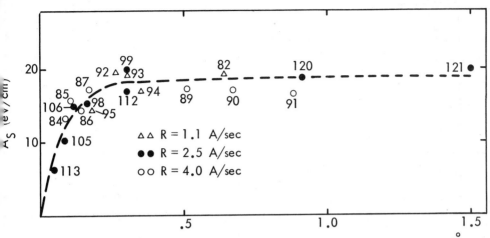

Fig. 3. Integrated infrared absorption as a function of P_H/R.

In the kinetic theory we have neglected thermal desorption of H from bonding sites, and assumed that the H and Si are far from thermodynamic equilibrium. This assumption can be checked by comparing the H content as a function of P_H, for films deposited at different substrate temperatures with other parameters held fixed. The results for two series of films, one deposited at 385°C and one at 225°C are shown in Fig. 4. The first thing to note is that the saturation H content at high P_H is higher for the low temperature films. A plausible explanation of this result is that the growing Si lattice anneals more at 385°C than at 225°C. At the high temperature the Si lattice is likely to be less defective and as a result may have fewer H bonding sites.

Although the data in Fig. 4 at low P_H is incomplete for the high temperature films, there is enough data to conclude that the sticking coefficient θ at high temperature (385°C) is about equal to or larger than the sticking coefficient at 225°C. This observation rules out a thermodynamic equilibrium interpretation of the data. In this interpretation the effective sticking coefficient at a given P_H would be determined by the ratio of the H flux onto the surface to the rate of thermal desorption. The desorption process will involve bond breaking and hence should be thermally activated and strongly temperature dependent. In this case, the apparent sticking coefficient would decrease dramatically from 225 to 385°C, contrary to the experimental results in Fig. 4, where if anything the sticking coefficient goes in the opposite direction. Thus we conclude that the system is far from thermal equilibrium and the kinetic model is appropriate.

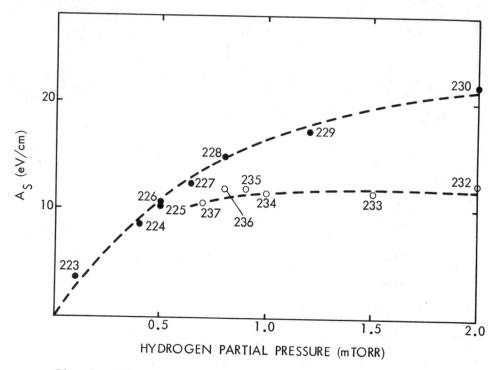

Fig. 4. Integrated infrared absorption as a function of hydrogen partial pressures for films produced at T_s = 225°C (●●) and T_s = 385°C (oo).

We thank R. Friedman, M. Hicks and Karen Rogers for sample preparations and measurements.

REFERENCES

1. T.D. Moustakas, J. of Electronic Materials 8, 391, (1979).

2. W.E. Spear, Adv. In Physics 26, 811 (1977).

3. A. Matsuda, K. Nakagawa, K. Tanaka, M. Matsumura, S. Yamasaki, H. Okushi and S. Izima, J. Non-Cryst. Solids 35-36, 183 (1980).

4. M.A. Paesler, T. Okumura and W. Paul, J. Vac. Sci. Technol. 17, 1332 (1980).

5. G.A.N. Connell and J.R. Pawlik, Phys. Rev. B 13, 787 (1976).

6. T. Tiedje, T.D. Moustakas and J.M. Cebulka, Phys. Rev. B (to be published).

7. W.A. Lanford, H.P. Trautretter, J.F. Ziegler and J. Keller, Appl. Phys. Lett. 28, 566 (1976).

COMPARISON OF a-Si:H PRODUCED BY rf SPUTTERING AND PLASMA DECOMPOSITION METHODS

G. Moddel, J. Blake, R. W. Collins, P. Viktorovitch,
D. K. Paul, B. von Roedern and William Paul

Gordon McKay Laboratory, Division of Applied Sciences,
Harvard University, Cambridge, MA 02138

ABSTRACT

We investigate the differences between sputter (S) produced and representative plasma decomposition (GD) produced a-Si:H in electron drift mobility activation energy, photoluminescence temperature quenching and peak energy, optical absorption extended by photoconductivity, and midgap state density from conductance/capacitance measurements. From these property measurements we conclude that for the GD material less modification of the bands occurs for the hydrogenation required to obtain a comparable midgap state density. This density, measured in both materials, is larger than that expected from an extrapolation of the band tails.

INTRODUCTION

A comparison of some of the electronic properties of a-Si:H produced by plasma decomposition of silane[1] and by rf sputtering of Si in an Ar-H_2 atmosphere[2] shows systematic differences between films produced by the two processes. We have studied a large number of samples sputtered under various conditions and contrasted them with a few silane decomposed samples whose properties are representative of those that appear in the literature. From the results we infer differences between the two types of material, at least as they are conventionally prepared at present, in the healing of defects by hydrogen.

SAMPLE PREPARATION

a-Si:H was prepared by rf sputtering (S) of a c-Si target in an Ar-H_2 atmosphere and by dc cathodic and rf plasma decomposition (GD) of SiH_4. The details are given elsewhere.[3]

EXPERIMENTAL METHODS AND RESULTS

We obtain drift mobility (μ_d) from the magnitude of photoconductivity per absorbed photon divided by the characteristic time of the initial slope of its decay upon the termination of illumination.[4] The temperature dependence of the photoconductivity magnitudes and decay times, measured at a constant incident photon flux of $\sim 10^{15}$ photons cm^{-2} s^{-1} at 1.96 eV, was corrected to account for the variation in the number of absorbed photons with temperature due to a shift in the absorption edge[5] of -4×10^{-4} eV K^{-1}. The results shown in Fig. 1 are consistent with published data for GD[6] and S[7] material

ISSN:0095-243X/81/730025-06$1.50 Copyright 1981 American Institute of Physics

in showing a larger variation of μ_d with temperature for the S material. The μ_d appears activated[8] with activation energies (E_{μ_d}) for the GD films of 0.12 and 0.15 eV and for the S films from 0.20 to 0.24 eV, roughly 0.1 eV higher.

The photoluminescence (PL) intensity (I) has been shown to obey the relation $(I_0/I)-1 \propto \exp(T/T_0)$ for a properly chosen[9] normalization constant I_0, yielding the parameter T_0. This parameter is proportional to the width and energy maximum in the distribution of activation energies for nonradiative recombination.[10] Data are shown in Fig. 2 for a typical S film and a GD film which shows similar PL *versus* T behavior to that reported elsewhere.[11] T_0 has been found to be proportional to E_{μ_d} in S and GD films.[12]

Measurement of the optical absorption coefficient (α) may be extended to low photon energies using properly normalized photoconductivity spectra[13] which yield accurate α spectra at least down to 1.2 eV.[14] Figure 3 shows α *versus* $h\nu$ for two different S samples and a GD sample exhibiting results consistent with those in the literature.[13] In the region of the edges about 1.6 eV, $\alpha(h\nu) \propto \exp[h\nu/E_\alpha]$. We have found that $\alpha(1.2$ eV) is proportional to the midgap density of states (DOS), determined from capacitance/conductance measurements of Schottky barriers at zero bias as a function of frequency.[15] In Fig. 4 this DOS is plotted as a function of E_{04}, the energy at which $\alpha = 10^4$ cm^{-1}. For S films the DOS varies exponentially with E_{04} down to $\sim 5 \times 10^{16}$ eV^{-1} cm^{-3}, where there is a saturation with scatter (10^{16}–10^{17} eV^{-1} cm^{-3}). The GD films exhibit an E_{04} which is roughly 0.15 eV smaller for a given DOS.

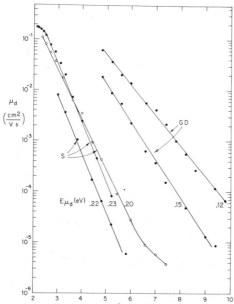

In Fig. 5 the PL peak energy (E_{pk}) is shown *versus* E_{04}. For the S samples $E_{04}(300$ K) - $E_{pk}(77$ K) $\simeq 0.6$ eV, and for the GD films it is as much as ~ 0.1 eV smaller.

DISCUSSION

It has been widely demonstrated that the incorporation of H into a-Si prepared both by S and GD is essential in compensating residual defects in the amorphous network leading to gap states,[2] and has been almost as widely noted that the quantities of incorporated H are far in excess of the number of states to be removed from the gap and hence must affect states elsewhere. Although properties related to gap

Fig. 1. Drift mobility μ_d vs $10^3/T$ for S and GD films with activation energy E_{μ_d}.

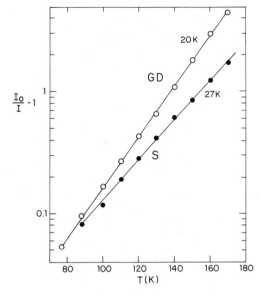

Fig. 2. Photoluminescence $(I_0/I - 1)$ vs T for S and GD films, where I is the intensity of luminescence. The indicated slopes (T_0) are typical of S and GD samples when measured under identical excitation conditions (5 mW/cm^2 at 2.33 eV).

cleanliness have shown dramatic improvement upon initial hydrogenation, increased H incorporation produces less unambiguous improvement. Aside from the possibility of H *induced* defects resulting in gap states,[16] the bands themselves are modified, as deduced from the shift of the absorption edge to higher energies.[5] With H levels of ~ 10% (~10^{22} cm^{-3}) it should be expected that band edge states (~10^{21} eV^{-1} cm^{-3}) are significantly affected.

In comparing the properties of S and GD a-Si:H, we consider those properties which are dependent on the gap DOS and induced alterations of the band edges, examining variations in S films and contrasting the differences with GD films which are representative of those described in the literature.

The μ_d activation energies shown in Fig. 1 may be associated with states below the conduction band edge with which photo-produced electrons in the band interact. The larger E_{μ_d} of the S films would therefore

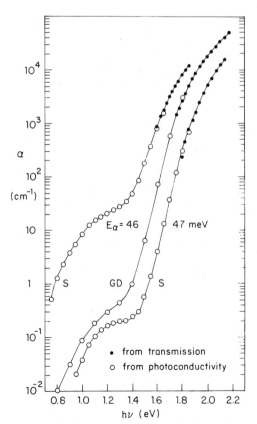

Fig. 3. Optical absorption coefficient α vs photon energy $h\nu$ for S and GD films from transmission measurements extended by photoconductivity. Values for the slope of the exponential region E_α are shown for the two films where it is most clearly definable.

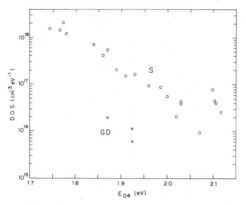

Fig. 4. Density of states DOS vs E_{04}, the energy where $\alpha = 10^4 cm^{-1}$, for S and GD films. The DOS have been deduced from the frequency dependence of the capacitance and conductance in Schottky diodes at zero bias.

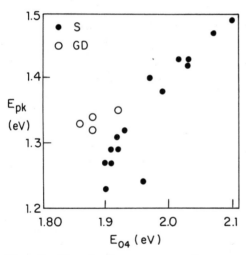

Fig. 5. Photoluminescence peak energy E_{pk}(77 K) vs E_{04}(300 K), the energy at which $\alpha = 10^4 cm^{-1}$, for S and GD films.

indicate that the states which perform this function extend deeper into the gap of S material. If the correlation between E_{μ_d} and the PL T_o results from the same states being involved in both processes,[12] then the initial states for radiative recombination lie farther below the conduction band in S films than in GD films.

The exponential region of the absorption edge has been attributed to exponential tails from the conduction and valence band whose overlap may determine the DOS in the middle of the gap.[17] The slope of the exponential is thought to equal the slope of the valence band tail[18] because there is evidence that this tail falls off more slowly than the conduction band tail. Using the observed value of $E_\alpha \simeq 0.05$ eV from Fig. 3, a distance from band edge to midgap of 0.9 eV and band edge DOS[19] of $10^{21} eV^{-1} cm^{-3}$, an exponential decrease to midgap would result in a DOS there of $10^{13} eV^{-1} cm^{-3}$. This is three orders of magnitude less than the value of the midgap DOS deduced from capacitance/conductance measurements. If the exponential absorption tails result from DOS tails, then the low energy α shoulder may be viewed as resulting from states just below midgap, which exist in far greater density than those from any exponential band tails. The shoulder appears to protrude farther from the exponential absorption tail in S material than in GD films.

The E_{04} is determined at sufficiently high α that it may be taken as a relative measure of the bandgap energy.[5] In spite of the midgap DOS not resulting from band tails, we find the relation between E_{04} and the DOS shown in Fig. 4 for S films in which there appears to be an intimate connection between the two. Thus we conclude that the process, probably hydrogenation, which has the effect of removing gap states has the quite separate but functionally related effect of shifting band edge states. The GD films have a gap which has been widened less for a given DOS than the S films. Therefore the GD process either creates fewer potential defects whose compensation requires hydrogenation during growth or H is more efficiently targeted to the defects by the GD process.

Finally, as shown in Fig. 5, the radiative transition energy is larger in the GD material for a given gap size. If the transition is associated with localized states in the gap with other parameters (phonon and Coulombic interactions) remaining constant, the states appear to fall off more slowly from at least one of the band edges, probably the conduction band edge,[12] in the GD *versus* the S material.

The S films used in this study are representative of the type generally produced by sputtering. That the few GD films we have studied are representative of the types of GD films generally discussed in the literature is evidenced by their similar photoconductivity,[6] photoluminescence[11] and absorption[13] properties, and by their Schottky diode characteristics discussed elsewhere.[20] In addition to the dc GD films deposited on to substrates on a cathodic platform, we have produced dc GD films on an anodic platform which have shown S-like properties.[12] If the similarity between the GD anodic films and S films correctly identifies electron bombardment as the source of the differences between S and conventional GD films, then it suggests that improvement in S material be sought through deposition conditions that reduce bombardment.

CONCLUSIONS

a-Si:H produced by the plasma decomposition of silane exhibits electronic properties which imply that it requires less modification of the bands by hydrogenation than sputter produced material for the healing of defects which produce states throughout the gap, and hence either the process creates fewer potential defects or H is more efficiently targeted to the defects by the decomposition process. In contrast to plasma decomposition produced films, sputter produced films exhibit: (i) an electron drift mobility activation energy for steady state photo-transport which is 0.1 eV larger; (ii) a photoluminescence temperature quenching coefficient which is larger and a peak energy which is smaller for a given bandgap; (iii) a midgap density of states for a given bandgap which is larger.

ACKNOWLEDGMENTS

We thank P. Ketchian for technical assistance in producing the S films and the Mobil Tyco Solar Energy Corporation for the rf GD films. This work was supported by the National Science Foundation under grant DMR78-10014 and by the Department of Energy under Subcontract XW-∅-9358-1 of Prime Contract EG-77-C-01-4042.

REFERENCES

1. R.C. Chittick, J.H. Alexander and H.F. Sterling, J. Electrochem. Soc. 116, 77 (1969), and W.E. Spear and P.G. Le Comber, Solid State Commun. 17, 1193 (1975).

2. W.Paul, A.J. Lewis, G.A.N. Connell and T.D. Moustakas, Solid State Commun. 20, 969 (1976).

3. Sputtering details appear in D.A. Anderson, G. Moddel, M.A. Paesler and William Paul, J. Vac. Sci. Technol. 16, 906 (1979). Our dc plasma decomposition parameters are described in D.K. Paul, B. von Roedern, S. Oguz, J. Blake and W. Paul, J. Phys. Soc. Japan 49, 1261 (1980). The rf GD films were produced by Mobil Tyco Solar Energy Corporation.

4. S.M. Ryvkin, Photoelectric Effects in Semiconductors (Consultants Bureau, New York, 1964).

5. E.C. Freeman and William Paul, Phys. Rev. B 20, 716 (1979).

6. W. Fuhs, M. Milleville and J. Stuke, Phys. Stat. Sol. B 89, 495 (1978).

7. T.D. Moustakas, J. Electron. Mater. 8, 391 (1979).

8. The meaning and validity of the μ_d magnitude determined this way are discussed in G. Moddel, P. Viktorovitch and W. Paul (unpublished). In this paper we focus only on the values for E_{μ_d}.

9. R.W. Collins, M.A. Paesler and William Paul, Solid State Commun. 34, 833 (1980).

10. M. Kastner, J. Phys. C 13, 3319 (1980).

11. See for example, C. Tsang and R.A. Street, Phys. Rev. B 19, 3027 (1979).

12. R.W. Collins and William Paul (unpublished).

13. G.D. Cody, B. Abeles, C.R. Wronski, B. Brooks and W.A. Lanford, J. Non-Cryst. Solids 35-36, 463 (1980).

14. G. Moddel, D.A. Anderson and William Paul, Phys. Rev. B 22, 1918 (1980).

15. P. Viktorovitch and G. Moddel, J. Appl. Phys. 51, 4847 (1980).

16. D.A. Anderson, G. Moddel, R.W. Collins and W. Paul, Solid State Commun. 31, 677 (1979).

17. M.H. Cohen, H. Fritzsche and S.R. Ovshinsky, Phys. Rev. Lett. 22, 1065 (1969).

18. R.S. Crandall, J. Non-Cryst. Solids 35-36, 381 (1980).

19. W. Paul, G.A.N. Connell and R.J. Temkin, Adv. Phys. 22, 531 (1973).

20. P. Viktorovitch, G. Moddel, J. Blake and William Paul (unpublished).

GROWTH CHARACTERIZATION OF a-Si:H FILMS BY IN SITU ELLIPSOMETRY IN A SILANE MULTIPOLE PLASMA

B. Drevillon, J. Huc, A. Lloret, J. Perrin, G. de Rosny and
J.P.M. Schmitt
Laboratoire de Physique Nucléaire des Hautes Energies and
Laboratoire de Physique des Milieux Ionisés
Ecole Polytechnique - 91128 Palaiseau, Cedex - France

ABSTRACT

Fast real time ellipsometry has been performed to follow the growth of a-Si:H films deposited in a low pressure D.C. discharge of silane. First results show that the growth is incompatible with a simple homogeneous layer by layer mechanism and suggest the presence of microstructure.

INTRODUCTION

Hydrogenated amorphous silicon (a-Si:H) films obtained either from glow discharge decomposition of silane or R.F. sputtering of a Si target in a $Ar-H_2$ mixture have been extensively studied in terms of electrical, optical and structural properties of the as-deposited or annealed material after removal from the deposition chamber. Nevertheless, no in-situ techniques have been yet employed, to our knowledge, to study the film growth which is known to lead to the formation of a columnar microstructure correlated with an essentially biphasic composition of the deposit evidenced by Knights[1]. In the case of amorphous material in a plasma environment, ellipsometry appears to be the only possible in situ and real time characterization. Using an automatic rotating polarizer ellipsometer, Hottier and Theeten[2] have already evidenced that the growth of a-Si deposited by low pressure C.V.D. of silane on Si_3N_4 is not a layer by layer one but can be interpreted in terms of nucleation. In order to follow the growth of silane glow-discharge a-Si:H, we have built a new type fast automatic ellipsometer and we present here our first results. We show that they cannot be explained by simple preliminary models of growth.

EXPERIMENTAL

The a-Si:H deposit is obtained from silane decomposition in a multipole D.C. discharge. We have already shown that such a reactor associated with various plasma diagnostics is a powerful tool to analyze silane dissociation mechanisms as well as an alternative device to produce a-Si:H[3].

The ellipsometer attached to the reactor is schematically described in Fig. 1. Its principle known as polarization modulated ellimpsometry was first proposed by Jasperson and Schnatterly[4]. The monochromatic light beam ($\lambda = 6328$ Å) is linearly polarized. It goes then through the photoelastic modulator which consists of a fused silica block cemented to an a.c. driven crystal quartz transducer

ISSN:0094-243X/81/730031-05$1.50 Copyright 1981 American Institute of Physics

(ω = 50kHz). The uniaxial standing strain wave established in the silica block generates an alternating relative retardation δ = A sin ωt. The beam is afterwards reflected by the sample and analyzed by a linear polarizer, its intensity being finally detected by a photomultiplier.

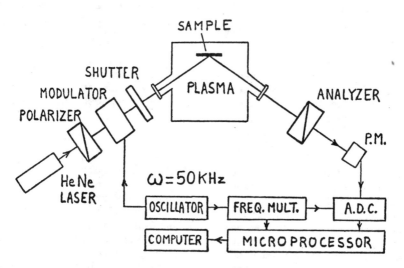

Fig. 1: Experimental Set-Up

The theoretical expression of the intensity appears as a linear combination of sin δ and cosδ:
$$I = I_0 + I_s \sin\delta + I_c \cos\delta.$$
I_0, I_s and I_c are related to the orientations of the optical components with respect to the plane of incidence on the sample and to the ellipsometric angles Ψ and Δ defined by the complex reflectance ratio: r_p/r_s = tg Ψ $e^{i\Delta}$, where r_p and r_s are the complex reflectance coefficients of the electric field components, respectively parallel and perpendicular to the incidence plan. The sine and cosine functions of δ can be expanded in the Bessel functions series:

$$\sin\delta = 2 \sum_{0}^{\infty} J_{2m+1} (A) \sin[(2m+1)\omega t]$$

$$\cos\delta = J_0(A) + 2 \sum_{1}^{\infty} J_{2m}(A) \cos[2m\omega t].$$

The signal is therefore the sum of a dc term $I_{dc} = I_0 + J_0(A)I_c$ and a modulated part. The entire information is obtained from the ratios R_ω and $R_{2\omega}$ of the a.c. amplitudes of the fundamental and second harmonic to the dc level. In operating conditions, A is adjusted so that $J_0(A) = 0$. Two convenient choices of the optical components orientations give then:

either $R_\omega = 2J_1(A)\sin2\Psi\sin\Delta$ $\qquad$ $R_{2\omega} = 2J_2(A)\cos2\Psi$

or $\qquad R_\omega = 2J_1(A)\sin2\Psi\sin\Delta$ $\qquad$ $R_{2\omega} = 2J_2(A)\sin2\Psi\cos\Delta$

which allows self-consistent calibrations.

To measure R_ω and $R_{2\omega}$ a fast analysis of the P.M. output is performed. The signal is sampled by a 8 bits A.D.C. (50 ns) triggered 256 times in one period of 20 μsec and monitored by a microprocessor (time cycle≃250 ns). To improve the lack of accuracy of the A.D.C. a small linear variable d.c. voltage is added to the signal during a sequence of 256 accumulated periods. The data are then transferred to a computer for an on-line Fourier analysis. The ultimate data acquisition rate is one point every ~ 5 msec. A detailed presentation of the system will be given elsewhere.

RESULTS AND DISCUSSION

A typical example of real-time ellipsometry on growing a-Si:H film on a fused silica substrate, heated at about 180°C, is presented. The plasma is established as follows: pure silane is sent into the reactor at a total pressure of 1.5 mTorr; the primary electron energy defined by the D.C. voltage between the hot cathode and the walls is 60eV and the discharge current is 400 mA. In such conditions, the deposition rate is 160 Å/mn and the deposit is due mainly to radicals[3].

The ellipsometric evolution is represented by a (Ψ,Δ) plot: in Fig. 2-a. The starting point of the curve corresponds to the uncovered substrate whereas the convergence point of the spiral due to the interference regime in the film is characteristic of the absorbing a-Si:H deposit. In the case of a semi-infinite medium/vacuum interface, the value of the complex refractive index ñ of the medium is deduced from the measured Ψ and Δ provided the angle of incidence Φ is known. On the contrary, if ñ is known a-priori, the value of Φ is obtained. For example, the actual angle of incidence has been measured in this way on the SiO2 substrate at room temperature using a refractive index of 1.46 - i 0.0; this gives $\Phi = 69°$. With this determination of Φ, the refractive index of the substrate at 180°C and of the a-Si:H film considered as a homogeneous medium are calculated from the (Ψ,Δ) of the starting and convergence points on each curve. Value of ñ thus obtained for a-Si:H on SiO_2 is 4.1 - i 0.36.

The growth process can now be analyzed from the trajectory followed by (Ψ,Δ) between both extreme points on the curve. At a first glance, Fig. 2-a shows that we do not deal with a simple layer by layer growth of a homogeneous material with an abrupt substrate/film interface since the curve has not the typical regular well-shaped spiral-like trajectory. To verify this observation we have plotted on Fig. 2-b the simulated curve assuming such a growth process of the film on SiO_2 with a three phase model[5] using the above determined value of the index for a-Si:H. A strong discrepancy between the experimental and simulated curve appears. This cannot be taken into account by the simple hemispherical nucleation model proposed by Hottier and Theeten[2] since the superimposition of the curves is never obtained

34

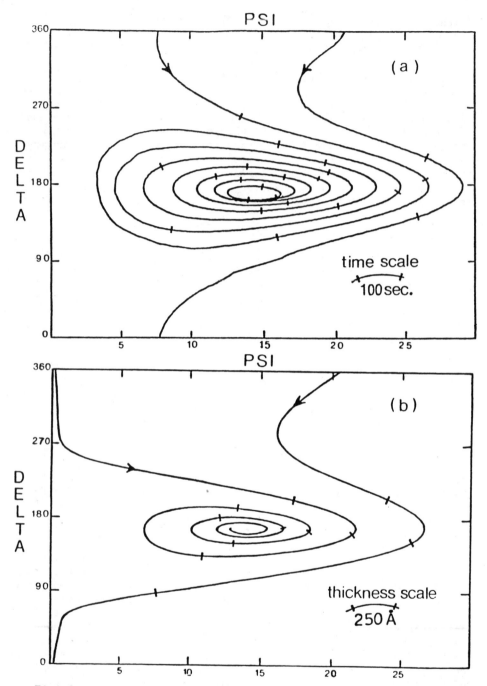

Fig. 2.: Variation of ellipsometric angles Ψ and Δ (in degrees):
(a) experimental curve for the growth of a a-Si:H film on a SiO$_2$
substrate; (b) theoretical curve for the growth of an homogeneous
film.

even after about 0.05 µm of deposit where the growth should become a layer by layer one. The fact that the convergence of the spiral is faster obtained in the simulation indicates that the actual imaginary part of the index of the material which is responsible for the damping of the oscillations is smaller than the calculated one. This difference, which is observed also for a deposit on a crystalline silicon substrate in the same plasma condition, can arise from the presence of bulk oriented microstructure or surface roughness; such hypotheses have to be tested, in particular with the help of spectroscopic ellipsometry which is in progress.

REFERENCES

1. J.C. Knights and R.A. Lujan, Appl. Phys. Lett. 35, 244 (1979).

2. F. Hottier and J.B. Theeten, J. Crystal Growth, 48, 644 (1980).

3. B. Drevillon, J. Huc, A. Lloret, J. Perrin, G. de Rosny and J.P.M. Schmitt, Appl . Phys. Lett. 37, 646 (1980).

4. S.N. Jasperson and S.E. Schnatterly, Rev. Sci. Instr. 40, 761 (1969).

   S.N. Jasperson, D.K. Burge and R.C. O'Handley, Surface Sci. 37, 548 (1973).

5. R.M.A. Azzam and N.M. Bashara, Ellipsometry and Polarized Light, North Holland (1977) p. 288.

INFLUENCE OF ELECTRIC AND MAGNETIC d.c. FIELDS ON THE ELECTRONIC TRANSPORT PROPERTIES OF a-Si:H ALLOYS PRODUCED BY r.f. GLOW DISCHARGE

R. Martins, A. G. Dias, L. Guimarães

Centro de Física Molecular das Universidades de Lisboa; U. N. L.
Complexo I (I. S. T.) Av. Rovisco Pais - 1000 LISBOA

ABSTRACT

This paper shows how electronic transport properties of a-Si:H alloys are modified through the application of electric and magnetic d.c. fields during the film formation. The films studied have been produced by capacitive and inductive r.f. glow discharge (3% SiH_4 in Ar). The photoconductivity and the density of defect states are greatly improved if a d.c. magnetic field is applied, perpendicular to the direction of electric d.c. field. A comparative study between the electronic transport properties of the films produced using the two techniques will be presented.

INTRODUCTION

There is a growing interest in knowing the role of deposition parameters on the properties of a-Si:H alloys produced by r.f. glow discharge for applications in photoelectric devices. The previous work done by Spear[1] shows that the subtrate temperature plays an important role on the electronic transport properties of films produced by that technique. Knights[2] and Tanaka[3] reported results showing that film properties are also influenced by r.f. power. Recent information about the role of electric and magnetic bias during film formation has also been reported (Knights[2] Tsai,[4] Fritzsche[5] Okamoto,[6] Taniguchi[7]). The influence of Ar in SiH_4/Ar mixtures has also been considered.[2,3] It was concluded that the films have high densities of defect states and high H concentrations except when a negative d.c. electric bias is used.[2] It was also observed that the degree of Ar incorporation in the films depends on the geometry configuration.[3] From these results it seems likely that improved film properties will be obtained if a well defined combination of substrate temperature, r.f. power and d.c. bias is achieved. It should then be possible to obtain films with low density of defect states ($10^{17} cm^{-3} eV^{-1}$) and low H concentration even when produced by using SiH_4 diluted in Ar. It is the purpose of this paper to present experimental data concerned with dark/photoconductivity properties of films produced by r.f. glow discharge capacitive or inductively coupled to a 3% SiH_4/Ar mixture under variable bias. Our results show that it is possible to obtain films with low density of defect states and high photoconductivities through suitable bias arrangement during film formation, which are as suitable for photodevice purposes as those obtained by decomposition of pure SiH_4.

EXPERIMENTAL DETAILS

Fig. 1 shows the r.f. capacitive and inductive-coupled glow discharge systems used in this work, which follow in a general way the Spear[1] and Knights[2] experiments. The pre-mixed 3% SiH$_4$/Ar is fed into the system at a flow rate of 100 c.c. min^{-1}. An expansion chamber with a quartz porous disc ($\emptyset$=50 μm) is used to increase the gas homogeneity. During film deposition, the substrate temperature, the pressure, power and frequency of the discharge are kept constant, respectively 260°C for inductive films (I.F.), 325°C for capacitive films, (C.F.), 1 torr, 20W and 12,9 MHz. For C.F. films, 7059 Corning glass substrates are placed in both sides of the heated pedestal (A and P films, fig. 1a). C1 and C2 provide a way to create an asymmetry in r.f. power distribution associated with each side of the discharge.

The d.c. electric bias applied during the deposition process (bias voltage in the range -200—+200V) was perpendicular to the substrate for I.F. films, having two components for C.F. ones, respectively parallel and perpendicular to the substrate surface. The d.c. magnetic field B was always parallel to the surface substrate, either for C.F. or I.F. films.

The samples used for measurements have 2mm spaced evaporated Al contacts in a gap cell configuration. Linear I-V characteristics were observed up to 10^{3}V cm^{-1} applied electric field. Dark and photoconductivity measurements as a function of the reciprocal temperature, T^{-1}, were performed under a vacuum better than 10^{-2} torr, using a field equal to 5X10^{2}V cm^{-1}. AM2 illumination was used for photoconductivity measurements. The growth rate is bias dependent irrespective of the deposition method used.[7,8]

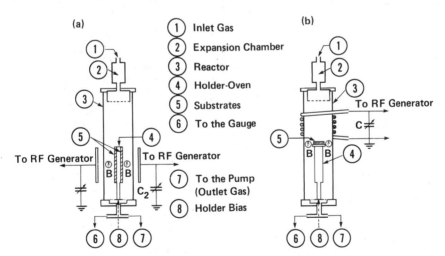

Figure 1 - Shows the apparatus used for a) capacitive-coupled r.f. glow discharge; b) inductive-coupled r.f. glow discharge.

RESULTS

Dark conductivity measurements, σ_D, versus T^{-1}, were made at different bias for both deposition methods described above. In general σ_D verus T^{-1} plots show well defined activation energies, ε_σ, except for a few samples produced without or at low fields. For such samples, we take as ε_σ value the asymptote to the σ_D versus T^{-1} curve containing the room temperature value. Indeed, here the conduction mechanism is hopping-assisted, so ε_σ might not be regarded as an activation energy.

Fig. 2 summarizes the ε_σ values as a function of d.c. electric bias, E_{dc}, with B=0 KG (fig. 2b) for both deposition methods. As it can be seen, ε_σ is lower for I.F. films than for C.F. films. Thus it can be associated with different T_s used[1,2] and with changes in sample composition due to plasma variation.[8] This difference will be observed through all the results presented below. In spite of this, curves ε_σ versus E_{dc} present similar shapes for C.F. and I.F. films produced with B=0 KG and different shapes when the films have been produced with B=1 KG. Thus, when B=0 KG (fig. 2a) the C.F. and I.F. films show that ε_σ is shifted upwards ~.25eV independent of the E_{dc} signal (from .45eV to .70eV for C.F. films and

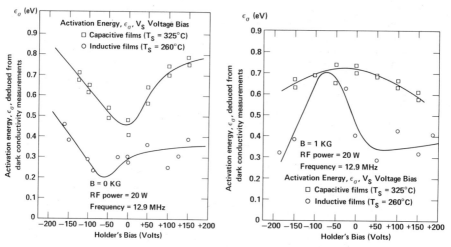

Figure 2 - Shows the dark activation energy ε_σ, for C.F. and I.F. films with a) B=0 KG; b) B=1 KG.

from .23eV to .48eV for the I.F. films). On the other hand, when B=1 KG, although ε_σ versus E_{dc} curves seem to decrease as E_{dc} changes, they don't have the same shape (fig. 2b). For C.F. films, the maximum is located E_{dc} ~0 (~.73eV) and ε_σ shifts ~.10eV independent of E_{dc}, while for I.F. films, ε_σ maximum is located at ~-75 voltage bias (~.70eV) and ε_σ shifts ~.35eV.

A further analysis of C.F. films shows that there is a slight difference in ε_σ values for A and P films (~.25eV) which can be explained by the different Ar and/or H contents in the films due

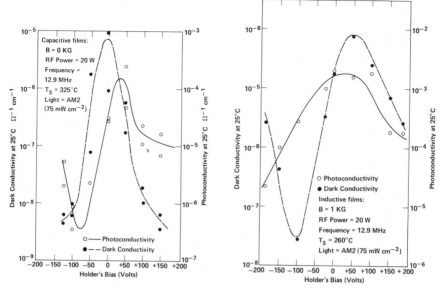

Figure 3 – Shows the dark and photoconductivities as a function of voltage bias for C.F. films a) with B=0 KG; b) with B=1 KG.

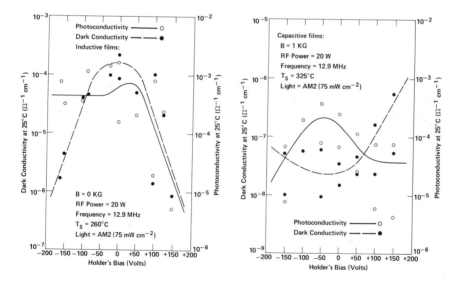

Figure 4 – Shows the dark and photoconductivities as a function of voltage bias for I.F. films a) with B=0 KG; b) with B=1 KG.

to the asymmetry created during film formation.[2,3,9] This difference is also observed in other results. Thus, the line drawn relating the different C.F. results represents the average of A and P films.

Figs. 3 and 4 shown σ_D at 25°C as a function of E_{dc} field with B=0 KG and B=1 KG for C.F. and I.F. films respectively. When B=0 KG, $(\sigma_D)_{25}$ shows a similar behaviour for C.F. and I.F. films (figs. 3a and 4a). But, when B=1 KG, while C.F. films (fig. 3b) shows a systematic $(\sigma_D)_{25}$ variation with E_{dc} ($\sim$3X10^{-8} Ω^{-1} cm^{-1} for negative bias increasing about one order of magnitude for postitive bias), the I.F. films don't show such systematic behavior [$(\sigma_D)_{25}$ changes between 7X10^{-4} Ω^{-1} cm^{-1} to 3X10^{-8} Ω^{-1} cm^{-1}—see fig. 4b.].

Figs. 3 and 4 also show the photoconductivity $\sigma_{ph}=\sigma_L-\sigma_D$ at 25°C as a function of E_{dc}, with B=0 KG and B=1 KG for C.F. and I.F. films. In general we observe that σ_{ph} is temperature activated[10] and that $(\sigma_{ph})_{25}$ doesn't exhibit any appreciable photoconductivity for films produced without or at low E_{dc} fields.[2,3,6,7] However bias during films formation will improve σ_{ph} as it can be seen in figs. 3 and 4. When B=0 KG, $(\sigma_{ph})_{25}$ presents a systematic change with E_{dc} (see fig. 4a) for I.F. films, while the C.F. films show a non-systematic change with E_{dc} (see fig. 3a). When B=1 KG the C.F. and I.F. films present similar $(\sigma_{ph})_{25}$ variations with E_{dc} (for C.F. films $(\sigma_{ph})_{25}$ decreases about one order of magnitude irrespect to the highest E_{dc} field used, while for the I.F. films it decreases about three orders of magnitude for the highest negative bias and only one order of magnitude for the highest positive bias - see figs. 3b and 4b).

The results described above show clearly that the conduction mechanism associated with C.F. and I.F. films changes with bias. Variations in the density and/or the nature of defect states into the films due to plasma composition might account for the differences observed.[2,9,10] Now the plasma kinetics are not only controlled by the r.f. signal and substrate temperature,[1,2,3,4,5] but also controlled by the electric and/or magnetic forces generated by the applied bias which will influence markedly the film's properties.[9,10]

CONCLUSIONS

The main conclusions that we can draw out of our results are:
—By suitable arrangement of d.c. electric field and/or d.c. magnetic field with substrate temperature and r.f. power during film's formation its possible to improve the electronic properties of a-Si:H alloys produced from SiH$_4$ mixed in Ar.
—When B=0 KG $(\sigma_{ph}/\sigma_D)_{25}$ ratio for I.F. films is improved up to $\sim$4X10^2 for a negative bias and it doesn't present any significant improvement when a positive bias is used. Thus it can be explained by changes in the kind of ions impinging the substrate.[2,3] On the other hand, for C.F. films $(\sigma_{ph}/\sigma_D)_{25}$ is improved about three orders of magnitude irrespect to E_{dc} signal.[9,10]

—When B=1 KG $(\sigma_{ph}/\sigma_D)_{25}$ ratio has a maximum ~10^4 at a voltage bias ~-100V for I.F. films and at a voltage bias ~-50V for C.F. films. After maxima $(\sigma_{ph}/\sigma_D)_{25}$ ratio decreases for both type of films. Such behaviour can be explained by changes in plasma kinetics.[9]

ACKNOWLEDGMENTS

We thank Joel Figueiredo for his technical support and I.N.I.C., U.N.L., J.N.I.C.T and D.G.E. for their financial support to the project.

REFERENCES

1. W. E. Spear and P. G. Le Comber, Solid State Commun. 17, 1193 (1975); Phil. Mag. 33, 935 (1976); 7th Int. Conf. on Am. and Liq. Semic., Edinburgh (]977) - ed. by W. E. Spear.
2. J. C. Knights, in Proc. of 10th Conf. on Solid State Devices (Tokyo, August, 1978), p. 101; in Proc. of 8th Int. Conf. on Am. and Liq. Semic. (Boston, 1979), p. 159 - ed. W. Paul and M. Kastner.
3. K. Tanaka, S. Yamasaki, K. Nakagawa, A. Matsuda, et al., in Proc. of 8th Int. Conf. on Am. and Liq. Semic. (Boston, 1979), p. 475 - ed. W. Paul and M. Kastner.
4. C. C. Tsai and H. Fritzsche, Solar Energy Materials 1 (1979) 29.
5. H. Fritzsche, 7th Int. Conf. on Am. and Liq. Semic. (Edinburgh, 1977), p. 3 - ed. by W. E. Spear.
6. H. Okamoto, T. Yamaguchi, Y. Nitta and Y. Hamakawa, in Proc. of 8th Int. Conf. on Am. and Liq. Semic. (Boston, 1979), p.201 - ed. W. Paul and M. Kastner.
7. M. Taniguchi, M. Hirose and Y. Osaka, in Proc. of 8th Int. Conf. on Am. and Liq. Semic. (Boston, 1979), p. 189 - ed. W. Paul and M. Kastner.
8. R. Martins, A. G. Dias and L. Guimarães, to be published.
9. R. Martins, Ph.D. Thesis.
10. L. Guimarães and R. Martins, to be published.

42

THE ROLE OF RF SUBSTRATE BIAS ON
THE GROWTH AND PROPERTIES OF PLASMA DEPOSITED a-Si:H

M. P. Rosenblum, M. J. Thompson,* and R. A. Street
Xerox Palo Alto Research Center, Palo Alto, CA 94304

ABSTRACT

The details of plasma characteristics, chemistry and its relationship to the nucleation and growth process of glow discharge a-Si:H remain unresolved. RF substrate bias is explored as a major influence on the deposition of amorphous Si:H. Recent investigations have revealed the importance of silane ion chemistry and surface chemical reactions in the process of film growth. Experiments, including those with various inert gas diluents, indicate the importance of various ionic and neutral Si_xH_y species in plasma-deposited a-Si:H films. The bias voltage on the substrate is induced by the r.f. plasma as a result of the difference in electron and ion mobilities in the plasma. The magnitude of the induced bias voltage is significantly dependent upon the geometry of the deposition system. Different substrate voltages are generated by tuning the r.f. substrate circuit and by feeding r.f. power directly through the substrate. Films have been grown under a wide range of bias voltages, both positive and negative, and in different gas mixtures of SiH_4/Ar, SiH_4/He, and PH_3 doped SiH_4. The effects of substrate bias on films characterized by their luminescence, I.R. spectra, optical absorption and morphology are discussed.

INTRODUCTION

In the past decade there has been a great quantity of research on glow discharge deposited amorphous silicon. The complexity of the deposition phenomena resulted in an empirical approach to process control and optimization. In recent years considerable effort has been made to analyze the deposition process. Experiments utilizing direct analysis of plasma species by mass spectroscopy[1] and various indirect observations[2] have demonstrated the importance of silane ion chemistry on the properties of the growing film. The critical nature of the interaction between the plasma species and the films surface can be inferred from the observations of film growth and etching in different plasma environments. The series of experiments we have performed are an investigation of the effects of induced substrate voltage, i.e., bias on the growth and properties of a-Si:H. Different substrate potentials will produce changes in the plasma surface interactions through changes in ionic bombardment and plasma characteristics.

EXPERIMENT

The films were deposited in two r.f. diode systems which have been described in detail elsewhere.[3] The geometry of the system will be discussed because of its importance in determining voltage levels induced on the electrodes. The deposition chamber is a vertically mounted steel cross with 8 centimeter diameter arms. Power is applied to the two electrodes through separate power supplies (a common exciter is used so that the r.f. to both electrodes has a constant phase shift). The close proximity of the grounded conducting walls results in considerable changes in the distributed capacitance with small changes in geometry. Different electrode configurations can therefore generate significantly different levels of induced voltage. The asymmetry of the voltages observed when equal power is applied to each electrode is due to differences in electrode geometry. In addition, the magnitude of the change in the induced voltage level depends strongly on gas composition being greatest for 5% SiH_4 in He and least with pure SiH_4. The term bias as used in sputter deposition terminology generally implies that only a small percentage of the total power is applied to the substrate. In the glow discharge deposition system all the power may be applied to the substrate electrode and still have film growth.

A series of depositions were done for three gas compositions, 5% SiH_4 in Ar, 5% SiH_4 in He, and SiH_4 doped with $10^{-3}PH_3$. Each set consisted of about six depositions in which the total power was kept constant but the distribution of power between the electrodes was varied between extremes. Comparisons are made with samples in which the substrate electrode was grounded. In each set the substrate electrode floats to a certain potential with respect to ground when 100% of the power is applied to the opposite electrode. As more of the power is applied to the substrate electrode, its potential decreases and becomes increasingly negative with respect to ground. The other deposition parameters were kept constant within the set of runs. Total power was held at 18 watts, 20 watts, and 10 watts for the 5% SiH_4/He, 5% SiH_4/Ar, and $10^{-3}PH_3/SiH_4$ respectively. Substrate temperatures were maintained at 230°C in all runs.

Measurements were made of the film thickness for deposition rate determination. Infrared transmission, optical absorption, and photoluminescence were measured on each sample. Fracture surfaces were observed in a scanning electron microscope. SIMS analysis was used in order to determine the phosphorous content of the doped films.

RESULTS

Results of the measurements on the Ar series are shown in Figure 1. The voltage induced on the substrate electrode varied from $+65$ to -45 volts as its share of power went from 0 to 100%. A monotonic shift downward is observed in the luminescence peak position and in the optical absorption edge as characterized by E_{04} (the photon energy at 10^4 cm^{-1} absorption), generally representative of a downward shift of the band gap. Infrared spectra show a decrease in the shoulder of the 2000cm^{-1} SiH bond stretching mode as substrate power is increased. This is accompanied by a reduction in absorption by bond bending modes at 845cm^{-1} and 890cm^{-1}. The band gap shift and the changes in H bonding in the sample are interesting in view of the fact that the hydrogen content of the films is rising with substrate power. The implication is that the hydrogen is being incorporated in small voids or clusters at higher substrate power levels while there is a reduction in the hydrogen distributed within the matrix. Observations of the fracture surface morphology are

44

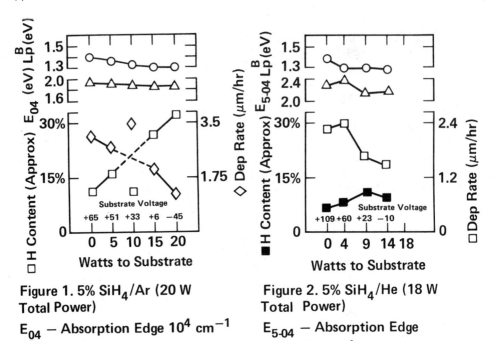

Figure 1. 5% SiH$_4$/Ar (20 W Total Power)

E$_{04}$ — Absorption Edge 10^4 cm^{-1}

Lp^B — Luminescence Peak Position (Band Edge)

Figure 2. 5% SiH$_4$/He (18 W Total Power)

E$_{5\text{-}04}$ — Absorption Edge 5×10^4 cm^{-1}

Lp^B — Luminescence Peak Position (Band Edge)

consistent with this interpretation. In samples prepared with greater than 50% of the power to the substrate, the fracture surfaces reveal little or no columnar structure in contrast to the strong columnar morphology seen in the other films prepared on grounded substrates.[4] Neutron and X-ray scattering experiments[5] on similar films deposited with 100% power to the substrate electrode indicate isotropic inhomogeneities on the order of ~60Å.

The deposition rates of this set were all lower than the rate when the substrate is grounded and decreased as more power was applied to the substrate. The films prepared with equal power to both electrodes exhibit some anomalous properties. This behavior was noted in other samples prepared under the same equal power conditions. It was generally observed that the plasma character was particularly sensitive to slight changes in tuning at this point. This may be responsible for sample variations.

The effects of substrate bias in the He series were the least dramatic (Figure 2). Films prepared from silane diluted in He (substrate grounded) have been shown[2] to have low ESR defect density, high photoluminesence intensity, and a very fine homogeneous microstructure. Few significant changes were observed. The luminescence peak shift is downward and the optical absorption edge, E$_{04}$, rises slightly as the substrate bias becomes less positive. Infrared spectra show no evidence of absorption at 2090cm^{-1},

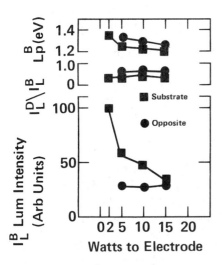

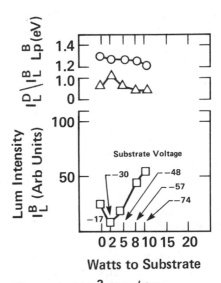

Figure 3. 10^{-3} PH$_3$/SiH$_4$
(Varying Power)

I_L^B — Band Edge Luminescence
Intensity

I_L^D — Defect Band Luminescence
Intensity

L_p^B — Luminescence Peak
Position (Band Edge)

Figure 4. 10^{-3} PH$_3$/SiH$_4$
(10 W Total Power)

I_L^B — Band Edge Luminescence
Intensity

I_L^D — Defect Band Luminescence
Intensity

L_p^B — Luminescence Peak
Position (Band Edge)

845cm^{-1} or 890cm^{-1}. Fracture surfaces of all the samples were smooth and featureless.

An additional set of conditions were used in deposition with 10^{-3} PH$_3$ doped SiH$_4$. Samples were prepared with increasing levels of power applied to each electrode while the other electrode was left floating. The luminescence intensity is plotted as a function of power to the substrate electrode for the constant and varying power series of depositions (Figures 3 and 4). The luminescence intensity remains constant at all power levels for samples prepared on a floating substrate electrode. The relative intensity of the defect band (~.9eV) luminescence remains constant in the two additional sets of depositions. This result suggests that changes in luminescence intensity are not primarily the result of changes in phosphorous concentration, since the defect band intensity should become much more prominent as the band edge luminescence decreases.[6] SIMS analysis also shows that the film with the highest luminescence intensity has among the highest total phosphorous content, contrary to the trend observed in films deposited on grounded substrates. A higher density of non-radiative recombination centers not directly associated with the phosphorous content would decrease the luminescence in such a manner. The results of the three sets of depositions show distinctly that the change in luminescence is not a simple result of either the bias or power dependence since neither description holds for all three series. However, the contrast between the two non-constant power series and the variation in the other set of runs definitively shows the critical importance of plasma interactions with the growing film surface.

CONCLUSIONS

These series of experiments have shown the critical importance of plasma-surface interactions in the growth and properties of a-Si:H. The results of the phosphorous doped series demonstrates that power and deposition rate are not sufficient to predict growth or properties of plasma deposited films. The high luminescence intensity observed in some at the doped films indicates potential for a method of modifying dopant incorporation and defect levels in a-Si:H. The Ar series links the film morphology and hydrogen incorporation to the interaction of ionic species with the film surface. Both the mechanical and chemical effects of ionic bombardment are enhanced by a negative potential on the substrate surface. Reduction in columnar morphology and $(SiH_2)_n$ incorporation in the Ar series may be a result of higher surface mobilities because of the kinetic energy transfer of impinging Ar^+ ions as well as possible etching effects of SiH_x^+ ions. The variations in the P doped series reiterate the complexity of the phenomena in glow discharge deposition.

REFERENCES

* Permanent Address: Department of Electronic Engineering, University of Sheffield, Sheffield, U.K.
1. G. Turban, Y. Catherine, and B. Grolleau, Thin Solid Films. 60, 147 (1979).
2. J. C. Knights, R. A. Lujan, M. P. Rosenblum, R. A. Street, D. K. Biegelsen, and J. A. Reimer, J. Appl. Phys., in press.
3. R. A. Street, J. C. Knights, and D. K. Biegelsen, Phys. Rev. B18, 1880 (1978).
4. J. C. Knights and R. A. Lujan, Appl. Phys. Lett. 35, 244 (1979).
5. A. J. Leadbetter, A. A. M. Rashid, R. M. Richardson, A. F. Wright, and J. C. Knights, Solid State Communications. 33, 973 (1980).
6. R. A. Street, Phys. Rev. B21, 5775 (1980).

THE GROWTH AND PROPERTIES OF BIAS-SPUTTERED a-Si-H

D. P. Turner, I. P. Thomas, J. Allison, M. J. Thompson*
Department of Electronic Engineering, Univeresity of Sheffield, UK

A. J. Rhodes, I. G. Austin, and T. M. Searle
Department of Physics, University of Sheffield, UK

ABSTRACT

a-Si-H films are sputtered from a Si target in an argon-hydrogen atmosphere. It has been found that the bias voltage induced on the heated substrate by the r.f. plasma influences film growth and has a profound effect on the properties of the a-Si-H. The photoconductivity of the films increase to a maximum and then decrease with increasing bias voltage applied to the substrate during growth. Although the hydrogen content of the films does not change significantly with bias, the variation in the relative magnitude of the vibrational stretching bands at 2000 and 2100 cm^{-1} appears to correlate with the photoconductivity bias dependence. The deposition rate and optical absorption edge decreases monotonically with increasing bias.

INTRODUCTION

The interactions between plasma and substrate during the growth of plasma deposited and sputtered a-Si-H is not well understood. In sputtering plasmas highly energetic atoms, ions and electrons are ejected from the target due to argon bombardment.[1] When sputtering a-Si-H, in an argon-hydrogen plasma both H and Si_xH_y ions are present in the plasma. The concentration of H appears largest near the target where it can etch and remove Si atoms.[2] Presumably the plasma species will also react with the growing films but the coupling between the plasma and the substrate is unknown. Various methods are available for influencing such interactions. At present, we are employing both magnetron and r.f. bias sputtering to control the ion flux to the substrate. This paper reports the growth and properties of bias sputtered a-Si-H films. R. F. power is applied to the substrate, as well as the target, resulting in an induced negative potential on the substrate due to the difference in mobility of ions and electrons. As the r.f. power and induced potential is increased the bombardment of Ar, Si_xH_y and H ions on the film increases. It is well known that Ar bombardment of sputtered metal films has a profound influence on film growth.[3,4] Loosely bound and impurity species can be selectively removed[3] and enhanced diffusion of atoms on the surface of the film can result from the momentum

*On sabbatical leave at Xerox Palo Alto Research Center, CA.

transfer from the bombarding sputtering gas ions.[5] Effects such as Ar implantation and changes in film morphology can occur at high bias voltages.[6]

In this paper we describe the properties of films grown under various bias conditions. The photoconductivity and dark conductivity of the a-Si-H are very sensitive to bias conditions during growth. The relative magnitude of the vibrational stretching modes show a similar dependence on bias as the photoconductivity however the hydrogen content remains constant. The deposition rate and optical absorption decreases monotonically with increasing bias. A discussion of the role of Ar bombardment in influencing the H bonding configuration, defects and electronic properties of the a-Si-H film is presented.

FILM PREPARATION

The a-Si-H films are deposited in a Nordiko r.f. sputtering system with a 20 inch diameter stainless steel bell jar containing two 8 inch targets and a 6 inch magnetron target. The base pressure of the system pumped by a turbomolecular pump is less than 10^{-6} torr. The sputtering conditions are similar to that used previously to obtain optimum material.[7] In particular the substrate is maintained at $240°C$ and the Ar partial pressure during sputtering is 6×10^{-3} torr. The r.f. power to the target is maintained at 100W resulting in a d.c. induced negative voltage of $-850V$. As this target voltage remains constant for all the runs the distribution in energy of species leaving the target should be identical for the growth of each film. R.F. power is applied to the substrate and varied

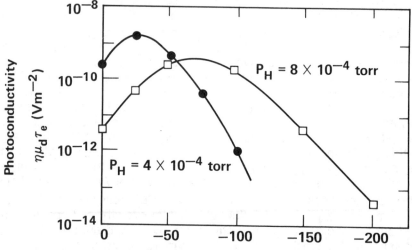

Fig. 1 Photoconductivity versus substrate bias for samples grown in P_H = 4×10^{-4} torr and 8×10^{-4} torr.

in order to induce different bias voltages on the substrate. Two sets of bias runs were made with hydrogen partial pressures (P_H) of 4×10^{-4} torr and 8×10^{-4} torr.

EXPERIMENTAL RESULTS

The photoconductivity of samples grown at various bias voltages and P_H are shown in Figure 1. The highest photoconductivity is obtained in samples grown in a $P_H = 4 \times 10^{-4}$ torr with a bias of $-25V$. However the photoconductivity of samples grown at this P_H is much more sensitive to bias conditions than those grown at a $P_H = 8 \times 10^{-4}$ torr. The maximum photoconductivity of samples grown at the high P_H is obtained in samples with a bias voltage between -50 and $-75V$. The room temperature dark conductivity and activation energy of the bias samples are shown in Figure 2. These are a maximum and minimum respectively for samples grown at the same bias voltages as these with maximum photoconductivity for $P_H = 4 \times 10^{-4}$ torr. However this is not the case with the samples grown at $P_H = 8 \times 10^{-4}$ torr. The I-R vibrational spectra were examined in all the samples. The ratio of 2000 cm^{-1}

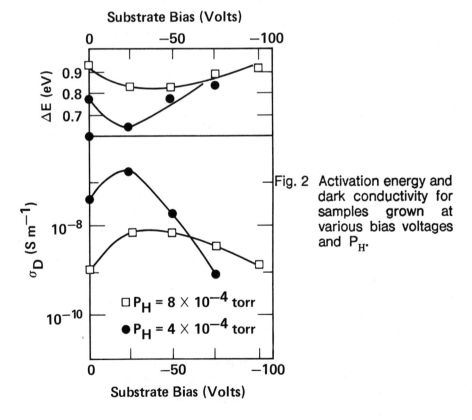

Fig. 2 Activation energy and dark conductivity for samples grown at various bias voltages and P_H.

absorption band over the total stretching band absorption (2000 cm⁻¹
and 2100 cm⁻¹) is shown in Fig. 3 as a function substrate bias voltage.
The stretching band strengths are calculated from the area under the
curves of two deconvoluted Gaussian distributions. Some correlation
exists between photoconductivity and I-R absorption variation with bias.
The 2000 cm⁻¹ peak is a maximum in samples with the highest
photoconductivity. However at high bias voltage the relative strength of
the stretching bands is a much more slowly varying function of bias than
the photoconductivity variations. Apart from the zero bias sample the
total strength of the stretch bands correlates with hydrogen content as
seen from a comparison of I-R and H evolution data. Figure 3 shows that
the total hydrogen content of the samples remains constant for samples
grown at greater than 0V bias. The optical absorption edge reduces
monotonically by 0.05 eV as the bias is increased from 0V to -100V. A
corresponding increase in refractive index of 10% is observed over the
same range of bias. The net deposition rate or accumulation rate
decreases from 0.21 μm/hr. to 0.20μm/hr. for 0 to -100V bias. However
at higher bias voltages the rate decreases more rapidly with bias.

DISCUSSIONS AND CONCLUSIONS

Until now it appeared that there was little correlation between the
relative magnitude of the vibrational stretching bands and the electrical
and device properties of sputtered a-Si-H. However here we have found
that the maximum photoconductivity appears in bias samples containing
the strongest 2000 cm⁻¹ SiH band. The dark resistivity and activiation

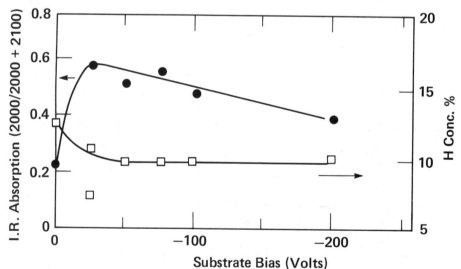

Fig. 3 The fraction of singly bonded hydrogen (2000/[2000 + 2100])
and hydrogen content for samples grown at various bias voltages
and $P_H = 4 \times 10^{-4}$ torr.

energy of this sample is lower than previously obtained in any of our unbiased samples. The increase in photoconductivity is partly due to a shift in Fermi energy towards the conduction band. This shift could be due to removal of deep defects in the material by ion bombardment. However for samples grown at higher bias voltages the reduction in photoconductivity appears to be due to more energitic Ar bombardment causing defect creation and reduced carrier lifetime.

We have previously shown that at low P_H all the hydrogen resides as SiH and no 2100cm$^-$ peak is observed. Above 4×10^{-4} torr the ratio of the 2000cm$^-$ to the total stretching band intensity remains constant (0.3) for increasing P_H despite the fact that the hydrogen incorportion in the film increases.[8] This implies that above 4×10^{-4} torr for every singly bonded H atom that is incorporated about 3 H atoms are incorporated elsewhere, possibly at SiH$_2$ sites around voids. As the photoconductivity is a maximum for samples with $P_H = 4 \times 10^{-4}$ torr this implies that above this pressure that some incorporated H is not compensating dangling bonds but possibly creating or modifying defects sites. The bias results supports this theory in that at a critical bias the defect sites associated with 2100cm$^-$ absorption (SiH$_2$) are removed by substrate bombardment and the photoconductivity increases. At the higher P_H the effect of bias is reduced as the number of SiH$_2$ sites is much larger. The slight reduction in optical absorption and increase in refractive index as the bias in increased is due to the decrease in SiH content of the film. It could be argued that the increases in photoconductivity is due to an increase in hole trapping. However the performance of solar cells is improved in the highly photoconductive samples; this is not consistent with an increase in hole trap density There is no evidence in our data for differences in stretching band oscillator strength between samples prepared in different bias conditions. Using S.E.M. analysis no columnar growth was observed in any of the samples.

REFERENCES

1. G. N. Jackson, Thin Solid Films, 5, 209 (1970).
2. A. Matsuda, K. Nakagaua, K. Tanaka, M. Matsumura, S. Yamasaki, H. Okustu, and S. Iizima, J. Non Cryst. Solids 35, 183 (1980).
3. J. Kay, J. Appl. Phys. 49, 4862 (1978).
4. A. G. Blackman Metal Trans. 2, 699 (1971).
5. A. H. Eltouky, J. Aply Phys. 51, 444 (1980).
6. E. Eser, R. E. Ogilvie, and K. A. Taylor, Thin Solid Films, 61, 265 (1980).
7. M. J. Thompson, M. M. Alkaisi, and J. Allison, Rev. de Phys. App., 13 625 (1978).

8. T. S. Nashashibi, T. M. Searle, I. G. Austin, K. Richards, M. J. Thompson, J. Allison., J. Non Cryst. Solids 35, 675 (1980).

FILM-PLASMA INTERACTIONS IN TRIODE-SPUTTERED a-Si:H*

P. M. Martin and W. T. Pawlewicz
Pacific Northwest Laboratory[+]
Richland, Washington 99352

The film-plasma interaction and its influence on total H content and SiH bonding in a-Si:H was studied using a dc triode (supported discharge) sputtering system. Use of the dc triode system allowed the influence of substrate bombardment energy (target voltage) for plasma species (electrons and neutral or ionize Ar, H, Si) to be studied independently from the influence of deposition rate (target current). As a result the mechanisms for H incorporation, whether by film bombardment or surface reactions and chemisorptive processes, were studied in greater detail than could be achieved in a diode sputtering system.

The energy of the plasma species bombarding the film was controlled by varying the target voltage (V_T). H. and Ar partial pressures (P_H and P_{Ar}), deposition rate (R_D) and substrate temperature (T_s) were held constant at 6.0 mtorr, 6.0 $\sim$ 2.0 Å/sec and 225°C respectively. TotalH content increased linearly from 5 to near 27 at.% with an increase in V_T from 100 to 2000 volts. Trapped Ar showed a concomitant linear increase from Ar/Si $\sim$ 0 to Ar/Si = 0.012, where Ar/Si is the ratio of the Ar and Si K_α emission lines in an electron-beam excited x-ray fluorescence spectrum. Because all other deposition conditions remained unchanged, the increase in H content was attributed to 1) an increase in trapped (implanted) H which could occupy interstitial positions or be chemically bonded in the network and 2) H bonded to broken Si-Si bonds resulting from the higher energy of plasma bombardment. The increase in implanted H is the primary effect attributed to the increase in energy of the plasma species.

The dominant Si-H bond type was always SiH_2 (infrared stretch mode at 2090 cm^{-1}) for films deposited with P_H = 6.0 mtorr, but SiH content increased from 0 to $\sim$ 6 at.% with the increase in V_T. This increase in SiH content may have resulted from the increase in trapping of energetic H ions and neutrals and/or from the stronger plasma bombardment of the film at high V_T.

The behavior of the electrical and optical properties of the triode-sputtered films can be explained by the increase in implanted H. Two regions are apparent for the electrical resistivity (ρ) and activation energy. For films with H content > 15 at.% (V_T > 800 volts), ρ increases from 30 Ω cm to 2.5 x $10^6 \Omega$ cm with the increase in trapped H from 15 to 27 at.%. ρ of these films correspond to rf diode-sputtered films with $\sim$ 10 at.% less H. This may have implications for Si-H bonding and passivation of dangling bond defects by H incorporated by implantation. The activation energy increases from $\sim$ 0.2eV (suggestive of dangling bond defects) to near intrinsic levels with the increase in H content. Films deposited with V_T < 800 volts were porous and display post-deposition oxidation and this increases ρ to $\sim$ 4 x $10^4 \Omega$ cm for V_T = 100 volts. The optical band gap increases and the refractive index decreases with increased H incorporated by trapping.

---

*Work supported by the Material Sciences Division of the Department of Energy - Office of Basic Energy Sciences
[+]Operated by Battelle Memorial Institute for the U.S. Department of Energy.

BOMBARDMENT EFFECTS IN a-Si:H SPUTTERED FILMS

R. C. Ross and R. Messier
Materials Research Laboratory
The Pennsylvania State University
University Park, Pennsylvania 16802

ABSTRACT

The substrate floating potential, V_s, was measured as a function of rf-sputtering conditions using an electrostatic probe. The large negative V_s induced at low P_{Ar} is responsible for energetic ion-bombardment at the growing film/plasma interface. This bombardment, when below a threshold potential $\sim$-20V, results in local atomic rearrangement and selective resputtering, leading to minimization of microstructural defects. Results on film characteristics vs. V_s, H-implantation in c-Si, and Si-H bonding vs. P_{H2} and T_s lead to a more complete picture of bombardment and thermal processes in a-Si:H film formation.

INTRODUCTION

Although a-Si:H films prepared by rf-sputtering and glow-discharge techniques are similar in structure and properties, the preparation-condition dependence of film characteristics for both cases, along with differences in the preparation parameters, makes comparison difficult. For rf-sputtered films the effect of bombardment processes has been related to film structure and bonding. Both Pawlewicz[1] and Anderson[2] et al. have suggested that bombardment effects are detrimental, due to defect creation. However, their proposed mechanisms for bombardment reduction differ in that Pawlewicz concludes that high pressures (>150mTorr) lead to thermalization of energetic particles while Anderson et al. suggest that film damage is due primarily to energetic Si atoms which are thermalized at much lower gas pressure (>10mTorr). Recently, we have shown[3] that bombardment effects are beneficial in producing films which have no observable microstructure, show no post-deposition degradation, are highly compressively stressed, and have predominant monohydride bonding. In the latter case, we related bombardment to a high negative self-bias, V_{sb}, induced on the growing film surface, in which the negative potential leads to Ar^+ bombardment with energy sufficient both to resputter deposited material and to implant into the growing film. The negative potential is inversely related to total gas pressure, P_T, of the sputtering gas. The relations between bombardment effects, structure, and resulting properties were found to be consistent with literature results in which the best photovoltaic sputtered a-Si:H films have been prepared only at low P_T[4,5]. Moustakas[6] has measured V_{sb} vs. P_T and obtains values almost identical to ours.

EXPERIMENTAL

The details of the rf-sputtering preparation and resulting film property measurements have been described previously[3]. In addition, films reported in the present study were prepared at elevated resistance-

ISSN:0094-243X/81/730053-05$1.50 Copyright 1981 American Institute of Physics

heater temperatures (T_h). Both T_h and T_s (film/substrate temperature) were measured, the latter with an Al/Ag thin film thermocouple.

The plasma potential, V_p, and the substrate self-bias potential (potential with respect to ground), V_{sb}, were taken from electrostatic probe I(V) characteristics as a function of Ar partial pressure, P_{Ar}, H_2 partial pressure, P_{H_2}, and rf-power level. The break in the characteristic at V_p (above which current is exclusively electronic) was distinct enough to determine ($\pm 2V$) by inspection. The probe was a 0.15mm diameter cylindrical W wire 7mm long and positioned 1cm above the substrate. The measuring circuit employed was as described by Eser et al.[7] The V_{sb} values agreed with previous measurements[3] in which V_{sb} was determined at the substrate/film surface. From these data the floating potential (substrate potential with respect to V_p), V_s, was calculated: $V_s = V_{sb} - V_p$. Obviously, film bombardment effects due to plasma induced biasing are related directly to V_s, and not V_{sb} as done previously[3,4].

RESULTS

Large differences between T_h and T_s were observed both in vacuum and at pressures below ∿1Torr. For $T_h=300°C$, $T_s=150°C$ (0W rf-power) and 190°C (100W rf-power) while for $T_h=30°C$, $T_s=75°C$ (100W rf-power). For the deposition conditions reported in this study V_s is almost a constant $-18V$ at $P_{Ar} >30$mTorr and becomes increasingly more negative for lower P_{Ar}, reaching $-50V$ at $P_{Ar}=7$mTorr.

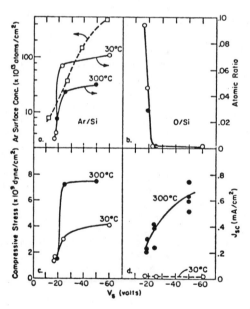

Figure 1. Threshold type dedendence of film properties upon the substrate floating potential, V_s: (a) Ar/Si atomic ratio, (b) O/Si atomic ratio, (c) intrinsic compressive stress, (d) J_{sc} at AM1 for Pd/a-Si:H/Cr/glass. Dashed line in (a) is Ar surface concentration in c-Si from low energy implantation studies (from reference 9). Data in (a-c) is for films prepared with no H: samples prepared at various P_{H_2} followed similar trends.

Fig. 1 shows a threshold type dependence upon V_s at ∿$-20V$ for several film properties. At more negative potentials the Ar content and compressive stress are greatly increased, the increase in Ar being larger for the low-T_h material and the increase in stress being larger for the high-T_h material. The oxygen content (primarily post-deposition) drops below detection at $V_s < -20V$, showing no clear temperature (T) dependence. At 300°C J_{sc} also increases at more negative V_s: at 30°C J_{sc} was not detectable.

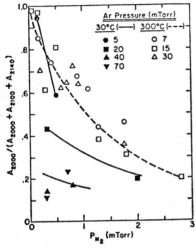

Figure 2

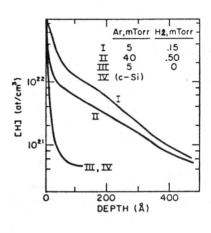

Figure 3

Figure 2.   Dependence of stretching mode intensity ratio, $A_{2000}/(A_{2000}+A_{2100}+A_{2140})$, upon P_{H_2} for $T_h=30$, 300°C and various P_{Ar}.

Figure 3.   SIMS H depth profiles of c-Si targets rf-sputtered at 100W and different P_{Ar} and P_{H_2}.

The ratio of the integrated absorption at 2000cm^{-1} to the total integrated absorption for all Si-H stretching modes is shown as a function of P_{H_2} in Fig. 2. For the 30°C films, the monohydride fraction increases strongly for lower P_{Ar} (and more negative V_s). At 300°C however, temperature appears to be more important than P_{Ar} or V_s in controlling the H bonding, in the range investigated.

H depth profiles of surfaces of single crystals of Si sputtered under several representative conditions are shown in Fig. 3. Quite clearly, during deposition large amounts of H$^+$ (up to 40 at %) are implanted in the target to substantial depths (several hundred angstroms).

DISCUSSION

The dramatic effects of V_s more negative than about $-20V$ appear to be due to energetic ion bombardment, probably Ar$^+$ and Ar^{++} [8]. In Fig. 1a Ar surface concentration in c-Si versus accelerating potential, as determined by Comas and Wolicki[9], is superposed on the Ar bulk concentration values for our samples. The surface concentration, and thus implantation, increases by a factor of 10 going from 15V to 30V. As we have discussed previously[3] this bombardment is a steady state process occuring at the growth interface and involves selective resputtering of weakly bonded species, and Ar^+ implantation accompanied by localized atomic rearrangement. Such bombardment processes minimize or remove the intercolumnar network of voids (i.e. low density regions) which are evident at high P_{Ar} and small V_s.

This picture is also consistent with the results presented above. For the films produced at V_S more negative than the threshold at $\sim-20V$, bulk Ar incorporation increases significantly (Fig. 1a) while post-deposition oxidation is reduced and compressive stress is increased (Fig. 1b and 1c), again due to void reduction.

The effects of T are also quite important, especially with regard to electronic properties. Carlson and Magee[10] have shown that energetic H^+ bombardment dramatically reduces a-Si:H MIS cell performance, but that performance can be restored by annealing at $T \gtrsim 200°C$. In the films produced at $T_S=75°C$ no photovoltaic response was observed, while for similar films prepared at $T_S=190°C$ there is appreciable response. In addition, T seems to govern electronic properties through the control of Si-H bonding. For example, at 75°C we observe that the monohydride fraction is greatly increased for conditions which favor Ar bombardment (i.e., low P_{Ar}; see Fig. 2). However, at higher T_S the monohydride fraction is maximized independently of P_{Ar} or V_s, at least for the range investigated. Here chemical kinetics at the growth front and/or thermal annealing effects are probably dominant.

Elevated T also tends to reduce the amount of Ar and H in the bombarded films, probably by reducing the sticking coefficient. That elevated T appears to increase the amount of intrinsic compressive stress indicates that T may also have some effect in reducing but not eliminating the void network. The post-deposition oxygen content appears to be independent of preparation T, indicating that V_S has the dominant effect on void minimization.

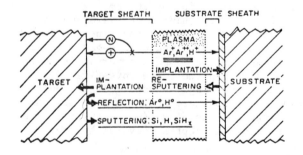

Figure 4. Schematic illustration of possible sources of bombardment and related processes in the rf-sputtering environment.

Aside from positive ion bombardment at the growing film surface due to negative V_S, several other bombardment processes possibly may be of importance in controlling film growth. These are indicated schematically in Figure 4 and discussed below.

The high level of H in the near surface of the target (see Fig. 3) leads to the consideration that it is actually hydrogenated a-Si, not c-Si, that is being sputtered. We may then speculate as to the importance of sputtered fragments. This could explain the substantial Si_xHy observed in the a-Si:H sputtering environment by optical emission studies[11], which is unlikely to be formed by plasma chemical reactions.

Ar bombardment of the growing film is due primarily to Ar^+ and Ar^{++} from the plasma accelerated by V_s, as discussed above. Because of the higher atomic mass of Ar as compared to Si, we may expect minimal back-reflection of Ar from the target.

There are four sources of energetic H impinging upon the film surface: (1) H^+ accelerated by V_s from the plasma across the substrate sheath; (2) H° elastically backscattered from the target at energies approaching the cathode potential; (3) H sputtered from the target surface; and (4) thermal H. For H^+ incident on the target, we can expect a total reflection coefficient of 0.25-0.50 for energies in the range 500-1000eV[12]. This reflected H could have an important role in energetic bombardment of the growing film, especially at low P_{Ar}.

We wish to acknowledge the assistance of Paul Moses in the IR data programming and Lee Eminhizer for microprobe measurements. This work was supported by the Solar Energy Research Institute under Sub-contract No. XG-0-9227.

REFERENCES

1. W. T. Pawlewicz, J. Appl. Phys. 49, 5595 (1978).
2. D. A. Anderson, G. Moddel, M. A. Paesler and W. Paul, J. Vac. Sci. Technol. 16, 906 (1979).
3. R. C. Ross and R. Messier, J. Appl. Phys. (accepted).
4. T. D. Moustakas, J. Elect. Mat. 8, 391 (1979); T. D. Moustakas, C. R. Wronski, and D. L. Morel, J. Non-Cryst. Solids 35-36, 719 (1980).
5. M. M. Al-Kaisi and M. J. Thompson, Solar Cells 1, 91 (1979/80).
6. T. D. Moustakas (private communication).
7. E. Eser, R. E. Ogilvie and K. A. Taylor, Thin Solid films 68, 381 (1980).
8. J. W. Coburn and E. Kay, J. Appl. Phys. 43, 4965 (1972); W. D. Davis and T. A. Vanderslice, Phys. Rev. 131, 219 (1963).
9. J. Comas and E. A. Wolicki, J. Electrochem. Soc. 117, 1197 (1970).
10. D. E. Carlson and C. W. Magee, 1979 Photovoltaic Solar Energy Conf., 312 (1979).
11. A. Matsuda, K. Nakagawa, K. Tanaka, M. Matsumura, S. Yamasaki, H. Okushi, and S. Iizima, J. Non-Cryst. Solids 35 and 36, 183 (1980).
12. W. Eckstein, F. E. P. Matschke and H. Verbeck, J. Nuc. Mat. 63, 199 (1976); O. S. Oen and M. T. Robinson, Nucl. Instr. Meth. 132, 647 (1976).

PROPERTIES OF AMORPHOUS SILICON PREPARED AT DIFFERENT TEMPERATURES BY PYROLYTIC DECOMPOSITION OF SILANE *

P. Hey[+], N. Raouf, D. C. Booth, and B. O. Seraphin
Optical Sciences Center, University of Arizona, Tucson, AZ 85721 USA

ABSTRACT

Over the range 525 < T_s < 650 C of substrate temperature T_s, the hydrogen content of amorphous silicon deposited by the pyrolytic decomposition of silane varies from 0.8 at% to 0.2 at%. This relatively small change is accompanied by order-of-magnitude variations in conductivity and field effect. The results are interpreted in terms of shifts of the Fermi level, density of states profiles, and change in the conduction mechanism.

INTRODUCTION

In amorphous silicon films deposited by pyrolytic decomposition of silane at substrate temperatures T_s, in the range 525 < T_s < 650 C, the hydrogen concentration varies from 0.8 at% to 0.2 at% respectively, as previously reported on the basis of SIMS measurements[1]. These values are much lower than those usually obtained in films deposited by glow discharge[2], or by sputtering and evaporation under hydrogen[3]. Previous measurements on CVD α-Si have consequently ignored the influence of variations of this small hydrogen concentration on the transport properties of the material[4]. The results reported here indicate, however, that conductivity as well as field induced current varies over orders of magnitude in response to very small differences of the hydrogen content, as generated by 25 C increments in T_s from 525 to 650 C.

SAMPLE PREPARATION

A horizontal, radiatively heated CVD reactor was used to prepare 0.5 and 1.0 μm thick α-Si films on ½x½" quartz substrates for conductivity measurements; similarly, 0.5 μm thick films were deposited on 100 Si wafers with a thermally grown (6700A) SiO_2 dielectric layer for field effect measurements. A flowrate of 22.5 cc/min silane in 4 1/min helium carrier gas was employed. Doping was accomplished by adding PH_3 and B_2H_6 to the gas phase at T_s = 650 C and 600 C, respectively. Impurity concentrations from 0.01 at% to 10 at% were obtained in the films. Microprobe analysis showed that three times as much phosphorous was incorporated as would be expected from the gas phase composition, while only 1/10 as much boron was found. Electrical contacts were made with CVD molybdenum or evaporated aluminum.

* Work supported by "Photo-Electric Properties of Amorphous Silicon Deposited by the Pyrolytic Decomposition of Silicon," DOE-SERI Subcontract XS-9-8041-8.

[+]Fulbright fellow to the Physics Department of the University of AZ.

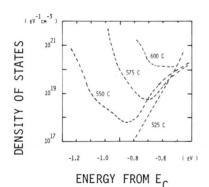

DENSITY OF STATES

$(\text{eV}^{-1}_{\text{cm}}{}^{-3})$

10^{21}

10^{19}

10^{17}

600 C

575 C

550 C

525 C

-1.2   -1.0   -0.8   -0.6   (eV)

ENERGY FROM E_c

Fig. 7. Density of states for the samples of Fig. 6 profiles.

The room temperature conductivity σ_{RT} is dominated by hopping conduction near the Fermi level; its decrease with T_s therefore suggests a reduction of gap states near the Fermi level with the incorporation of hydrogen. This is supported by the results of field effect measurements performed at about 60 C. The field induced conductance changes by two orders of magnitude over the deposition temperature range (Fig. 6), and is very sensitive to variations of Ts. Note that negative fields yield a small but measurable change in the field effect response, indicating contributions from hole conduction. These variations have not been observed in related work[8]. The evaluation of these measurements in terms of the density of states in the gap as shown in Fig. 7 is based on a derivation that does not involve the explicit solution of Poisson's equation[9]. The resulting N(E) profiles support the assumption that the hydrogen terminates gap states around the Fermi level, with midgap densities increasing from less than 10^{17} to about 10^{20} per eV per cm^{+3}, as Ts increases from 525 to 650 C. This result correlates well with the fact that only a small fraction of the hydrogen incorporated in amorphous films produced by glow-discharge actually saturates dangling bonds[10]. The Fermi level position for the N(E) curves was determined assuming the relation

$$(E_c - E_f)_T = (E_c - E_f) - \gamma T \qquad (T)$$

where $\gamma = 2.0 \times 10^{-4}$ eV/K is the temperature coefficient of the Fermi level[5].

Substitutional doping at 650 C for phosphorous and at 600 C for boron above a threshold impurity concentration of 1.0 at% for phosphorous and 0.1 at% for boron, reduces the activation energy to 0.2 eV. The room temperature conductivity goes up by five to six orders of magnitude over σ_{RT} for undoped samples, in agreement with related work[4]. A maximum relative increase of $(\sigma_{ph} - \sigma_d)/\sigma_d = 80$ in photoconductivity over the dark conductivity is found for 2 at% P and 0.1 at% B in the white light of a 500 W light bulb.

CONCLUSIONS

It is concluded that the changes in the very small hydrogen content of amorphous Si films deposited by CVD at high temperatures suffice to produce order-of-magnitude modifications in the transport properties. It may consequently be possible to optimize the photo-electrical properties of the material within the wide range of these modifications.

60

EXPERIMENTAL RESULTS AND DISCUSSION

The deposition temperature T_s for undoped α-Si was varied from 525 to 650 C in steps of 25 C. The incorporated hydrogen concentration as determined by SIMS[1] shows a decline from less than 1 at% at T_s = 550 C to 0.2 at% at 650 C (Fig. 1). The 1/T profile of the dc conductivity σ consists of the two semilogarithmic parts usually assigned to hopping versus extended-state mechanism[5]. Size and slopes of these profiles respond sensitively to variations of the hydrogen concentration. The conductivity at room temperature is plotted in Fig. 2. Activation energy $(E_c - E_f)_0$ and pre-exponential factor σ_0 for the high-temperature branches are shown in Figs. 3 and 4, respectively.

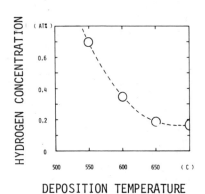

Fig. 1. Hydrogen concentration of CVD silicon deposited at different deposition temperatures T_s.

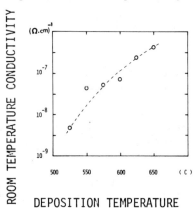

Fig. 2. Room temperature conductivity of undoped CVD α-Si as a function of T_s.

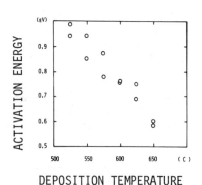

Fig. 3. Activation energy of the high temperature conductivity for undoped CVD α-Si.

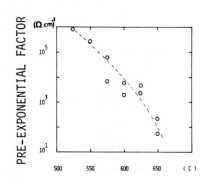

Fig. 4. Pre-exponential factor of the high-temperature conductivity for undoped CVD α-Si.

The variation of the hydrogen concentration with T_s demonstrated in Fig. 1. may be solely responsible for the changes shown in Figs. 2, 3 and 4, although other reasons such as structural variations cannot be excluded[6]. The change in activation energy indicates a displacement of the Fermi level towards the conduction band edge as the hydrogen content decreases. A smaller amount terminates fewer dangling bonds, and the density of states in the gap increases.

This trend appears to be confirmed by the ESR spin density profile[7] shown in Fig. 5, although the small variations, uncertain in the face of the large error bars, may not be able to account fully for the order-of-magnitude changes of the transport properties shown in Figs. 2-4.

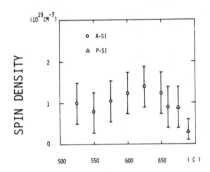

DEPOSITION TEMPERATURE

Fig. 5. Spin density of amorphous (A-Si) and polycrystalline (P-Si) silicon prepared by CVD.

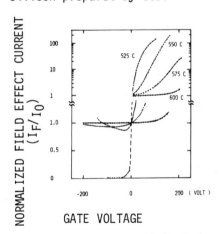

GATE VOLTAGE

Fig. 6. Normalized field induced current of undoped CVD α-Si samples deposited at different temperatures T_s.

Note in particular that a spin density of 10^{19} cm^{-3} is not reflected in the field effect measurements plotted in Fig. 6. Independent of the analysis of these measurements which lead to the density-of-state profiles of Fig. 7, it is evident that the strong variation of the field effect response of Fig. 6 could not be observed on the basis of a density of states in the order of the spin density. This suggests that the two measurements probe the density-of-state profile in different regions of the gap. We wish to draw attention to this difference, although at present we do not have an explanation for it.

The decrease of σ_0 by three orders of magnitude upon increasing T_s can be related to a change in the transport mechanism. At a lower density of dangling bonds, conduction occurs through extended states with high mobility[5], leading to a high σ_0. At higher deposition temperatures, corresponding to less hydrogen, and presumably more dangling bonds, hopping conduction through localized states with their low mobility becomes more important, resulting in a lower σ_0.

ACKNOWLEDGEMENTS

The authors would like to thank Dr. J. Fordemwalt and Mr. J. Homoki in the Electrical Engineering Department, University of Arizona, for their support in producing microcircuits for the field effect measurements.

REFERENCES

1. D. C. Booth, D. D. Allred and B. O. Seraphin, Solar Energy Mater., 2, 107 (1979).
2. H. Fritzche, M. H. Tanielian, C. C. Tsai, P. J. Gaczi, J. Appl. Phys. 50 (5), 3366 (1979).
3. A. K. Malhotra, G. W. Neudeck, Appl. Phys. Lett. 28 (1), 47 (1976).
4. M. Hirose, M. Taniguchi, T. Nakashita, Y. Osaka, T. Suzuki, S. Hasegawa, T. Shimizu, J. Non-Cryst. Solids, 35-36, 297 (1980).
5. P. G. Lecomber, A. Madan, W. E. Spear in "Electronic and Structural Properties of Amorphous Semiconductors," (Academic Press, London and New York, 1972), p. 373.
6. R. Messier, S. V. Krishnaswamy, L. R. Gilbert, P. Swab, J. Appl. Phys. 51 (3), 1611 (1980).
7. P. J. Gaczi, D. C. Booth, Solar Energy Mater. 4, 297 (1981).
8. T. Nakashita, M. Hirose, Y. Osaka, Jpn. J. Appl. Phys., 18 (2), 405 (1979).
9. M. Gruenewald, P. Thomas, D. Wuertz,, Phys. Stat. Sol. (B), 100, K139 (1980).
10. T. D. Moustakas in "Amorphous Silicon/Materials Subcontractor Review," SERI/SP-614-1056, Denver, Col., Feb. 1981.

PREPARATION OF AMORPHOUS SILICON FILMS BY CVD OF HIGHER ORDER SILANES Si_nH_{2n+2} for n ≥ 2

S. Gau, B. R. Weinberger, M. Akhtar, Z. Kiss and A. G. MacDiarmid
CHRONAR CORP.
P.O. Box 177
Princeton, N.J. 08540

ABSTRACT

We have prepared amorphous silicon films by chemical vapor deposition (CVD) using higher silanes Si_nH_{2n+2}(n ≥ 2) in the temperature range of 380° - 500°C. The films show electrical properties comparable to those prepared by glow discharge of silanes. Optical absorption spectra both in the visible and Far I.R. regions differ substantially from those obtained for hydrogenated amorphous silicon. Gold Schottky devices were fabricated with short circuit currents of 13mA/cm^2 under AM-1 illumination over an area of 5 mm^2.

INTRODUCTION

In recent years, substantial progress has been made in the developement of efficient, thin film photovoltaic devices based upon amorphous silicon (a-Si). Solar conversion efficiencies in the range of 5% have been achieved.[1]. The breakthrough which precipitated this progress was the realization that alloying a-Si with hydrogen[2] resulted in a drastic reduction of the density of states in the a-Si energy gap. It was found that the electronic properties of a-Si:H could be controlled over a wide range by substitutional doping and that the photosensitivity of the films was dramatically improved, presumably due to the elimination of photocarrier recombination centers.

Device quality a-Si:H films have been deposited from the plasma discharge[3] of monosilane (SiH$_4$) or the sputtering[4] of silicon in a hydrogen atmosphere. a-Si may also be produced by the pyrolytic decomposition of SiH$_4$. However, due to the high temperatures required to achieve appreciable deposition rates (500°C - 750°C)[5], bonded hydrogen in the resulting films is limited[6] (∿ 1% compared to 15-50% in glow discharge a-Si). Consequently, the defect density and density of gap states for such films produced by chemical vapor deposition (CVD) from monosilnae is orders of magnitude larger than from glow discharge a-Si. This makes CVD a-Si from SiH$_4$ unsuitable for photovoltaic device applications without post-deposition treatment[7].

We, therefore, propose an alternate CVD process for the formation of a-Si with appreciable hydrogen alloying, based on the pyrolytic decomposition of higher order silanes.

TECHNICAL DISCUSSION

Silane, SiH$_4$, is just one of a homologous series of compounds (Si_nH_{2n+2},n=1,2...). Like monosilane, the higher order silanes decompose when heated to yield silicon hydrides and hydrogen gas[8].

ISSN:0094-243X/81/730063-04$1.50 Copyright 1981 American Institute of Physics

64

However, the higher order silanes decompose at successively lower
temperatures and consequently the CVD of a a-Si from these higher
silanes should be possible at lower temperatures than for SiH_4
with greater inclusion of bonded hydrogen resulting. Recently,
the deposition of highly photosensitive a-Si:H from the plasma
discharge of disilane (Si_2H_6) has been reported.[9] In this paper we
present initial results of our study of the CVD of a-Si from higher
silanes. Included is preliminary characterization of higher silane
CVD Schottky devices.

We have successfully deposited a-Si films by CVD of higher
silanes at temperatures as low as 375°C in a flow system using
argon as a carrier gas, and in a stationary system using the higher
order silanes only. Silanes were produced in a reactor flask by
the addition of Mg_2Si to dilute HCl.[10] In this reaction approximately 25% of the silicon is converted to a mixture of silanes containing 40% SiH_4, 30% Si_2H_6, 15% Si_3H_8, 10% Si_4H_{10} and 5% higher
silanes.

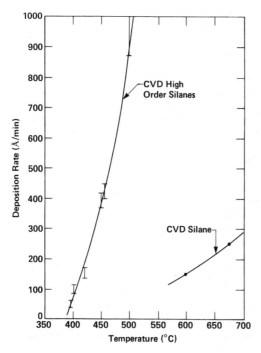

Fig.1 deposition rate as
a function of temperature

Figure 1 summarizes the rate of deposition as a function of
temperature. For comparison, the deposition rates for CVD of monosilane is also shown[10,11]. The difference between the CVD of mono-
and higher order silanes lies not just in the deposition rates
alone. More importantly, the large photoconductivities observed for
the films deposited from the higher order silanes are not observed
for those deposited from mono-silanes. The deposition rates shown

in Figure 1 were observed at pressures of 50 torr of the silanes. The film thicknesses were initially measured by both weighing the deposited films and by measuring the thickness with a Sloan thickness gauge. After this initial calibration the thickness was determined by measuring the film transmission using 6329Å laser light.

Figure 2 shows the visible absorption spectra of the CVD films and those prepared by glow discharge, using the same higher order silanes in both preparations. The CVD films show several broad absorption bands in the 0.7 to 2.5 micron range.

The dark conductivity of the CVD films is between $10^{-8} - 10^{-7}$ (Ω-cm)$^{-1}$ over the temperature range studied. The photoconductivity varies between 6×10^{-5} to 10^{-6} (Ω-cm)$^{-1}$, depending on temperature and deposition parameters. The films were doped to both p and n type conductivity. To reach a given conductivity, relatively high percentages of dopant gases PH_3 and B_2H_6 have to be used, since the breakdown of these gases is not very efficient at the low deposition temperatures.

DEVICE CHARACTERISTICS

Experimental gold Schottky devices were fabricated both on conductive glass and metallic substrates (steel and molybdenum). The device configuration and the I-V curve is shown on Figure 3 The Isc and η quoted on the Figure represent internal conversion efficiencies. We have obtained Isc=12 mA /cm^2 external current on a 0.65 cm^2 area device under 3.3 AM-1 illumination with 30% transmission of the gold film.

In conclusion, we have demonstrated a novel deposition process for amorphous silicon, which lends itself well to manufacturing flow processstechniques. The material obtained has differing

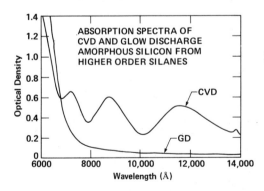

Fig.2 Optical absorption

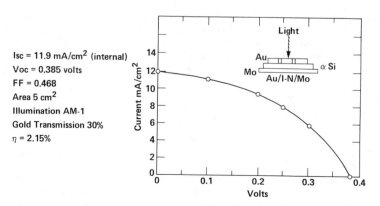

Isc = 11.9 mA/cm² (internal)

Voc = 0.385 volts

FF = 0.468

Area 5 cm²

Illumination AM-1

Gold Transmission 30%

η = 2.15%

Figure 3   I-V Performance of an Au-i-n-Mo

Schottky device

optical properties from the glow discharge deposited hydrogenated amorphous silicon. Further work is required to delineate the nature of the compensating complex.

Acknowledgements: We wish to thank Prof. D. S. McClure for valuable consultations, and Dr. K. R. Ramaprasad for important contributions to various aspects of this work.

REFERENCES

1.   D. E. Carlson and C.L. Wronski, J. Electron. Mater. 6, 95 (1977).

2.   W. E. Spear and P. G. Le Comber, Sol. St. Commun. 17, 1193 (1975).

3.   H. F. Sterling and R.C.G. Swann, Sol. St. Electron 8, 653 (1965).

4.   W. Paul, A. J. Lewis, G.A.N. Connell, and T. D. Moustakas, Sol. St. Commun. 20, 969 (1976).

5.   M. Taniguchi, M. Hirose, and Y. Osaka, J. Cryst. Growth 45, 126 (1978).

6.   D. C. Booth, D. D. Allred, and B. O. Seraphin, J. Non. Cryst. Sol. 35, 213 (1980).

7.   N. Sol, D. Kaplan, D. Dieumegard, and D. Dubreuil, Sol. 35, 291 (1980).

8.   E. M. Tebben and M. A. Ring, Inorg. Chem. 8, 1787 (1969).; J. H. Purnell and R. Walsh, Proc. Roy. Soc. A293. 543 (1966).

9.   B. A. Scott, M. H. Brodsky, D. C. Green, P. B. Kirby, R. M. Plecenik and E. E. Simonyl App. Phys. Lett. 37, 725 (1980).

10.   A. Stock and C. Somieski, Chem. Ber. 49, 111 (1916); A. Stock Hydrides of Boron and Silicon, Cornell University Press, New York, (1933).

11.   M. Taniguchi, M. Hirose, and Y. Osaka, J. Crys. Growth, 45, 126 (1978).

NMR STUDIES OF SPUTTERED AND GLOW DISCHARGE DEPOSITED a-Si:H*

W.E. Carlos** and P.C. Taylor
Naval Research Laboratory, Washington, D.C. 20375

S. Oguz and W. Paul
Division of Applied Sciences
Harvard University, Cambridge, MA 02138

ABSTRACT

Nuclear Magnetic Resonance has recently been used to establish the existence of two separate hydrogen environments in glow discharge deposited a-Si:H. Here we compare our results for sputtered films with those obtained for glow discharge samples. The sputtered films have more hydrogen in the highly clustered environments than do the glow discharge films. In addition, films prepared with a low partial pressure of hydrogen in the sputtering gas show no minimum in the spin lattice relaxation time T_1 as a function of temperature, unlike the glow discharge films where a minimum in T_1 is observed. This minimum, which is attributed to relaxation via disorder modes, is also seen in a sputtered film prepared under a high partial pressure of hydrogen.

INTRODUCTION

Hydrogenated amorphous silicon (a-Si:H) films of high quality may be prepared in a number of ways. The two most successful methods are the glow discharge of silane and RF sputtering in an atmosphere containing hydrogen. These processes produce films having similar electrical and optical properties. In this paper we will emphasize results of our ^{1}H NMR studies of the lineshapes and spin lattice relaxation rates for samples prepared by the sputtering technique.

EXPERIMENTAL DETAILS

The glow discharge samples, with which the sputtered samples will be compared, were obtained from several different laboratories. All were "device grade" materials containing ~10% hydrogen. Further details have been published elsewhere.[1] Three samples designated A, B and C were prepared by sputtering in an argon/hydrogen atmosphere with a partial pressure of argon of 5 milli Torr. The partial pressures of hydrogen were 0.4 milli Torr for samples A and B and 4 milli Torr for sample C. Substrate temperatures were 325°C for samples A and C and 250°C for sample B. The Hydrogen content of all three samples was approximately 12 at.% and ESR measurements indicated that the spin density was approximately $10^{17} cm^{-3}$ in all samples.

The NMR data were taken using a standard pulsed NMR spectrometer operating at a frequency of 42.3 MHz. The temperature was varied

*Work supported by SERI under D.O.E. Contract #DEAIO2-80CS83116.
**NRC/NRL Postdoctoral Research Associate.

68

between 4K and 300K. The lineshapes were obtained by Fourier trans-
forming the free induction decay (FID) while spin lattice relaxation
times, T_1, were obtained using the repetition rate technique.[2]

LINESHAPE RESULTS

In all samples which we have studied the NMR line is composed
of a broad Gaussian line superimposed on a narrow Lorentzian line.
These two Gaussian and Lorentzian components are manifested in the
free induction decay shown in Fig. 1 as a rapid fall off at short
times and an exponential tail at long times, respectively. "Hole
burning" experiments by Reimer, Vaughan and Knights[3] and our own solid
echo measurements[1] show that these two lines are due to two separate
hydrogen bonding sites and that there is little spectral diffusion
between the two sites. Reimer et al.[3] have also shown that both linewidths are due to dipolar broadening. Furthermore, both linewidths
are large enough to indicate that the hydrogen atoms are probably
clustered at both sites.

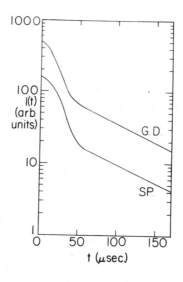

Fig. 1. The free induction decays of a glow discharge (GD) and a
sputtered (SP) a-Si:H film. The relative intensities are arbitrary.

In Fig. 1, the free induction decays for a glow discharge film
obtained from RCA and for a sputtered film (A) are compared. These
two samples are representative of those prepared by the two processes.
As can be seen from the figure the lines are quite similar. For
films prepared in either manner the narrow component is Lorentzian
and has a full width at half maximum of about 3.7 kHz with a variation from sample to sample of about ±0.5 kHz. This variation implies
a variation from sample to sample of only about ±4% in the average

proton-proton separation in these less clustered sites, regardless of the method of preparation. However, there are distinct differences between the sputtered and glow discharge samples as far as the broad line is concerned. Firstly, for the glow discharge samples the ratio of broad to narrow component is between 2 and 3 to 1, while in the sputtered films the ratio is between 6 and 8 to 1 for comparable hydrogen concentrations. Secondly, the broad line is about 18 kHz wide for sputtered films as compared with about 25 kHz for the glow discharge films. This fact indicates that although there are more protons in the more highly clustered environments of the sputtered material the average proton-proton separation in these clusters is about 10% larger than for the broad line seen in the glow discharge material.

Although the narrow line is probably predominantly due to an isolated monohydride species, the broad line undoubtedly results from several different, clustered environments including configurations such as SiH_2, SiH_3, polymeric $(SiH_2)_n$, and hydrated or partially hydrogenated vacancies, divacancies, or larger voids. Because of this ambiguity it is difficult to draw any specific conclusions concerning the structural implications of the observed linewidth changes of the broad line. Qualitatively, one can say that those sites which give rise to larger dipolar broadening (such as fully hydrated, unrelaxed vacancies or divacancies where $\sigma \sim 100$ kHz) are less prevalent in the sputtered films. On the other hand, the presence in the sputtered films of larger voids which yield internal surfaces approaching those of a crystalline Si(111) surface ($\sigma \sim 8$ kHz) cannot be excluded. In addition, partially hydrated vacancies or divacancies are also consistent with the linewidths observed in the sputtered films. A third possible contribution to the broad line in the sputtered films is that from polyhydride species, although the infrared results indicate that there is not enough hydrogen on these sites to account fully for the intensity of the 18 kHz line.

Relaxation effects will tend to narrow the predicted dipolar width for a given configuration, but the magnitude necessary to fit the observed linewidth is probably too large for the cases of fully hydrated vacancies and divacancies. In order to fit the observed linewidths, the hydrogen atoms on a vacancy must move away from their unrelaxed vacancy positions by $\sim 0.5 \text{\AA}$ in either the sputtered or glow discharge films.

SPIN LATTICE RELAXATION

The spin lattice relaxation time, T_1, provides a measure of the coupling between the nuclear spin system and the amorphous lattice. In Fig. 2 we present T_1 as a function of temperature for a glow discharge sample (RCA) and a sputtered sample (C) prepared with a high partial pressure of hydrogen. Although the details of the curves differ somewhat from sample to sample, all glow discharge films we have investigated show a T_1 minimum at about 40K. The sputtered sample C follows a similar trend.

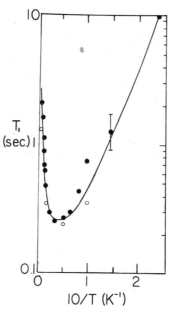

Fig. 2. The spin lattice relaxation time, T , for a glow discharge sample (filled circles) and a sputtered sample (C) prepared under a high partial pressure of hydrogen (open circles). The curve is calculated using equation 2.

We have previously explained[1] this behavior using a model based on disorder modes which are associated with a small fraction of the hydrogen atoms ($\sim 10^{17} cm^{-3}$). At these disorder modes the hydrogen atoms can hop over a potential barrier ΔE which separates two positions of local equilibrium. This motion modulates the dipolar field felt by nearby hydrogen atoms. Atoms further away are relaxed via spin diffusion. For simplicity we assume a rectangular distribution of barrier heights from E_{min} to E_{max}. With these assumptions the average relaxation rate is given by

$$<R>=kT\gamma^2 h_o^2/[w_o(E_{max}-E_{min})]\{\tan^{-1}[w_o\tau_o\exp(E_{max}/kT)]$$
$$- \tan^{-1}[w_o\tau_o\exp(E_{min}/kT)]\} \qquad (1)$$

where γ is the gyromagnetic ratio for protons, h_o is the fluctuating field due to the disorder mode, w_o is the angular NMR frequency, and τ_o is the exponential prefactor for thermally activated hopping. When the effects of spin diffusion are included, then T_1 is given by

$$T_1^{-1} = \alpha[-1-S+(1+6S+S^2)^{\frac{1}{2}}] \qquad (2)$$

where $\alpha = 2\pi W(a/d)^3$, $S = <R>/2\alpha$. The parameter W is the probability of a spin flip between nearest neighbors ($\cong 2x10^3 sec^{-1}$), a is the average H-H separation and d is the distance between disorder modes. This model provides a reasonable fit to T_1 data for glow discharge samples with slight adjustments of parameters from sample to sample.

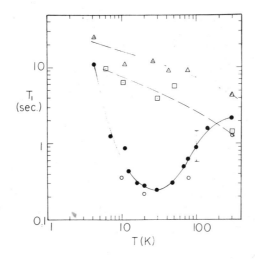

Fig. 3. T_1 for the glow discharge film (filled circles) and the sputtered films (A - triangles, B - squares and C - open circles).

However, as can be seen in Fig. 3, no T_1 minimum is seen for sputtered samples A and B prepared with a low partial pressure of hydrogen. At $T \cong 40K$ the relaxation rates differ by one to two orders of magnitude from the glow discharge or high hydrogen pressure sputtered samples. This behavior clearly indicates that the density of disorder modes is much smaller in these samples. In fact, in these two samples T_1 is determined by relaxation via the paramagnetic dangling bond spins which are present in all a-Si:H samples on the order of 10^{15}-$10^{17} cm^{-3}$. To account for the rates at 4K for samples A and B in Fig. 3 we require $\sim 10^{17} cm^{-3}$ and $\sim 2 \times 10^{17} cm^{-3}$ spins. These numbers are in quite good agreement with the ESR results which give $9 \times 10^{16} cm^{-3}$ and $3 \times 10^{17} cm^{-3}$ spins for samples A and B, respectively. The weak temperature dependence of T_1 for samples A and B is also as expected for relaxation via paramagnetic spins such as the Si "dangling bonds." At low temperatures where a direct relaxation of the electronic spins dominates the temperature dependence, the nuclear relaxation rate goes as $T^{\frac{1}{4}}$ while at higher temperatures an increasing slope ($\lesssim T^2$) is expected. The dashed curves in Fig. 3 are drawn with low temperature asymptotes proportional to $T^{\frac{1}{4}}$. Thus it is clear that not only the magnitude of T in samples A and B, but also the temperature dependences are consistent with our proposed relaxation mechanism (via paramagnetic Si dangling bonds).

The question remains as to why, of all the sputtered and glow discharge films investigated with hydrogen content near 10 at.%, only those sputtered films prepared under low partial pressure of hydrogen ($P_H \ll 1$ m Torr) show no evidence for the presence of disorder modes

($T_\perp$ minimum)? At present there is no definitive answer to this question, although the ultimate solution probably involves some of the hydrogen atoms which replace strained silicon-silicon bonds. It could be that at low partial pressure, the hydrogen in the sputtered films is not as effective in relieving an important, but as yet undetermined, subset of the strained Si-Si bonds as it is in the sputtered films at higher partial pressures and in all the glow discharge films for all the conditions so far studied.

ACKNOWLEDGEMENTS

The authors are grateful to D.E. Carlson and J. Dresner (RCA), H. Fritzsche and C.C. Tsai (University of Chicago), R.W. Griffith (Brookhaven National Laboratory) and P. Reid (Naval Research Laboratory) for supplying well-characterized glow discharge samples. W.M. Pontuschka is gratefully acknowledged for assistance with the ESR measurements.

REFERENCES

1. W.E. Carlos and P.C. Taylor, Phys. Rev. Lett. 45, 358 (1980).
2. S. Alexander and A. Tzalmona, Phys. Rev. 138, A845 (1965).
3. J.A. Reimer, R.W. Vaughan and J.C. Knights, Phys. Rev. Lett. 44, 193 (1980) and Phys. Rev. B (to be published).
4. In the original equation published in ref. 1 the factor $kT/(E_{max}-E_{min})$ was erroneously omitted.

NUCLEAR SPIN-LATTICE RELAXATION BY DIFFUSION IN AMORPHOUS SI:H

B. Movaghar and L. Schweitzer
Fachbereich Physik, Universität Marburg, Renthof 5
F.R. Germany

ABSTRACT

Spin diffusion and relaxation is considered in the framework of the Master equation. The formalism is applied to nuclear spin lattice relaxation in disordered systems. We consider the model of relaxation at local modes proposed recently by Carlos and Taylor for a Si:H. In contrast to these authors we find that the data require a density of 10^{19}–10^{20} cm^{-3} local relaxation centers.

INTRODUCTION

Proton nuclear magnetic resonance (NMR) has proven to be a powerful tool in elucidating the influence of hydrogen on both, electronic and structural properties of glow discharge amorphous silicon [1,2]. Proton spin lattice relaxation measurements in a-Si:H have also been reported recently [3,4] and were explained by postulating the existence of hydrogen containing disorder modes. Carlos and Taylor [3] conclude that paramagnetic dangling bond centers are not the cause for the relatively short spin-lattice relaxation time T_1 observed in these materials. Moreover, Reimer et al. [4] showed that there is essentially no correlation between dangling bond spin density and T_1 by investigating a number of samples containing up to $6 \cdot 10^{18}$ spins/cm^3.

The idea of the model proposed by Carlos and Taylor is that structural relaxation modes modulate the dipolar interaction between two closely spaced hydrogen nuclei. The latter act as spin relaxation centers to which the rest polarization is transmitted by spin-diffusion. They have applied de Gennes's solution method [5] to their model with modified boundary conditions. Unfortunately, however, this method fails unless the relaxation rate is much faster than the diffusion rates in the neighborhood of the center. This applies generally to paramagnetic spins with short spin-lattice relaxation times. In case of hydrogen nuclei acting as relaxation centers, however, due to the smaller nuclear moment, the relaxation rate is reduced by six orders of magnitude compared to the diffusion rate. On the other hand, if diffusion were the rate limiting process, as assumed in the theory, the nuclear spin-lattice relaxation time would not depend on temperature, hence, the minimum of T_1 observed at about 30 K could not be explained. Thus, the theory employed by Carlos and Taylor does not apply to the model they have proposed.

MASTER EQUATION APPROACH

For that reason we consider the problem of diffusion and relaxation of spin polarization in the framework of the master equation. This description is more general than the diffusion equation method and unlike the latter, is not restricted to high density situations.

ISSN:0094-243X/81/730073-05$1.50 Copyright 1981 American Institute of Physics

We shall apply our result to the local mode relaxation model of Carlos and Taylor.

Consider for example the nuclear spin polarization $p_i(t)$ at a site "i" in a general network of "sites". The physical situation we wish to investigate is described by the Master equation

$$\frac{d}{dt} p_i(t) = - \sum_j W_{ij} \, p_i(t) + \sum_j W_{ji} \, p_j(t) - \varepsilon_i(p_i(t) - p_o) - 2A \, p_i(t) \qquad (1)$$

The first two terms on the R.H.S. describe the polarization flowing away from site i and the polarization transmitted to site i, respectively. The third term denotes the relaxation process at i with rate ε_i and the last term is the spin-flip rate induced by the external microwave field. Now, we do not follow the usual procedure and transform the Master equation into a diffusion equation, since this is not valid in general. We tackle the discrete problem given by eq. (1) by using the tight binding analogy, since eq. (1) is equivalent to a tight binding Hamiltonian in the presence of diagonal disorder. This has in detail been shown elsewhere [6].

Now we have to consider the relaxation rate ε_i, which in general is determined by the model adopted. If the effective range R_c of the relaxation rate about a site "i" does not exceed the average nearest neighbour distance a ($R_c \leq a$), we can neglect correlations of the $\{\varepsilon_i\}$ so that the probability distribution function P reads

$$P\{\varepsilon_i\} = P(\varepsilon_i) \, P(\varepsilon_j) \ldots P(\varepsilon_n) \qquad (2)$$

This is exact if the relaxation is completely local (δ-function potentials). On the other hand, when $R_c \gg a$, we cannot neglect the correlations and we have to solve the full scattering problem with "potentials" of finite range [7]. In the model we wish to describe, relaxation is caused by mutual dipolar interaction of two closely spaced hydrogen atoms, as proposed by Carlos and Taylor, so that we are clearly in the regime $R_c \leq a$ and eq. (2) applies.

The solution of the Master equation (1) is given by [6]

$$p(t) = < 1/N \sum_{ij} G_{ij}(t) > \qquad (3)$$

where G_{ij} is the probability of finding an excitation at time t at site j, provided at t = 0 it started from i. For long times ($t \to \infty$)

$$p(t) \sim p_o(1 - e^{-t/T_1}) \qquad (4)$$

with

$$\frac{1}{T_1} = \int_0^\infty \frac{P(\varepsilon_i) \, d\varepsilon_i}{\varepsilon_i^{-1} + \Sigma(o)^{-1}} \qquad (5)$$

$\Sigma(o)$ is a direct measure of the diffusion rate, and on a cubic lattice

$$\Sigma(o) = \frac{6\ D}{1.52\ a^2} \tag{6}$$

where D is the diffusion constant and a the lattice constant.

Equation (5) has a simple physical interpretation. Consider for example a situation where a concentration x of sites has $\varepsilon_i = \infty$ and $(1-x)$, $\varepsilon_i = 0$. In this case the spin-lattice relaxation is always diffusion limited and given by

$$\frac{1}{T_1} = x\ \Sigma(o) = x\ \frac{6D}{1.52 \cdot a^2} \tag{7}$$

On the other hand if $\varepsilon_i \ll \Sigma(o)$, we get

$$\frac{1}{T_1} = \int P(\varepsilon_i)\varepsilon_i\ d\varepsilon_i \tag{8}$$

and T_1 is limited by the relaxation rates ε_i.

It is obvious, that the diffusion limited case, with $\varepsilon_i = \infty$, gives the shortest T_1. Inserting the values as given by Carlos and Taylor for D and a, we find

$$T_1 = 1/x\ 0.25 \cdot (3\mathring{A})^2 \cdot 5 \cdot 10^{11} cm^{-2} s = 1/x\ 1.14\ 10^{-4} s \tag{9}$$

Putting $x = 4.5 \cdot 10^{-4}$, we obtain the experimentally observed value of $T_1 \cong .25$ s. One should note, that even in the favorablest situation with infinitely fast relaxation centers, at least .04% of the sites must be such centers. Thus, in case of the much slower hydrogen containing relaxation centers, we clearly need a larger concentration.

Turning now to the disordered system where the corresponding equations read [7]

$$\frac{1}{T_1} = \int_o^\infty \frac{P(\varepsilon_i)d\varepsilon_i}{\varepsilon_i^{-1} + \sigma_1(o)^{-1}} \tag{10}$$

and

$$\sigma_1(o) = n\ a_p \int \frac{d\vec{R}_{ij} W(\vec{R}_{ij})\sigma_1}{\sigma_1 + W(\vec{R}_{ij})} \tag{11}$$

where n is the site density and a_p a connectivity factor, which takes care of the correct counting of the paths. $W(\vec{R}_{ij})$ is the transition rate.

LOCAL RELAXATION MODEL

In the model of local relaxation centers proposed by Carlos and Taylor [3], $\varepsilon_i < \sigma_1$, and the ε_i are given by

$$\varepsilon_i = \frac{\gamma_N^2 h_o^2 \, \tau_i}{1 + \omega_o^2 \tau_i^2} \; ; \quad \tau_i = \tau_o \exp \{E_i/kT\} \tag{12}$$

where γ_N, h_o and ω_o denote the nuclear magnetic moment, the amplitude of the fluctuating local magnetic field and the NMR resonance frequency, $\omega_o = 2\pi\nu$, respectively. The τ_i describe the modulations, which are due to strucural relaxations involving barriers of height E_i. Within this model, we get

$$\frac{1}{T_1} = x \, kT\gamma_N^2 h_o^2 \, \tau_o \int \frac{N(E)dE \, e^{E/kT}}{1+(\gamma_N^2 h_o^2\tau_o/\sigma_1)e^{E/kT}+\omega_o^2\tau_o^2 e^{2E/kT}} \tag{13}$$

and with $N(E) = \text{const.}/(E_{max}-E_{min})$, we finally obtain

$$\frac{1}{T_1} = x \, \frac{\gamma_N^2 h_o^2 \, kT}{(E_{max}-E_{min})} \, \frac{2}{\Delta^{1/2}} \, [\text{arctg}\{\frac{\gamma_N^2 h_o^2/\sigma_1+2\omega_o^2\tau_o \, e^{E_{max}/kT}}{\Delta^{1/2}}\}$$
$$- \text{arctg}\{\frac{\gamma_N^2 h_o^2/\sigma_1+2\omega_o^2\tau_o \, e^{E_{min}/kT}}{\Delta^{1/2}}\}] \tag{14}$$

which holds for $\Delta = (4\omega_o^2 - \gamma_N^4 h_o^4/\sigma_1^2) > o$, and the effective diffusion rate is given by

$$\sigma_1 = \frac{1}{20} \, \gamma_N^4 \, \hbar^2 \, \frac{4\pi^4}{9e^2} \, T_2 \, n^2 \tag{15}$$

Both, the spin-spin relaxation time T_2 and n can be determined from experiment . We find for the lorentzian line, $T_2 = 8.3 \cdot 10^{-5}$ s with $n = 4.1 \cdot 10^{21} \text{cm}^{-3}$, and hence $\sigma_1 \simeq 250 \text{s}^{-1}$. Taking the experimental parameters it follows, that $4\omega_o^2 >> \gamma_N^4 h_o^4/\sigma_1^2$ so that the expression for $1/T_1$ approximately reduces to

$$\frac{1}{T_1} = x \, \frac{\gamma_N^2 h_o^2}{\omega_o} \, \frac{kT}{E_{max}-E_{min}} \, [\text{arctg}(\omega_o\tau_o \, e^{E_{max}/kT})-\text{arctg}(\omega_o\tau_o e^{E_{min}/kT})] \tag{16}$$

And with the parameters of ref.1, we find a minimum of T_1 at $T \simeq 30$ K, $T_1 \simeq \frac{0,22}{x}$ s, so that $x \simeq 1$ to account for the experimental value T_1 = 0.25 s. Even if we increase the amplitude of the fluctuating field up to 5 gauss, we find that at least 10% of the hydrogen sites have to be identified as relaxation centers, which must contain clustered hydrogen. This brings the model in serious difficulties, since such clusters should be seen in the resonance spectrum. Therefore, we suggest that there is only one nuclear spinsystem, which is distributed inhomogeneously in space. The clustered hydrogen is mainly located at the grainboundaries and internal surfaces, coupled to local modes and acting as relaxation centers to which the spin polarization diffuses from the more dilute regions. These numerous clusters must show up in the wings of the NMR resonance line and are probably responsible for the broad line observed experimentally.

REFERENCES

1. J.A. Reimer, R.W. Vaughan and J.C. Knights, Phys.Rev.Lett.44,193(1980)
2. J.A. Reimer, R.W. Vaughan and J.C. Knights, Sol.St.Comm. 37,161(1981)
3. W. E. Carlos and P.C. Taylor, Phys. Rev.Lett. 45,358 (1980)
4. J.A. Reimer, R.W.Vaughan, J.C. Knights, to be published
5. A. Abragam, "The Principles of Nuclear Magnetism"(Claredon Press, Oxford, 1961)
6. B. Movaghar, J. Phys. C, 13, 4915 (1980)
7. B. Movaghar and L. Schweitzer, to be published

PROTON MAGNETIC RESONANCE STUDIES OF PLASMA DEPOSITED a-Si:H FILMS*

Jeffrey A. Reimer
IBM T.J. Watson Research Center, Yorktown Heights, NY 10598

John C. Knights
Xerox Palo Alto Research Center, Palo Alto, CA 94304

ABSTRACT

Proton magnetic linewidth data for sixteen different plasma-deposited amorphous Si:H films are presented. The microstructural information obtained from these data is interpreted in terms of H gettering at high strain regions in the growing film. In addition, changes in microstructure with deposition conditions is shown to furnish new evidence for the role SiH_2 and SiH_x^+ ions have in models for gas phase reactions leading to film growth.

INTRODUCTION

It has been established recently that proton magnetic resonance lineshapes and linewidths are a sensitive structural probe of a-Si:H films.[1-4] Linewidth and lineshape data have shown[1] direct evidence for two-phase compositional inhomogeneity. Modeling of proton distributions led to the conclusion that the high H density domain could be due to local clustering on silicon atoms [e.g. $(SiH_2)_n$ "polysilane" regions] or monohydride clustering on internal surfaces. Monohydride clustering was confirmed by further proton NMR studies[2] of annealed a-Si:H films. In those studies we showed that upon annealing, H in the less clustered domain (predominantly monohydride) diffuses internally (prior to evolution) concomitant with the reduction in paramagnetic center density.[5] Further combined NMR and infrared studies on the effects of inert gas dilution on film formation and growth[6] have shown that high deposition rates achieved with He and N diluent gases are associated with levels of H incorporated in the form of heavily clustered monohydride configurations. Thus, inhomogeneous microstructure occurs not only when $(SiH_2)_n$ is present but when clustered SiH are present as well. The purpose of this work is to examine the microstructural implications, via proton magnetic resonance lineshapes, of changing deposition parameters. Specifically, we wish to show that the spatial isolation of the two proton domains may be understood in terms of strain in the film during

*This research was supported in part by NSF DMR-7721394 and SERI XJ-0-9079-1.

deposition and that gas phase chemistry in the discharge influences the microstructural properties of the films.

EXPERIMENTAL

Proton magnetic resonance data were taken at 56.4 MHz with an NMR spectrometer described previously.[7] The spectra were obtained by Fourier transformation of the free induction decay (FID) of the magnetization following a 90° preparatory pulse. The 90° pulse lengths were always less than 2 μseconds. In all experiments, the FIDs were signal averaged prior to Fourier transformation with 500 acquisitions typically accumulated. Full spin-lattice relaxation was allowed between acquisitions in order to obtain accurate counts of proton spins. The H content of the films was determined from proton spin counts and sample weight. All spectra were least-squares fitted to the sum of a Gaussian component (broad line) and a Lorentzian component (narrow line). The resulting fits were excellent and, based on values of χ^2 resulting from a variety of initial starting parameters, the errors are $\pm$ 1 kHz in the FWHM (full width at half maximum) of the broad component ($\pm$ 0.3 kHz narrow component) and = $\pm$ 0.3 atom percent in the distribution between broad and narrow components. The samples were prepared in an rf-diode deposition described elsewhere.[8] The samples were deposited on ~ 2-inch diameter aluminum foil substrates in thicknesses of ~ 0.1 to 100 μ resulting in sample masses in the range of ~ 0.5-100 mg after removal of the substrates with a dilute hydrochloric acid etch. Tables 1 and 2 detail (i) the deposition conditions for a variety of samples, (ii) the H content, distribution and linewidths from the FID spectra.

RESULTS AND DISCUSSION

The observation of two-phase compositional homogeneity presents an interesting question: Is the structure of these films determined by surface/bulk processes during deposition or by gas phase reactions? We shall argue that, in fact, both factors influence film microstructure. However, the persistence of the two-phase structure as seen by NMR, regardless of the deposition conditions, would imply a bulk or surface rearrangement of the film after nucleation. To test this hypothesis, we prepared a high unpaired spin density ($>$ 10^{19} cm^{-3}, by depositing from 5% SiH_4/Ar at 25°C with an rf power of 18 watts) sample and recorded the NMR spectrum just after deposition and then recorded the spectrum with the same sample allowed to stand in dry air for approximately six months. As deposited, the NMR spectra yields the H content to be 23.8% with 18.1% broad (25.8 kHz FWHM), 5.0% narrow (1.65 kHz FWHM), and ~ 1.5% very narrow (~ 1 kHz FWHM). The proton spectrum of the "aged" sample yields 29.5 atom% H with 20.9%

broad (26.8 kHz FWHM) and 3.7% narrow (2.8 kHz FWHM). It has been shown previously[9] by NMR relaxation data that the H content of this fresh sample, as determined by NMR lineshapes, is artificially low (~ 8 atom%) because of the large dipolar broadening of the H spins by the abundant unpaired electrons. Nonetheless, we propose that the "stabilization" process (vide supra) may serve as a model for what may happen during film growth, namely hydrogenation of dangling and strained bond interfaces by diffusion of H from other regions in the lattice. We then picture areas of high strain during film growth as "gettering" the H out of the immediately surrounding lattice and forming a hydrogenated void, thereby stabilizing the lattice and spatially isolating the H in the void from that in the bulk. It is worth noting that during growth of films in which there are $(SiH_2)_n$ polymer phases, the same process may occur with the polymer phase playing the same role as the hydrogenated void; a mechanism by which the strain in the continuous random network is relieved.

TABLE 1: ANODE FILMS

SAMPLE	POWER[1]	T_S	GAS[2] COMP.	ATOM % HYDROGEN: TOTAL[3]	NARROW	BROAD	LINEWIDTH (KWHM, khz) NARROW	BROAD
A	18	RT	5%/Ar	32.3	2.6	29.7	4.7	25.4
D	2	230°C	100%	7.8	3.4	4.4	3.8	26.3
F	1	230°C	5%/Ar	11.6	3.8	7.8	2.0	26.2
G	18	230°C	5%/Ar	12.9	4.5	8.4	1.0	22.4
H	11	RT	5%/Ar	30.1	2.4	27.7	1.3	26.3
L	18	230°C	5%/He	15.8	4.1	11.7	3.0	24.2
N	2	RT	100%	29.0	3.6	25.4	3.6	27.7
AA	1	230°C	100%	7.8	3.6	4.2	3.1	31.5
DD	1	230°C	5%/He	15.1	4.7	10.4	3.5	23.4
KK	18	230°C	100%	12.6	2.8	9.8	2.8	26.5

TABLE 2: CATHODE FILMS

SAMPLE	POWER[1]	T_S	GAS[2] COMP.	ATOM % HYDROGEN: TOTAL[3]	NARROW	BROAD	LINEWIDTH (KWHM, khz) NARROW	BROAD
B	18	RT	5%/Ar	16.3	2.2	14.1	3.9	22.1
C	1	RT	5%/Ar	12.6	3.5	9.1	4.7	29.5
I	18	RT	5%/Ar	15.4	2.0	13.4	2.9	22.2
M	2	RT	100%	23.1	4.6	18.5	5.4	24.0
S	18	RT	5%/He	16.5	4.0	12.5	2.3	19.4

(1) RF power (watts) net in matching network.

(2) Percentage silane in diluent gas.

(3) Determined from integrated proton spin density and sample weight.

While all the samples reported herein have two-component proton NMR spectra, there are considerable variations between the samples as to the atom% H, particularly the atom% H contained within the broad component. We wish to point out the trends in these proton data may be understood in terms of some gas phase reactions and mechanisms for film growth. Two recent proposals for film growth from $SiH_2(g)$ species[10] and subsequent modification by ionic species[6] are:

$$(SiH_2(g))_n \rightarrow SiH_x(s) + SiH_4(g) + H_2(g) \tag{1}$$

$$SiH_x^+(g) + ((SiH_2)_n)_{surface} \rightarrow Si_xH_y^+(g). \tag{2}$$

We propose that Equations (1) and (2) are sufficient to explain the trends observed herein.

Consider the data for films AA, F and DD (Table 1) which compare the effects of deposition from pure silane, 5% in Ar, and 5% silane in He. The deposition rates for these films are in the order of 100% SiH_4 < 5% SiH_4/Ar < 5% SiH_4/He. Inspection of Equation 1 shows that more $SiH_2(g)$ or less $H_2(g)$ will provide for faster growth of the film. Mass spectroscopic studies[10,11] have shown the concentration of $H_2(g)$ to be higher in the pure SiH_4 deposition than deposition from Ar, consistent with Equation 1 and the deposition rates. The observed increase in H content in the films over this same trend may be the result of trapping of H in the growing film, i.e., faster film growth implies more H is trapped in the growing film. This faster growth implies a more strained a-Si lattice which in turn is relaxed by the formation of divacancies or other microstructural features. Accordingly, faster deposition rates would imply an increase in the broad component in the NMR spectra, consistent with the observed data. Whether or not the broad component corresponds to divacancies or to $(SiH_2)_n$ regions, larger voids, cracks, etc., depends on the availability of ions (SiH_x^+) to "scour" the surface. As discussed previously,[6] deposition in He or pure SiH_4 results in higher ion densities (more scouring) than deposition in Ar because Ar has a metastable energy less than the ionization potentials of SiH_x, (x = 1.3) and thus absorbs most of the plasma electron energy. Hence, films deposited in He and pure SiH_4 have only monohydride signature in their vibrational spectra and finer scale inhomogeneities as seen by electron microscopy (broad component = di, tri-vacancies, etc.).

In summary, we have presented proton NMR spectra for a-Si:H films under a variety of deposition conditions. The spatial separation of the broad and narrow component protons may arise from regions of high strain during film growth "gettering" H nuclei out of the neighboring a-Si lattice and forming hydrogenated voids which in turn relieve local strain. We have shown that this is the case in at least one sample which, as deposited, was "metastable" and microstructural changes, via the NMR lineshapes, were found to occur with time. Furthermore, changes in the details of the NMR lineshapes as a function of deposition conditions have been described in terms of film formation from SiH_2 gas phase species and film scouring due to the presence of SiH_x^+ ions.

REFERENCES

1. J.A. Reimer, R.W. Vaughan and J.C. Knights, Phys. Rev. Lett. 44, 193 (1980).
2. J.A. Reimer, R.W. Vaughan and J.C. Knights, Solid State Comm., *in press*.
3. W.E. Carlos and P.C. Taylor, Phys. Rev. Lett. 45, 358 (1980).
4. M.E. Lowry, R.C. Barnes, D.R. Torgeson and F.R. Jeffrey, Conf. Materials Research Society, November 16-21, 1980, Boston, MA (Elsevier, 1981).
5. D.K. Biegelsen, R.A. Street, C.C. Tsai and J.C. Knights, Phys. Rev. B 20, 4839 (1979).
6. J.C. Knights, R.A. Lujan, M.P. Rosenblum, R.A. Street, D.K. Biegelsen and J.A. Reimer, Appl. Phys. Lett. *in press*.
7. R.W. Vaughan, D.D. Elleman, L.M. Stacey, W.K. Rhim and J.W. Lee, Rev. Sci. Instrum. 43, 1356 (1972).
8. R.A. Street, J.C. Knights and D.K. Biegelsen, Phys. Rev. B 18, 1880 (1978).
9. J.A. Reimer, R.W. Vaughan and J.C. Knights, Phys. Rev. B, *in press*.
10. G. Turban, Y. Catherine and B. Grolleau, Thin Solid Films 67, 309 (1980).
11. G. Turban, Y. Catherine and B. Grolleau, Thin Solid Films *submitted*.

CHARACTERIZATION OF THE PROTONIC DISTRIBUTION AND ENVIRONMENT IN AMORPHOUS SILICON-HYDROGEN ALLOYS USING PROTON NMR AND ESR

F. R. Jeffrey, M. E. Lowry, M. L. S. Garcia, R. G. Barnes, and
D. R. Torgeson
Ames Laboratory-USDOE* and Department of Physics
Iowa State University, Ames, Iowa 50011

ABSTRACT

We present magnetic resonance data from a series of a-Si(H) samples deposited under varied hydrogen partial pressures. This parameter has been shown to be directly related to the sample-wide average proton density. The other sputtering parameters were maintained such that no dihydride bonding (as determined by the 890 cm^{-1} ir bending mode) is present. Measurements presented are the NMR absorption spectrum (from the Fourier transform of the free induction decay), relaxation time T_1, and ESR absorption. The NMR absorption spectrum identifies two distinct forms of H incorporation. One is a tightly clustered form, such as H bonded on the inner surface of a microvoid of maximum dimension 5Å, while the other is a randomly distributed phase with local H density of $3.5 \times 10^{21} cm^{-3}$. The distributed phase H density is independant of the sample-wide average, indicating a fixed composition phase which occupies a larger percentage of the sample as H pressure is increased during deposition. This phase appears to extend to a maximum of 88% of the sample. The protonic spin-lattice relaxation time (T_1) measures the coupling of the spin system to its environment, "the lattice". For the series of samples, we find that T_1 first increases from 2.8 s to 44.8 s with increasing H content and then decreases to 8.1 s as H density is further increased. In an effort to understand this unusual relaxation behavior, we have made temperature dependant T_1 and ESR measurements. Utilizing these results, the protonic relaxation mechanism is discussed in terms "disorder mode" and electronic state models.

INTRODUCTION

Considerable effort is being made to unveil the structure of amorphous silicon-hydrogen alloys (a-Si:H) and the nature of the variation from one method of preparation to the next. Infrared absorption studies[1,2] have identified bonding configurations where one, two or three H atoms are bonded to a Si atom. It has been empirically shown[1,3] that material with only one H per Si atom (SiH bonding) possesses the prefered semiconductor properties, thus most studies have concentrated on this type of material.

More recently, NMR studies on both glow discharge produced[4] and reactively sputtered[5] a-Si:H have shown that at least two types of H

*Operated for the U.S. Department of Energy by Iowa State University under contract No. W-7405-Eng-82. This research was supported by the Director for Energy Research, Office of Basic Energy Sciences, WPAS-KC-02-02-02.

distribution occur in the SiH bonded material. It is apparent that one of these distributions is more tightly clustered than the other, however, the exact nature of these formations is still unclear. The work reported here approaches the problem through NMR studies on a series of a-Si:H samples with differing H content. The dependence of the relative proportions of the two types of distributions, the NMR linewidths, and spin-lattice relaxation time (T_1), on the overall H density are used to deduce a structural model for certain aspects of the system.

EXPERIMENTAL

The samples for this study were produced by reactive sputtering of a high purity crystalline silicon target in an Ar-H atmosphere. The partial pressure of Ar during deposition was held at 30 mTorr while the partial pressure of H was varied between samples in order to achieve a range of H density in the films. Substrate-target separation during deposition was 1.5 cm for all samples, with the rf power being held at 3.1 W/cm^2. Details of the sputtering system and collection technique for the samples are given elsewhere.[6] Depositions under identical conditions were made on single crystal silicon substrates for ir measurements. These measurements yielded no SiH_2 scissors-bending mode at the 890 cm^{-1} position, which was taken to indicate the absence of appreciable SiH_2 bonding.

The NMR data may be broken down into 3 categories: proton spin counting, Fast Fourier Transformed free induction decay (FFT) spectra, and spin-lattice relaxation time (T_1) measurements. All measurements were made at an operating frequency of 35 MHz. Details of the experimental method and instrumentation will be found in Ref. 7.

RESULTS AND DISCUSSION

FFT proton NMR spectra were accumulated for each of the samples as referenced. As has previously been observed,[4,5] the spectra appeared to be a superposition of more than one absorption line. A computer fitting program was used to optimize the width, amplitude and position of the components. The optimum fit in all cases was obtained with a superposition of Lorentzian and Gaussian shape functions. This combination indicates that two distinct types of H distribution exist in the films.

It will be argued that the Lorentzian is due to dilute, randomly distributed SiH groups while the Gaussian arises from some form of hydrogen clustering. The observed full width at half maximum (FWHM) linewidths for the two components are plotted vs. the total sample wide average H density (TSWAHD) in Fig. 1. Both linewidths are constant within experimental precision, indicating little change in the local characteristics of the two types of distribution.

Sample wide H density averages of each component were also calculated for all the samples. This was done by determining the percentage of the area due to each component and multiplying that by the TSWAHD determined from the spin count. Figure 2 is a plot of these sample wide averages for each component vs. the TSWAHD. The average H density in the Lorentzian associated component can be seen to initially rise most rapidly but then reach a maximum. The Gaussian associated distribution, however, rises through the entire range.

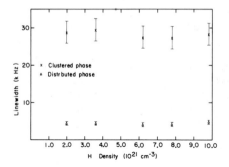

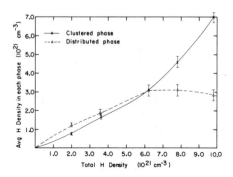

Fig. 1. The optimized linewidths of the Gaussian (clustered phase) and the Lorentzian (distributed phase) vs. the total sample wide average H density.

Fig. 2. The sample wide average H density for each of the two types of H distribution plotted against the total sample wide average H density

ESR spin density vs. the overall H density for the series of samples is shown in Fig. 3. The electron spin density (widely considered to be a measure of the number of dangling bonds) drops dramatically as the first small amount of H is added. This is in the range where most of the H is being incorporated in the distributed phase. The amount of H incorporated is still an order of magnitude greater than the number of dangling bonds being eliminated. Therefore, any correlation between the dangling bond density and the distributed phase only should be drawn cautiously.

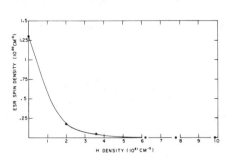

Fig. 3. The ESR spin density plotted against the total sample wide average H density.

For a system of spins on a lattice, a Lorentzian lineshape will be obtained when the site occupancy is dilute (less than 1%) and the spins are randomly distributed.[8,9] This leaves the majority of the spins well separated such that their relatively weak interactions will produce a large central peak, while a few spins will be very close and will give the wide low wings that complete the Lorentzian lineshape. For an a-Si:H sample with 10 at. % H, 2.5% of the possible Si bonding sites will be occupied. This would appear to not be a dilute system. However, because the material is amorphous with bond lengths and angles varying, a continuum of spin spacings is possible. Hence, we believe that the amorphous network affords the same "randomness" at moderate spin concentrations as is found in the crystal lattice at the dilute limit. Then the Lorentzian lineshape should prevail for the supposed randomly distributed phase. The other likely source of a Lorentzian lineshape is motional narrowing. Measurements have been taken from 4K to 300K with no apparent change in linewidth, thereby eliminating motional narrowing as the possible cause of the Lorentzian component.

That the Lorentzian linewidth is a constant for all samples, indicates the randomly distributed form of H is a distinct phase with a constant local H density. Changes in the fraction of the spectrum that is Lorentzian with changing TSWAHD must then be due to changes in the proportion of the sample containing that phase.

An estimate of the local H density in the dilute phase can be obtained from the linewidth of the Lorentzian. The relationship between density in a dilute spin system and the FWHM of the Lorentzian is given by:[9]

$$ FWHM = \frac{\pi}{\sqrt{3}} \left(\frac{M_2^2}{M_4} \right)^{1/2} \qquad \Delta = 10.6 \ \gamma^2 \hbar D $$

where M_2 and M_4 are the second and fourth moments of the lineshape and Δ is the rms width. This calculation assumes a truncated Lorentzian in order to have finite moments. This is physically reasonable. There is obviously a minimum separation between spins which would impose a maximum on the wings of the Lorentzian. The calculation yields a local density of $3.5 \times 10^{21} cm^{-3}$ for the observed linewidth of 4.2 kHz. Comparing this to the sample wide averages shown in Fig. 2, it appears that at the maximum sample wide average of distributed phase, $3.1 \times 10^{21} cm^{-3}$, 88% of the sample volume is devoted to the distributed phase. This leaves 12% for the clustered phase volume, which is in reasonable agreement with previous calculations.

A Gaussian lineshape may arise when the spins all "see" similar environments. This would be the case with spins on a regular lattice (all sites occupied) or a system of nearly identical spin cluster formations. The density of spins on a regular lattice required to give the observed linewidth can be estimated by using the formula for the second moment on a cubic lattice:[9]

$$ M_2 = 5.1 \ \gamma^4 \hbar^2 \ I(I+1) \ \frac{1}{d^6} = \left(\frac{FWHM}{2.35} \right)^2 $$

where I is 1/2 for the proton and d is the spacing between lattice sites. This yields a density higher than the density of Si in the samples and is therefore inconsistant with the absence of SiH$_2$ bonds. A number of cluster configurations can, however explain the linewidth. The simplest models are a broken Si-Si bond terminated with two H atoms and Si atom void in the network terminated by four H atoms. Other void models requiring yet other numbers of H atoms would also be reasonable on the basis of the linewidth. For each model, an average H separation can be calculated to match the observed linewidth using the relationships for second moment:[9]

$$ M_2 = \frac{3}{5} \ \gamma^4 \hbar^2 \ I(I+1) \ \sum_k \frac{1}{r_{jk}^6} $$

where r is the distance between protons. Although the present NMR data allows determination of the separation required for each model, it does not allow distinction between the models. Future work may clarify this point.

Spin-lattice relaxation time, T_1, is plotted vs. the sample wide average H density in Fig. 4. This is a measure of the rate at which energy from the spin system may be tranferred to lattice. It is seen that T_1 starts relatively low for low H density, rises to a maximum, $T_1=44$ sec. at an H density of about $6 \times 10^{21} cm^{-3}$ and then falls again as more H (principally in clusters) is added. To better understand the mechanisms controlling relaxation, the temperature dependence of T_1 was measured for one sample on each side of the maximum. This data is presented in Fig. 5.

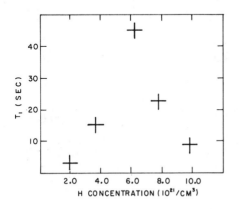

Fig. 4. Relaxation time, T_1 vs. the TSWAHO, at room temperature.

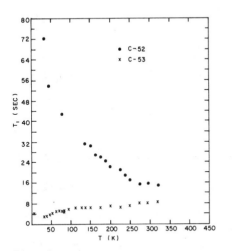

Fig. 5. The temperature dependence of the relaxation time for sample C-52 which has a low H density and sample C-53 which has a high H density.

For the low H density sample, C-52, the relaxation is thermally activated. This would be the case if localized electronic states were acting as relaxation centers. An appreciable number of dangling bonds still exist in this H density region and may be the relaxation centers. A careful analysis of the thermally activated relaxation behavior will lead to approximations of the density of localized states and the degree of localization. This and correlation with detailed ESR studies in the same sample will give us a much clearer picture of the nature of these electronic states. These details will be given in a separate publication.

For the high H density sample, C-53, an entirely different relaxation mechanism is apparent. T_1 decreases slowly with decreasing temperature to an apparent minimum in the vicinity of 30K. This behavior is characteristic of disorder mode relaxation and has been observed in glow discharge deposited a-Si:H.[10] Briefly, in this mechanism the spin energy relaxes via the interactions produced when a proton hops between two approximately equal potential wells. The clusters added after the maximum room temperature T_1 is reached are supposed to provide this more efficient relaxation center. A moderate number of clusters

added before the maximum room temperature T_1 is reached do not
contribute significantly to the relaxation. This could mean that a
different sort of clustered configuration appears at a threshold H
content. However, it seems more likely that a low H content the disorder mode centers are at such low concentration that their
contribution is masked.

CONCLUSIONS

Evidence has been presented for the existence of two types of
SiH bond distribution in a-Si:H. The first is a distinct phase of
randomly distributed H with an average local H density of
$3.5 \times 10^{21} \text{cm}^{-3}$. The second is a clustered phase. The details of the
clustering architecture are not clear; it is supposed that these
clusters are in some way connected with the onset of disorder mode
relaxation. As the H content of the film increases, the volume
occupied by the distributed phase grows and diminishes greatly the
concentration of ESR active electrons (dangling bonds). In this series of samples, a maximum of 88% of the film contains the distributed
phase with the remaining portion apparently containing clusters.
Spin-lattice relaxation for the a-Si:H with low H density is thought
to be due predominantly to localized electronic states (possibly
dangling bonds). In contrast, for higher H density relaxation is
primarily through disorder modes. The onset of the disorder mode
relaxation is considered to be due to either a slightly modified
cluster incorporation or an unmasking of an intrinsic disorder mode
relaxation due to the centers increased concentration. Further work
on the localized electronic state relaxation phenomena may lead to
information about the degree of the localization and the relative
energies of the states involved.

REFERENCES

1. M. H. Brodsky, Manuel Cordona, and J. J. Cuomo, Phys. Rev. B 16, 3556 (1977).
2. G. Lucovsky, R. J. Nemanich, and J. C. Knights, Phys. Rev. B 19, 2064 (1979).
3. R. C. Chittick, J. H. Alexander, and H. F. Sterling, J. Electro-chem. Soc. 116, 77 (1969).
4. J. A. Reimer, R. W. Vaughan, and J. C. Knights, Phys. Rev. Lett. 44, 193 (1980).
5. M. Lowry, F. R. Jeffrey, R. G. Barnes, and D. R. Torgeson, In press, Sol. State Commun.
6. F. R. Jeffrey, H. R. Shanks, and G. C. Danielson, J. Appl. Phys. 50, 7034 (1979).
7. F. R. Jeffrey and M. E. Lowry, submitted to J. Appl. Phys. (Feb. 1981).
8. Charles W. Myles, C. Ebner, and Peter A. Fedders, Phys. Rev. B 14, 1 (1976).
9. A. Abragam, the Principles of Nuclear Magnetism (Clarendon, Oxofrd, England, 1961).
10. W. E. Carlos and P. C. Taylor, Phys. Rev. Lett. 45, 358 (1980).

RELATION BETWEEN SILICON-HYDROGEN COMPLEXES
AND MICROVOIDS IN AMORPHOUS SILICON FILMS FROM IR ABSORPTION[†]

D. E. Soule,[*] G. T. Reedy, E. M. Peterson and J. A. McMillan
Argonne National Laboratory, Argonne, IL 60439

ABSTRACT

A line shape analysis was made of IR absorption bands observed by reflection mode measurements to 400 cm^{-1} on hydrogenated amorphous silicon a-Si:H films. Individual Gaussian absorption lines were resolved through a least-squares deconvolution of multiple stretch mode bands. Emphasis is made on the structural and optical trends toward low-temperature deposited films, with their relaxed open a-Si network containing microvoids. The vibrational behaviors of Si-H, Si-H$_2$ and Si-H$_3$ complexes were studied over a wide range of deposition temperatures $T_D = 350°C$ to $-121°C$. Systematic vibrational frequency shifts were resolved for all complexes due to a shift in bond angle distortion with T_D. Frequency shifts and line broadening effects identified the Si-H$_3$ complex as distinct in behavior within microvoids from Si-H and Si-H$_2$. In the limit of low T_D, the observed frequencies approached closely those of representative substituted silane molecules establishing the identification of Si-H$_n$ complexes and their corresponding structural relation to the bond angle distortion model.

INTRODUCTION

An investigation was made of hydrogenated amorphous silicon a-Si:H films as deposited by RF glow discharge decomposition of silane.[1,2] The transition in the optical and structural properties of these films with deposition temperature T_D was studied from the high T_D regime to that at low T_D where a wide structural change occurs. At high T_D, the films have hard reflective surfaces R(visible) $\simeq 0.44$ with a refractive index of 4.7 and density of 2.3 g/cc, essentially that of x-Si. At low T_D, on the other hand, the films become soft and spongy with a density of 1.2 g/cc. Their surfaces are rougher with a reflectance of $R \simeq 0.05$ and a refractive index of 2.3. Thus, while the high-temperature form is dense having a tight-knit structure with distorted tetrahedral bond angles ($\Delta\theta \simeq 10°$), the low-temperature form has a loose stress-released structure with a high microvoid concentration. Particular emphasis was made in the present study on this latter type of structure and what it would explain about the role of Si-H$_n$ complexes in microvoids. The structure contains $\simeq 50$ At.%H in the form of higher polymeric Si-H$_n$ complexes. Si-H$_2$ and Si-H$_3$ dominate, with Si-H playing a lesser role. The deconvolution of IR absorption bands giving higher resolution has revealed new evidence about the detailed behavior of individual types

[†]Work supported by the U. S. Department of Energy
[*]Present address: Department of Physics, Western Illinois University, Macomb, IL 61455

of Si-H$_n$ complexes through relative frequency shifts, line broadening and integrated absorption strengths. The observed dependence of Si-H$_n$ vibrational modes on bond angle distortion has provided a model for the microstructural relationship between Si-H$_n$ bonding in the a-Si network with microvoids.

EXPERIMENTAL

Amorphous silicon films 0.5-2µm thick were deposited by RF glow discharge from 3% and 10% mixtures of silane in argon at 0.1 Torr pressure. Films were deposited on zero-biased polished tungsten substrates over a range of substrate temperatures T$_D$ from 350°C down to -125°C. The deposition was carried out usually at 1.0W power, though studies have also been made over a range of powers from 0.25W up to 5W. Infrared absorption measurements were made in the reflection mode[1,3] along with the refractive index over frequencies from 3900 cm^{-1} to 400 cm^{-1} with an FTS-14 Fourier transform spectrometer. Most of the optical measurements were made at room temperature, though a limited investigation was extended down to 10°K. A Gaussian fitting procedure was developed[1] to deconvolute absorption bands using a least-squares computer program (VA02A) analysis to resolve individual absorption lines. This was applied primarily to stretch mode bands, where the resulting increased resolution revealed new frequency shifts and line broadening effects.

RESULTS AND DISCUSSION

Reflectance traces for a series of 10% silane films are shown in Fig. 1 as approximately normalized for different film thicknesses. The transition with T$_D$ in the character of the Si-H$_n$ vibrational spectra can be seen, where the stretch modes S grow steadily with decreasing T$_D$ along with the bend mode doublet B. The wag mode W, however, decreases in amplitude. This behavior is seen in more detail in Fig. 2, where the different vibrational mode bands are shown. The S band (primarily due to Si-H$_2$ below room temperature T$_D$) grows steadily with decreasing T$_D$ similar to the total H content, as determined from H$_2$ evolution measurements.[4] The dramatic difference between the trends in the W and S bands suggests quite different local oscillator strengths controlling wagging and stretching vibrations in the a-Si network. A verification of this point, however, is complicated by the fact that the W band is believed to be multiple[5,6] containing components of all of the Si-H$_n$ complexes and therefore may not give an overall trend comparable to any one component. The B band doublet is well resolved for 10% silane films and the 845 cm^{-1} B$_1$ band closely follows the S band, undoubledly due to an Si-H$_2$ band mode as previously established.[5,6] The 890 cm^{-1} B$_2$ band, however, though perhaps attributable to Si-H$_2$ or (Si-H$_2$)$_n$ complexes,[6] does not follow this general trend and is therefore uncertain. There is a switching of the two peaks of the B doublet, where the 890 cm^{-1} peak dominates at high T$_D$ and the 845 cm^{-1} peak dominates at low T$_D$. A similar behavior was observed with increasing RF power from 0.25W up to 5W for 3% silane films. In 3% silane films a higher relative concentration of Si-H$_3$ complexes was observed, as demonstrated by the S band deconvolution. Correspondingly, an additional satellite doublet at about 860 cm^{-1} and 900 cm^{-1}

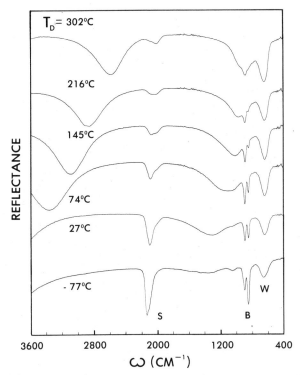

Fig. 1. Reflectance traces with deposition temperature T_D of 10% silane films on W.

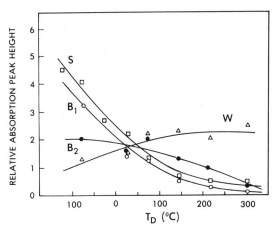

Fig. 2. Observed multiple absorption band amplitudes with deposition temperature T_D for 10% silane films.

appeared, that became more prominant with increasing $Si-H_3$ concentration at lower T_D and at higher RF power. This correlation with $Si-H_3$ is in general agreement with the Lucovsky, Nemanich and Knights[6] results.

A systematic least-squares deconvolution was carried out on the multiple stretch mode S bands.[1] A fitting of individual lines with frequency ω_i, amplitude A_i and half-width $\Delta\omega_i$ could be made typically to within 1% of the observed integrated line strength. The resolution achieved allowed us to study for the first time the behavior of individual lines for specific $Si-H_n$ complexes. These individual lines were established as Gaussian in shape, that remained invariant down to a measurement temperature of $10°K$. This form of line broadening is consistent with a random distribution of bond angles and lengths. The behaviors of individual Si-H, $Si-H_2$ and $Si-H_3$ stretch mode lines were studied over a wide range of T_D from $350°C$ down to $-125°C$. Representative fits to stretch mode bands for 10% silane films are shown in Fig. 3, where the Si-H complex at A is seen to dominate at high T_D rising to about 400 cm^{-1}. At low T_D, the $Si-H_2$ complex at B dominates rising to about 2500 cm^{-1}. As mentioned above, the overidingly dominant complex below room temperature T_D is clearly seen to be $Si-H_2$, dominating the overall S band intensity shown in Fig. 2. In addition, $Si-H_2$ can clearly be followed as one band with

92

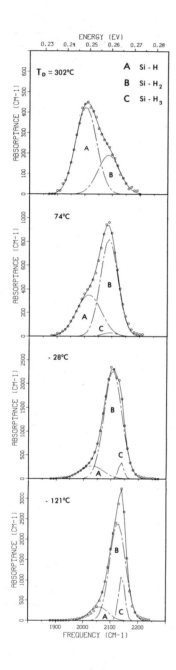

ENERGY (EV)

0.23 0.24 0.25 0.26 0.27 0.28

A   Si - H
B   Si - H$_2$
C   Si - H$_3$

T_D = 302°C

74°C

- 28°C

- 121°C

1900   2000   2100   2200
FREQUENCY (CM^{-1})

Fig. 3. Gaussian fits to stretch mode absorption bands with deposition temperature T_D.

a smooth transition over the whole T_D range, implying that it is a single type of complex for the Si-H bond stretching vibration, unaffected by possible chain effects. The Si-H$_3$ complex at C first appears near room temperature T_D and grows toward low T_D, consistent with an increase in polymeric forms located in the more open microvoids of the a-Si network.

Increased resolution of the individual Si-H$_n$ stretch mode terms by deconvolution revealed for the first time[2] a systematic frequency shift with T_D in these a-Si:H films as shown in Fig. 4 for the 3% and 10% silane films. The Si-H and Si-H$_2$ complexes show a similar rise in frequency with decreasing T_D of the order of 2%. The Si-H frequency shifted from 2002 ± 8 cm^{-1} at high T_D to 2059 ± 8 cm^{-1} at -121°C, while the Si-H$_2$ frequency shifted from 2082 ± 8 cm^{-1} to 2124 ± 8 cm^{-1}. The shift for Si-H$_3$ is distinctly different, varying only slightly from 2137 ± 8 cm^{-1} at 75°C to 2144 ± 8 cm^{-1} at -121°C. For Si-H and Si-H$_2$, this frequency shift is qualitatively consistent with a model where the tetrahedral Si-Si-Si bond angle distortion decreases with decreasing T_D to the more relaxed a-Si network causing a shortening of the Si-H bond. The effective local dielectric constant[7] will also be affected by this juxtaposition of Si-H$_n$ complexes within a microvoid, hence affecting the coupling between the electric field of incident radiation and the local dipole moments; accounting for the divergent behavior between the stretch and wag mode amplitude dependence on the a-Si network structural change, where the wagging vibration encompasses a wider volume than the stretching vibration making it more sensitive to nearest-neighbor proximity effects.

The observed line broadening for these Si-H$_n$ complexes is again consistent with the above bond angle distortion model. The average line width $\overline{\Delta\omega}$ for the Si-H line is 94 cm^{-1}, for Si-H$_2$ is 78 cm^{-1} and for Si-H$_3$ is 25 cm^{-1}. Both Si-H and Si-H$_2$ lines are broad and both are intimately bonded to the distorted a-Si network. The Si-H$_3$ line, on the other hand,

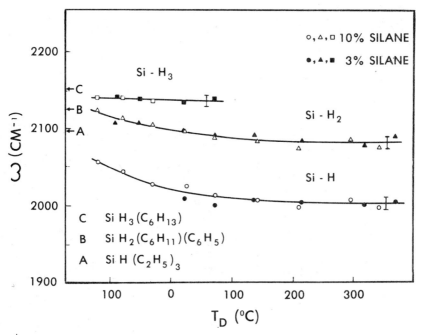

Fig. 4. Stretch mode frequency dependence of Si-H_n complexes with deposition temperature T_D for 3% and 10% silane films.

is very narrow--a factor of three smaller than that of the Si-H_2 line, for example. This is consistent with the expected second-order effect resulting from the isolation from the nearest neighbor in the network. A structural comparison of the possible Si-H_n complexes shows that only Si-H_3 has this bond isolation characteristic. A further justification for this model is the relatively slight shift in the Si-H_3 stretch mode frequency shown in Fig. 4, corresponding to an insensitivity to the structural change of the a-Si network with T_D. This combined evidence strongly supports the existence of Si-H_3 complexes in these films.

In the limit of low T_D, the loose relaxed network allows the Si-H_n complexes to approach their true tetrahedral configuration. Several molecular approximations to the Si-H_n complexes in an a-Si network have been studied[5,6,8] with a range of substituted silanes that give rise to distinctive Si-H stretch mode vibrations in the 2000-2200 cm^{-1} region.[9] One form of substituted silane of particular interest involves primarily extended organic alkyl chains with tetrahedral bonding containing at least two nearest neighbor C atoms, with electronegativity close to that of tetrahedrally bonded Si (Si(te^4) 7.3 eV and C(te^4) 8.0 eV).[10] Representative molecules of this type[9,8] are triethyl silane SiH$(C_2H_5)_3$ as an approximation to the Si-H complex in a-Si, phenyl cyclohexyl silane SiH$_2$ (C_6H_{11}) (C_6H_5) for Si-H_2 and n-hexyl silane SiH$_3$ (C_6H_{13}) for Si-H_3. In the low T_D limit of an open a-Si network, we would expect the Si-H_n stretch mode vibrational frequencies to approach these substituted silane molecular approximations, as shown by the arrows A, B and C, respectively in Fig. 4. A comparison in the figure and in Table I shows good agreement. This agreement gives strong evidence for the identification of the Si-H$_n$ complexes in these films and supports the high degree of structural relaxation of the a-Si network at low T$_D$.

TABLE I

a-Si:H (T$_D$ = -121°C)		Substituted Silane	
Complex	ω_s(cm^{-1})	Compound	ω_s(cm^{-1})
≡Si-H	2059 ± 8	SiH (C$_2$H$_5$)$_3$	2097
=Si-H$_2$	2124 ± 8	SiH$_2$ (C$_6$H$_{11}$)(C$_6$H$_5$)	2125
-Si-H$_3$	2144 ± 8	SiH$_3$ (C$_6$H$_{13}$)	2152

Comparison of low deposition temperature T$_D$ stretch mode frequencies with substituted silane structural models.

REFERENCES

1. D. E. Soule, G. T. Reedy and E. M. Peterson (to be published).
2. D. E. Soule and J. A. McMillan (to be published).
3. D. E. Soule and G. T. Reedy, Thin Solid Films 63, 175 (1979).
4. J. A. McMillan and E. M. Peterson, Jour. Appl. Phys. 50, 5238 (1979).
5. M. H. Brodsky, M. Cardona and J. J. Cuomo, Phys. Rev. B 16, 3556 (1977).
6. G. Lucovsky, R. J. Nemanich and J. C. Knights, Phys. Rev. B 19, 2064 (1979).
7. H. Shanks, C. J. Fang, L. Ley, M. Cardona, F. J. Demond and S. Kalbitzer, Phys. Stat. Sol. B 100, 43 (1980).
8. G. Lucovsky, Solid State Com. 29, 571 (1979).
9. A. L. Smith and N. C. Angelotti, Spectrochim. Acta 15, 412 (1959).
10. R. S. Mulliken, J. Chem. Phys. 2, 782 (1934); 3, 573 (1935).

STRUCTURAL INHOMOGENEITIES AND THE INTERPRETATION
OF IR ABSORPTION FOR a-Si:H FILMS

G. Lucovsky and R. A. Rudder

Dept. of Physics, North Carolina State Univ., Raleigh, NC 27650

ABSTRACT

The IR absorption is calculated for an inhomogeneous thin film with a columnar morphology similar to that reported in a-Si:H. We conclude that IR absorption measurements must be complemented by both direct structural characterization (TEM and/or SEM), and a determination of the hydrogen concentration by a primary technique (nuclear reaction techniques), if the interpretation of IR features in terms of different local Si-H bonding configurations is to be meaningful.

INTRODUCTION AND BACKGROUND

There is direct evidence from both TEM and SEM micrographs that a-Si:H films can exhibit macroscopic structural disorder in the form of a columnar morphology.[1,2] This occurs in films produced by the glow-discharge-decomposition of silane,[1,2] and by sputtering,[3] with the degree of the columnar structure varying with the deposition parameters. For films produced on substrates at 200 to 300°C, the diameters of the columns are of the order of 50-100 Å,[2,3] and the columns are in the direction of the film growth. The spacing between columns, i.e., the extent of the so-called "connective tissue", varies between dimensions of the same order as the column diameters, to dimensions that are barely resolved in the TEM micrographs (<10Å).[1,2,3] Other experimental probes, NMR,[2,4] Raman scattering and IR absorption,[5] have demonstrated that the hydrogen concentration and the local Si-H bonding are different in the columns and the connective tissue. We have calculated the optical absorption for thin films having a columnar structure using a model in which the absorption constant (α) and reflectivity (R) of the material in the columns and connecting tissue are different. We have applied these calculations to a-Si:H films to demonstrate the way the inhomogeniety effects the qualitative and quantitative interpretations of the IR spectra.[6,7]

CALCULATION OF THE THIN FILM TRANSMITTANCE

Figure 1(a) is a schematic representation of a typical columnar structure.[1,2] In the TEM micrographs, the columnar material, A, appears dark and has dimensions of about 50-100 Å, and the connecting tissue, B, appears light. The ratio of the surface area of the columns to the connecting tissue ranges from about 1:1 to 1:50.[1,2,3] For comparison, Fig. 1(b) also shows a thin film structure with a different type of inhomogeneity, a layer morphology.

For the geometry in Fig. 1(a), we assume: (1) that the columns have a long dimension that is perpendicular to the film surface, (2) that the laterial dimensions of the columnar regions and the connective tissue are much larger than the wavelength of the radiation,

ISSN:0094-243X/81/730095-05$1.50 Copyright 1981 American Institute of Physics

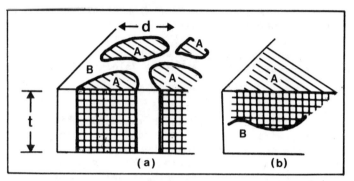

Fig. 1 Schematic representation of (a) columnar morphology and (b) layer morphology. The diameter of the columns, d, is typically 50-100Å, and the film thickness, t, may vary from about 0.5 μm to 10μm.

and (3) that the material in the columnar and connective regions is different, but also homogeneous so that we may assign to each different values of the optical absorption constant, α_A and α_B and the reflectance, R_A and R_B. The transmittance, T_C is then given by

$$T_C = \frac{I_t}{I_0} = F_A \frac{(1-R_A)^2 e^{-\alpha_A t}}{1-R_A^2 e^{-2\alpha_A t}} + F_B \frac{(1-R_B)^2 e^{-\alpha_B t}}{1-R_B^2 e^{-2\alpha_B t}} \qquad (1)$$

I_0 is the incident radiation, I_t the transmitted radiation, and F_A and F_B are respectively the fractional surface areas of the columnar material, and the connecting material. R_A and R_B are generally different, but neither is a function of the photon wavenumber whereas, α_A and α_B are of strong functions the wavenumber through the characteristic frequencies of the various stretching, bending and wagging modes. We consider the application of Eq. (1) for the case where the absorption is strong, i.e., $R_j^2 e^{-2\alpha_j t} \ll 1$. We also neglect any small differences between R_A and R_B, taking them both equal to the same value of R. The absorption constant is the product of an absorption cross-section, σ_j and the volume density of absorbing centers, N_j, $\alpha_j = \sigma_j N_j$. Substituting this definition into Eq. (1) and dividing the transmittance T_C by $(1-R)^2$ to define an effective transmittance T_C', we have, for the columnar morphology

$$T_C' = F_A e^{-\sigma_A N_A t} + F_B e^{-\sigma_B N_B t} \qquad (2)$$

For a layer morphology (Fig. 1(b)) the corresponding transmittance T_L' is given by

$$T_L' = e^{-(\sigma_A N_A t_A + \sigma_B N_B t_B)} \qquad (3)$$

where $t_A + t_B = t$.

IR ABSORPTION IN a-Si:H FILMS

There are two aspects of the IR absorption that have received a considerable study: (1) the use of IR as a tool to identify different local atomic configurations, SiH, SiH_2, $(SiH_2)_n$, etc., through their characteristic vibrational frequencies,[6,7,8] and (2) the use of the integrated absorption to determine the total amount of incorporated hydrogen.[9] Other studies have used IR to describe changes in the hydrogen incorporation following the evolution of hydrogen via an-nealing at elevated temperatures,[10] and following sequences of ion-bombardment and thermal annealing cycles.[11]

To obtain the total hydrogen concentration, the film is assumed to be homogeneous so that the effective transmittance is given by

$$T' = e^{-\sigma N t} \tag{4}$$

The integrated absorption is then calculated for either the bond-stretching (1950 - 2150 cm^{-1}) or bond-bending (500 - 700 cm^{-1}) regimes, and this is assumed to be proportional to the number of Si-H bonds, and hence, the hydrogen concentration.[9,12] The proportionality fac-tor is obtained by determining the hydrogen concentration via a pri-mary technique, resonance nuclear reactions.[9] This allows one to compare absorption cross-sections for the various Si-H vibrations in a-Si:H with cross-sections of similar vibrations in silane molecules. These comparisons indicate large differences between these cross-sections, which have been related to differences in the partial charges on the Si and H atoms of the particular Si-H group.[8,12]

If a film is homogeneous, and the value of σ has been determined via a primary technique, then the value of N obtained from Eq. (4) is the Si-H concentration that contributes to that vibration. If the film is inhomogeneous, the value of N so obtained can be in serious error. For the layer morphology, application of Eq. (4), yields

$$N = \frac{\sigma_A N_A t_A + \sigma_B N_B t_B}{\sigma t} \tag{5}$$

If the <u>same</u> species contributes to the vibrations in both regions A and B, so that the two layers differ only in the concentration, then N is given by

$$N = \frac{N_A t_A + N_B t_B}{t} \tag{6}$$

and is the correct average value of the concentration of Si-H bonds. If two different species, e.g., SiH and SiH_2 groups, contribute to the absorption, as in the bond-rocking regime at 630 cm^{-1} and if each local configuration has a different value of σ, then Eq. (5) applies and the calculated value of N in general is not equal to the hydrogen concentration. For the columnar morphology, the situation is differ-ent in as much as the value of N calculated by assuming a homogeneous medium (Eq. (4)) is <u>never</u> a correct measure of the hydrogen content. For the columnar morphology, this general result of this analysis is

$$N = -\frac{1}{\sigma t} \ln \left(F_A e^{-\sigma_A N_A t} + F_B e^{-\sigma_B N_B t} \right) \tag{7}$$

It is established that the material in the columns contains pre-dominantly SiH groups with ν_{S1} = 2000 cm^{-1}, ν_{R1} = 630 cm^{-1}, whereas the material in the connecting tissue is predominantly $(SiH_2)_n$ with $\nu_{S2} \approx 2100$ cm^{-1}, $\nu_{B2} \approx 850\text{-}900$ cm^{-1} and $\nu_{R2} = 630$ cm^{-1}. Figure 2 contains schematic representations of spectra for a situation in which the concentration of hydrogen in A and B are essentially equal, i.e., the area under S_1 in (a) is approximately equal to the area under S_2 in (b). The spectrum shown for an aspect ratio of $F_A/F_B = 9:1$ in (c), is dominated by the absorption of the SiH group. Application of Eq. (7), in which the B-contributions are neglected yields the result that $N \approx N_A$ or an error of about a factor of two! Similarly, the situation in which $F_A = F_B$, (d) gives about the same error for the calculation of the total hydrogen content.

From the TEM micrographs reported[1,2] for films produced by glow-discharge decomposition of silane, and deposited at temperatures between 250° and 300°C, we observe that the areas of the columnar and connective materials are very nearly equal. These films usually exhibit comparable IR absorption in the stretching vibrations assigned to SiH and $(SiH_2)_n$ groups.[2,6,7] From the analysis given above and based on the use of the absorption in the stretching regime, we conclude that a calculation of either the total hydrogen concentration or the fraction of hydrogen in the either SiH or $(SiH_2)_n$ configurations that assumes homogeneity will be in serious error, of the order of a factor of two. Any estimate of the hydrogen concentration based

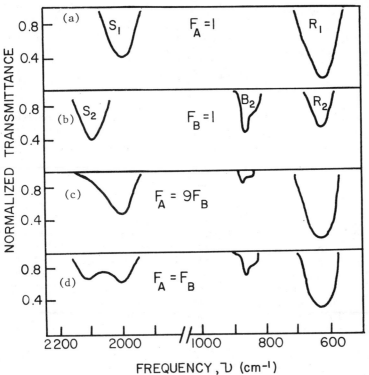

Fig. 2 Schematic representations of IR spectra. (a) SiH spectrum: S_1 = Stretch; R_1 = Rock. (b) SiH_2 spectrum: S_2 = stretch; B_2 = Scissors Bend and R_2 = Rock. (c), (d) are Spectra for inhomogeneous columnar material with different column/tissue aspect ratios.

on the rocking modes near 630 cm^{-1}, R_1 and R_2, also leads to comparable errors. Films produced by magnetron sputtering on the other hand, display a larger ratio of dark to light areas in the TEM micrographs.[3] Therefore, the $(SiH_2)_n$ contributions can effectively be <u>invisible</u> in the bond-stretching and bond-rocking regions of the IR, but are in evidence through a weak contribution due to bending modes[6,7,8] near 850-900 cm^{-1}. Hydrogen evolution occurs preferentially from the $(SiH_2)_n$ in connecting tissue of these films, and hence, may not always be detectable through changes in the IR. Evolution, without charges in the IR absorption can therefore be a result of inhomogeneous incorporation of hydrogen in the a columnar morphology, rather than an indication of large amounts of non-bonded hydrogen.[10]

SUMMARY

We have calculated the absorption for a model thin film structure with a columnar morphology with different incorporations of hydrogen in the two regions, SiH in the columns and $(SiH_2)_n$ in the connecting tissue. Subsequent interpretation of IR data, <u>without</u> a knowledge of the film morphology, can lead to serious errors in both qualitative and quantitative interpretations of the spectra. We conclude that in order to interpret IR spectra correctly, films should be studied by TEM and/or SEM to determine the homogeneity, and by nuclear reactions to determine the hydrogen concentration. These measurements combined with the IR, can then give a meaningful model of the microscopic aspects of the hydrogen incorporation.

The authors acknowledge helpful discussions with Dr. M.A. Paesler, and support for this work through SERI subcontract No. HZ-0-9238 under EG-77-C-01-4042.

REFERENCES

1. J.C. Knights and R.A. Lujan, Appl. Phys. Lett. <u>35</u>, 244 (1979).
2. J.C. Knights, J. Non-Cryst. Solids <u>35-36</u>, 159 (1980).
3. G. Lucovsky, R.A. Rudder, T.M. Donovan and T. McMahon (to be published).
4. J.A. Reimer, R.W. Vaughan and J.C. Knights, Phys. Rev. Lett. <u>44</u>, 193 (1980).
5. R.J. Nemanich, D.K. Biegelsen and M.P. Rosenblum, J. Phys. Soc. Japan <u>49</u> (suppl. A), 1189 (1980).
6. M.H. Brodsky, M. Cardona and J.J. Cuomo, Phys. Rev. <u>B16</u>, 3556 (1977).
7. G. Lucovsky, R.J. Nemanich and J.C. Knights, Phys. Rev. <u>B19</u>, 2064 (1979).
8. G. Lucovsky (these proceedings).
9. C.J. Fang, K.J. Gruntz, L. Ley, M. Cardona, F.J. Demond, G. Müller and S. Kalbitzer, J. Non-Cryst. Solids <u>35-36</u>, 255 (1980).
10. S. Oguz, R.W. Collins, M.A. Paesler and W. Paul, J. Non-Cryst. Solids <u>35-36</u>, 231 (1980).
11. S. Oguz, D.A. Anderson, W. Paul and H.J. Stein, Phys. Rev. <u>B22</u>, 880 (1980).
12. G. Lucovsky, Solar Cells <u>2</u>, 431 (1980).

CHEMICAL BONDING EFFECTS ON THE LOCAL VIBRATIONS
IN FLUORINATED AND HYDROGENATED AMORPHOUS SILICON

G. Lucovsky

Dept. of Physics, North Carolina State Univ., Raleigh, NC 27650

ABSTRACT

We extend calculations of vibrational frequencies based on the bond induction approach to the stretching and wagging modes of $(SiH_2)_n$, and the stretching modes of SiF, SiF_2 and $(SiF_2)_n$. This provides the quantitative basis for a structural assignment of features in the IR absorption spectra films of a-Si:H and a-Si:F.

INTRODUCTION

The frequencies of Si-H stretching vibrations in substituted silane molecules vary systematically with the electronegativities of the other atoms or groups bonded to the central Si-atom. This type of induction effect has been applied to a-Si where it provides a quantitative explanation for (1) the relatively low frequency of the stretching vibration of the SiH group[1,2]; (2) the changes in the frequency of this mode induced by neighboring oxygen atoms[3]; and (3) the frequencies of stretching vibrations of SiH_2 and SiH_3 groups.[1,2] This paper extends the study to other configurations of interest in a-Si: (1) to an inclusion of remote inductive effects[4] in polysilane, $(SiH_2)_n$; (2) to bond-bending forces associated with the H-Si-Si configuration; and (3) to bond-stretching vibrations of SiF and SiF_2 groups. This approach provides an assignment for the local mode frequencies ($\nu > 500$ cm^{-1}) reported in the IR spectra of glow-discharge deposited, and sputtered a-Si:H and a-Si:F.[5] Changes in the spectra by annealing at temperatures sufficiently high to evolve H[6], or via ion-bombardment followed by annealing[7], may in some cases be associated with defect configurations not considered in this study.

a-Si:H ALLOYS

The frequencies of the SiH stretching vibrations in silane molecules, $HSiR_1R_2R_3$ vary according to the empirical relation,[1,2]

$$\nu = 1740.7 + 34.7 \ \Sigma Xj \pm 13 \ \text{cm}^{-1} \qquad (1)$$

where Xj is the stability ratio electronegativity of the Rj atom or group.[8] Rj is either a halogen atom, or an organic group, CH_3, C_2H_5, etc., but may not be H or D. For the same vibration in a-Si:H or another amorphous solid, a generalization of Eq. (1) applies; i.e.,

$$\nu = \nu_o + a^{(1)} \ \Sigma Xj + a^{(2)} \ \Sigma X_k + a^{(3)} \ \Sigma X_\ell \ \ldots \qquad (2)$$

where inductive effects associated with more distant neighbors are included in the sums over $k, \ell, \ldots$, etc.[2] From arguments in Ref. 2, and in Ref. 4, we find that the coefficients of these more distant sums

ISSN:0094-243X/81/730100-06$1.50 Copyright 1981 American Institute of Physics

decrease systematically

$$a^{(1)} > a^{(2)} > a^{(3)} \ldots \text{etc.} \tag{3}$$

and to within the uncertainty in the empirically determined constants in Eq. (1), $a^{(2)}$, $a^{(3)}$, etc. can be neglected so that Eq. (1) applies to amorphous solids as well.

The physical basis of the induction effect is demonstrated by re-casting Eq. (1) in terms of the partial charge on the Si-atom.[8,9] This approach derives from an observation that many properties of molecular systems, e.g., NMR, core level shifts, can be understood in terms of the electron density, or equivalently the partial charge on the constituent atoms. This paper extends these relationships to vibrational frequencies of groups involving terminal or univalent atoms. We have calculated partial charges using the Sanderson method[8] including the modifications in Ref. 4 and have found that for silane molecules the partial charge on the Si-atom, e_{si}, is a function of ΣXj,

$$\Sigma Xj = 6.77 + 18.77\, e_{si} \tag{4}$$

Substituting Eq. (4) into Eq. (1), we have

$$\nu = 1975.5 + 651.2\, e_{si} \pm 13 \text{ cm}^{-1} \tag{5}$$

The frequency of the bond-stretching vibration of the SiH group increases as e_{si} <u>increases</u>, and results from an associated <u>decrease</u> in the Si-H bond length.[2,9]

A relationship parallel to Eq. (1) also applies to the stretching frequencies of the SiH_2 group

$$\nu = 1956.3 + 25.4\, \Sigma Xj \pm 12 \text{ cm or } \nu = 2035.3 + 489.9 e_{si} \pm 12 \text{ cm}^{-1} \tag{6}$$

where the sum is over two atoms or groups (see Fig. 1). The difference between the symmetric and asymmetric stretching frequencies of this group is smaller than the uncertainty in the empirical relation so the same relation applies to both modes.

Figure 1 includes three local bonding configurations associated with the SiH_2 group. Configuration (b) is an isolated SiH_2 group

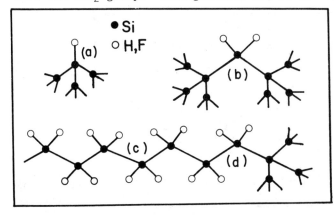

Fig. 1 Local atomic configurations in a-Si:H and a-Si:F. (a) SiH and SiF; (b), (c) and (d) SiH_2 and SiF_2.

where all of the neighbors to the H-atoms are Si-atoms. Configuration (c) indicates the local environment in the interior portion of $(SiH_2)_n$ segment, where the near neighbors are other SiH_2 groups. Configuration (d) is at the junction between an $(SiH_2)_n$ chain and an amorphous network of Si-atoms. For the configuration shown in (b), $\Sigma X_j = 5.24$ and the calculated frequency is 2089 cm^{-1}. Lucovsky, Knights and Nemanich[2] (LKN) have associated IR absorption centered at 2090 cm^{-1} with an isolated SiH_2 group. For configurations (d) and (c), the values of ΣX_j are 5.83 and 6.42 respectively; these correspond to frequencies of 2104 cm^{-1} and 2119 cm^{-1}. LKN have associated the onset of a doublet absorption band at 845 cm^{-1}, 890 cm^{-1} with the development of polysilane environments. A shift in the stretching absorption from 2090 cm^{-1} to about 2100 cm^{-1} is associated with the observation of this doublet. A further shift in the doublet from 845 cm^{-1}, 890 cm^{-1} to 867 cm^{-1}, 905 cm^{-1} has been attributed by LKN to SiH_3, and is accompanied by a further shift in the stretching vibration from 2100 cm^{-1} to 2120 cm^{-1}. The calculations here suggest that <u>both</u> pairs of doublets, and the <u>accompanying changes</u> near 2100 cm^{-1} are due to polysilane configurations; e.g., Fig. 1 (c) and (d). Alternatively, both pairs of doublets may be associated with interior SiH_2 groups, (c), but with different degrees of stereo-regularity.[5]

The exact nature of the doublet-structure near 850-950 cm^{-1} has long been a question. Knights, Lucovsky and Nemanich[10] suggested that it was associated with polysilane-like environments, specifically with coupled scissors vibrations, whilst LKN suggested that the lower frequency component was due to a bond-wagging motion and the higher frequency component to a scissors motion. This question is resolved by considering induction effects associated with bond-bending force constants.

Bond-bending motions are associated with triads of atoms and two such triads are relevant to the SiH_2 configuration. The first involves H-Si-H, the triad that participates in the scissors motion.[2] Comparisons based on substituted silane molecules with SiH_2 groups indicate that the bond-bending force constant, $k_\theta^{(1)}$ associated with this triad is <u>insensitive</u> to the electronegativities of R_1 and R_2. On the other hand the bond-bending force constant, $k_\theta^{(2)}$ associated with the triad H-Si-Si (see Fig. 2) is <u>sensitive</u> to the local chemistry. For the SiH

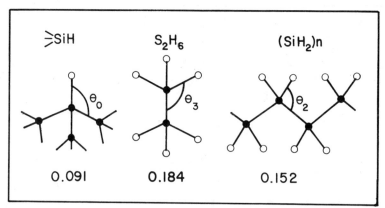

$\geqslant$SiH S_2H_6 $(SiH_2)n$

0.091   0.184   0.152

Fig. 2 H-Si-Si triads. Values of $k_\theta^{(2)}$ in units of 10^5 dyne/cm The subscripts 0, 3 and 2, indicate the number of H-atoms bonded to the end Si-atom.

configuration (θ_o), $k_\theta(2) = 0.091 \times 10^5$ dyne/cm, whereas for the configuration (θ_3) in disilane (Si_2H_6), $k_\theta(2) = 0.184 \times 10^5$ dyne/cm. We propose an induction relationship of the following form

$$k_\theta^{(2)} = a\Sigma Xj + b \qquad (7)$$

where the sum is over the neighbors to the end Si atom, i.e. over three Si-atoms for the Si-H group (7.86), and three H-atoms for S_2H_6 (10.65). For the interior SiH_2 configuration in $(SiH_2)_n$, ΣXj is over two H-atoms and one Si-atom (9.72). From the values of $k_\theta(2)$ for Si-H and Si_2H_6, we find a = 0.0333 and b = -0.171. This in turn yields a value of $k_\theta(2) = 0.152 \times 10^5$ dyne/cm for the $(SiH_2)_n$ configuration. For an isolated SiH_2 group, as in Fig. 1 (b), $\Sigma Xj = 7.86$ and $k_\theta(2) = 0.091 \times 10^5$ dyne/cm. Applying these force constants, we obtain the results shown in Table I.

Table I SiH_2 Frequencies

| Mode | Isolated SiH_2 | | Interior SiH_2 - $(SiH_2)_n$ | |
	Calculated (cm^{-1})	IR Absorption (cm^{-1})	Calculated (cm^{-1})	IR Absorption (cm^{-1})
Stretching	2087	2090	2120	2100, 2140
Scissors	880	875	910	890, 907
Wagging	650	630	821	845, 867

The calculated changes in the stretching, scissors and wagging frequencies going from an isolated SiH_2 group to an interior SiH_2 group in $(SiH_2)_n$ are consistent with the changes observed in the IR absorption. This implies that all of the IR structure can be explained in terms of SiH, SiH_2 and $(SiH_2)_n$ configurations. The large change in the wagging frequency between an isolated SiH_2 group and the $(SiH_2)_n$ interior group is a result of the large induction effect calculated from Eq. (7).

a-Si:F ALLOYS

The mass of F(19.0) with respect to H(1.01), and relative to that of Si(28.1) produces two important effects in the vibrational spectra: (1) the only modes with frequencies in excess of the highest frequency of an a-Si network are stretching vibrations; and (2) the frequency of the asymmetric vibration of an SiF_2 group, ν_a, is 10% higher than that of the symmetric vibration, ν_s.[5]

Absorption measurements have yielded five distinct absorptions between 800 cm^{-1} and 1025 cm^{-1}.[11,12,13] These are attributed to stretching vibrations.[5] There has been disagreement with regard to the origin of the strong and sharp absorption at $\sim$1010 cm^{-1}. It has been attributed by one group to SiF_3[12] and by another to SiF_4 molecules trapped within the amorphous phase.[13] We have used induction arguments to resolve this question.

Figure 3 gives the induction relationship for SiF modes. The straight line is a fit to molecular data, SiF vibrations in fluorosilane molecules. The relationship can also be cast in terms of the

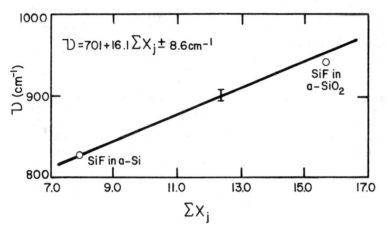

Fig. 3 Bond Induction relation for the SiF group.

partial change on the Si-atom, i.e.,

$$\nu = 789.1 + 272.7 \, e_{si} \qquad (8)$$

Similar induction relations can be derived for the asymmetric and symmetric modes of the SiF_2 group;[5]

$$\nu_s = 698 + 24.7 \, \Sigma Xj \quad \text{or} \quad \nu_s = 720.7 + 367.8 \, e_{si}$$

$$\nu_s = 815 + 21.0 \, \Sigma Xj \quad \text{or} \quad \nu_a = 834.3 + 312.7 \, e_{si} \qquad (9)$$

Table II includes calculations of ν_s and ν_a for the three SiF_2 groups shown in Fig. 1 (b), (c) and (d). These computations are the basis of the structural assignment contained in the table.

Table II SiF and SiF_2 Stretching Vibrations

Configuration	e_{si} (e)		Vibrational Frequency (cm^{-1}) Calculated	IR Absorption
SiF	.132		825	830
Isolated SiF_2	.287	ν_s	826	827
		ν_a	924	930
Terminal SiF_2:$(SiF_2)_n$	.405	ν_s	870	870
		ν_a	961	965
Interior SiF_2:$(SiF_2)_n$	.536	ν_s	918	925
		ν_a	1002	1012

CONCLUSIONS

We have extended the induction approach to $(SiH_2)_n$ configurations, to bending motions of the triad H-Si-Si, and to stretching vibrations of SiF, SiF_2 and $(SiF_2)_n$. This provides a quantitative basis for the

assignment of local modes in the IR spectra. In particular, we identify the nature of the modes which have been subject to the most controversy: (1) modes near 850 cm^{-1} in a-Si:H are wagging motions of
the SiH$_2$ group in (SiH$_2$)$_n$ and (2) the mode at $\sim$1010 cm^{-1} in a-Si:F
is the asymmetric stretching mode of an SiF$_2$ group in the interior of
an (SiF$_2$)$_n$ chain.

Our calculations do not include downshifts in frequency, $\Delta\nu$, associated with the polarizability of the a-Si host ($\varepsilon\approx12$). For an SiH
vibration in an a-Si host, $\Delta\nu$ can be estimated from the expression
given in Ref. 14,

$$\Delta\nu = \frac{3\ (\varepsilon-1)\ (e_M^*)^2}{2\ (\varepsilon+3)\ \mu V_M \omega_M c} \tag{10}$$

where e_M^* is the effective charge[9] for an Si-H vibration in SiH$_4$ ($\sim$0.15e),
μ is the reduced mass ($\sim$1.7 x 10^{-24}g), V_M is a characteristic molecular
volume ($\sim$2.5 x 10^{-23} cm^3), ω_M is the "molecular" frequency calculated
from Eq. (1), and c is the speed of light. Substitution into Eq. (10)
yields $\Delta\nu \approx 12$ cm^{-1}, with comparable values estimated for SiH$_2$, SiF
and SiF$_2$ vibrations. However, it should be noted that $\Delta\nu$ is comparable
to the uncertainty in ν as calculated from Eq. (1), so that neglect
of effects associated with the medium polarization will not alter, in
any significant way, the conclusions drawn in the body of this paper.

The author acknowledges partial support for this work through
SERI subcontract No. HZ-0-0238 under EG-77-C-01-4042.

REFERENCES

1. G. Lucovsky, Solid State Commun. 29, 571 (1979).
2. G. Lucovsky, R.J. Nemanich and J.C. Knights, Phys. Rev. B19, 2064 (1979).
3. J.C. Knights, R.A. Street and G. Lucovsky, J. Non-Cryst. Solids 35-36, 279 (1980).
4. J.C. Carver, R.C. Gray and D.M. Hercules, J. Amer. Chem. Soc. 96, 6851 (1974).
5. G. Lucovsky, Kyoto Summer Institute 1980, Springer-Verlag (in press).
6. S. Oguz, R.W. Collins, M.A. Paesler and W. Paul, J. Non-Cryst. Solids, 35-36, 231 (1980).
7. S. Oguz, D.A. Anderson, W. Paul and H.J. Stein, Phys. Rev. B22, 880 (1980).
8. R.T. Sanderson, Chemical Periodicity (Reinhold, New York 1960).
9. G. Lucovsky, Solar Cells 2, 431 (1980).
10. J.C. Knights, G. Lucovsky and R.J. Nemanich, Philos. Mag. B37, 467 (1978).
11. A. Madan, S.R. Ovshinsky and E. Benn, Philos. Mag. B40, 259 (1979).
12. T. Shimada, Y. Katayama and S. Horigome, Jap. J. Appl. Phys. 19, 265 (1980).
13. L. Ley, H.R. Shanks, C.J. Fang, K.L. Gruntz and M. Cardona, J. Phys. Soc. Japan 49 (Suppl. A), 1241 (1980).
14. H. Wieder, M. Cardona and C.R. Guarnieri, Phys. Status Solidi (b) 92, 99 (1979).

BEHAVIOR OF FLUORINE ATOMS IN a-Si:H:F ALLOY INVESTIGATED BY GAS EVOLUTION

S. Usui, A. Sawada and M. Kikuchi
Sony Corporation Research Center, 174 Fujitsuka-cho, Hodogaya-ku
Yokohama, 240 Japan

ABSTRACT

The behavior of fluorine atoms in a-Si:H:F film produced by the glow-discharge method was investigated using a mass spectrometer. Fluorine atoms leave the film in the form of SiF_4 which evolves moderately at 120°C and abruptly at 750°C. The moderate evolution at 120°C is caused by water adsorption. Infrared transmission spectra for the annealed film showed that the $\equiv SiF$ and $=SiF_2$ in the network change to SiF_4 at temperatures above 400°C. The result differs from that on hydrogenated amorphous silicon for which the evolved gas is hydrogen only.

INTRODUCTION

Although fluorinated amorphous silicon has been proposed by Madan et al.[1] as an excellent material for photovoltaic applications, to date only Fang et al.[2] have reported on the behavior of fluorine atoms in a-Si:H:F alloy. Further work in this area may prove to be important if it can be established that Si-F bonds yield an amorphous silicon more stable than hydrogenated silicon. We are going to report on the results of our investigation on the behavior of fluorine atoms by gas evolution, infrared (ir) absorption, EPMA and conductivity measurements. We conclude that $\equiv SiF$ and $-SiF_3$, when they coexist with hydrogen atoms, do not remain stable in the bonding network at temperatures above 400°C.

EXPERIMENTAL

Samples were prepared in an inductively-coupled glow-discharge by decomposition of four different gas mixtures, $SiF_4/SiH_4/Ar$, $SiF_4/SiH_4/H_2$, $SiF_4/H_2/Ar$ and SiF_4/H_2. Table I shows the deposition conditions, the fluorine content determined from EPMA and the hydrogen content determined from the Si-H stretching absorption peak in the ir spectrum of film prepared in each gas mixture.

For the gas evolution experiment, films were deposited on a tungsten substrate held at 300°C. The substrate was prebaked at 1000°C to minimize adsorbed gases which otherwise would be released from the tungsten substrate during deposition and evolution. The deposited films were transferred to a 400 ml evolution chamber to which were connected a capacitance manometer and a quadrupole mass spectrometer. The variation in the mass spectrum and the total pressure of the evolving gas were measured as the temperature of the film was raised to 800°C. The temperature was monitored a thermocouple attached to the film. The heating rate

ISSN:0094-243X/81/730106-05$1.50 Copyright 1981 American Institute of Physics

Table I Deposition Conditions for four different gas mixtures

Sample	I	II	III	IV
Gas mixture	$SiF_4/SiH_4/Ar$	$SiF_4/SiH_4/H_2$	$SiF_4/H_2/Ar$	SiF_4/H_2
$SiF_4/(SiH_4$ or $H_2)$	1.00	0.72	0.67	1.00
Pressure (Torr)	0.12	0.07-0.08	0.16-0.17	0.06-0.07
rf power (W)	200	270	250	250-300
Sub. temp. (°C)	300	300	300	300
H content (at %)	10-15	20-27	19-20	8-10
F content (at %)	2.5-3.0	9-12	8-10	9-11

was held at about 400°C/min. in order to eliminate the influence of gases from the chamber wall during the measurement.

Infrared transmission and EPMA measurements were made on the samples prepared under the same condition on a c-Si substrate.

The temperature dependence of conductivity of the film deposited on the glass substrate (Tempax 8330) was measured in a vacuum. Aluminum electrodes with a 0.5 mm gap were formed on the film and the current through the film was measured using logarithmic picoammeter (Keithley 26000) at a constant voltage of 3 V. A thermocouple dipped in a gallium droplet placed on the film surface was used to measure the exact temperature of the film.

EXPERIMENTAL RESULTS

Figure 1 shows typical evolution curves for the samples prepared from the $SiF_4/SiH_4/H_2$ mixture. Mass spectroscopic analysis showed that the evolved gases were H_2, H_2O, SiF_4, HF and F. At 350°C the large amount of hydrogen evolved caused the chamber pressure to begin to rise. The amount of other gases evolved was very small between 100°C and 750°C.

SiF_4 evolution was confirmed by comparing the spectrum of the evolving gas with the spectrum observed when pure SiF_4 was introduced. Actually, the SiF_3^+ peak was the highest of all fragments of SiF_4, followed by SiF^+ and SiF_2^+. Figure 1 shows that SiF_4 evolves moderately at 120°C and in an abrupt and explosive manner between 750°C and 800°C. This is characteristic of all four kinds of samples.

In Fig.2, the evolution curve of the film exposed to moisture at 50°C for 30 minutes is compared with the curve of the film kept in dry air. Notice that the low temperature evolution of SiF_4 from the sample exposed to moisture occurs in the narrow range between 100°C and 200°C, whereas SiF_4 from the dry sample evolves over the wider range between 100°C and 700°C. Hydrogen evolution from the sample exposed to moisture seems to be retarded by water adsorption.

The Si-F bond in the film was also investigated using ir absorption. The spectrum for the unannealed sample has peaks at 830 cm^{-1} caused by SiF stretching, at 920 cm^{-1} caused by SiF_2 stretching and at 1010 cm^{-1} caused by SiF_4 stretching.[3,4]

108

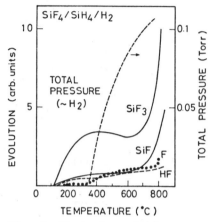

Fig. 1. Typical evolution
curves. SiF$_4$ evolution was
monitored by referring to SiF$_3^+$
peak intensity.

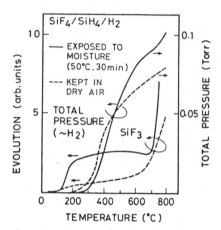

Fig. 2. The variation in
evolution curves for dry and
wet samples prepared under
the same condition.

Figure 3 shows the ir spectra of samples prepared in an SiF$_4$/H$_2$/Ar
glow discharge observed after annealing at different temperatures.
The samples deposited in gas mixtures I, II and IV showed similar
variations in their spectra, but the SiF, SiF$_2$ and SiF$_4$ peaks
looked relatively weak and broad because they were masked by
strong Si-H bending absorption. As the temperature was raised
above 400°C, The absorption caused by SiF and SiF$_2$ decreased,
while the SiF$_4$ peak increased slightly. At 850°C the SiF$_4$ peak
suddenly disappeared.

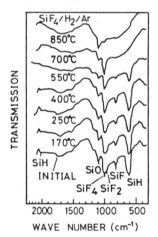

Fig. 3. Variations in ir
spectra with annealing
temperatures.

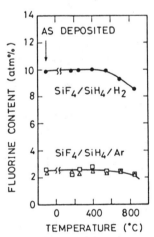

Fig. 4. Fluorine concentration
in a-Si:H:F film plotted
against annealing temperatures.

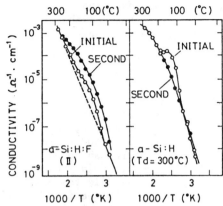

Fig. 5. Temperature dependence of conductivity for a-Si:H:F film and a-Si:H film. The latter was deposited at 300°C in a capacitively coupled glow-discharge of SiH$_4$/Ar.

The fluorine concentration in the film prepared from the SiF$_4$/SiH$_4$/Ar and SiF$_4$/SiH$_4$/H$_2$ mixtures determined by EPMA is plotted against the annealing temperatures in Fig. 4. The fluorine concentration was constant at temperatures below 700°C, but it began to decrease rapidly at 750°C, corresponding to the abrupt increase in evolving SiF$_4$, as can be seen in Fig. 1.

Figure 5 shows the temperature dependence of conductivity for a-Si:H:F film prepared from the SiF$_4$/SiH$_4$/H$_2$ mixture. For comparison, it also shows temperature dependence of conductivity of a-Si:H film. In the first measurement run (and only in the first measurement run), there appears a hump on the conductivity curve at about 120°C, the temperature at which SiF$_4$ evolves. The basic shape of the conductivity curve for a-Si:H:F varies with successive measurement runs. A similar hump was observed in the first measurement run for a-Si:H film, but, in contrast to a-Si:H:F film, the basic shape of the conductivity curve did not vary with successive measurement runs, although the hump disappeared after the first run.

DISCUSSION

It is clear from Fig. 2 that the adsorption of water is associated with SiF$_4$ evolution at 120°C. The typical evolution curves in Fig. 1 suggest that our films' exposure to moisture in air when they were transferred from the plasma reaction chamber to the evolution chamber may have been the occasion for this adsorption.

We are interested in the relation between the conductivity curves in Fig. 5 and the SiF$_4$ evolution curves in Fig. 1. The temperature dependence of the dark conductivity of a-Si:H:F film in Fig. 5 seems to have some correlation with the low temperature evolution of SiF$_4$. At about 120°C the curve for the first measurement run has a hump. We believe that this hump may be caused by an ionosorption process in which water molecules act as donors. At temperatures above 120°C we can speculate that a reaction between water molecules and -SiF$_3$ such as the following may take place: Si-SiF$_3$+H$_2$O → Si-OH+SiHF$_3$. SiHF$_3$ may possibly decompose to SiF$_4$ and HF on the film surface. In fact, HF gas evolution was observed at the same temperature as SiF$_4$ evolution. The varying of the basic shape of the conductivity curves with successive measurement runs suggests that -SiF$_3$ in the surface region changes to SiF_4 at low temperatures. The basic shape of the a–Si:H conductivity curve, however, does not change with successive measurement runs and there seems to be no change in the surface.

EPMA measurements of the annealed samples established that SiF_4 evolved abruptly at high temperatures also. The decreased amount of fluorine incorporated in the film at temperatures above 700°C agrees with the results of the evolution experiments, as can be seen in Fig. 1. These EPMA measurements show that there is little gas evolution below 750°C. The ir spectra, however, show variations occurring between annealing temperatures of 400°C and 750°C. The fact that hydrogen evolves at temperatures above 350°C (as can be seen in Fig. 1) suggests that hydrogen atoms in the film contribute to the breaking of the Si–Si bond in this temperature range. If this is true, $Si–SiF_3$ bonds, when they coexist with a sufficient amount of hydrogen, are unstable above 400°C. This is in sharp contrast to the results on a–Si:F in which SiF and SiF_3 peaks in ir spectra do not change up to 700°C.[5] We can, therefore, conclude from the decreasing SiF and SiF_2 peaks and from the fact that SiF_4 only evolves moderately below 750°C but evolves abruptly at that temperature, that $\equiv SiF$ and $=SiF_2$ change to SiF_4 in our material. This is not contradicted by our finding no change in the ir spectra at 120°C, because ir absorption cannot detect the very small number of fluorine atoms which evolve at this temperature.

CONCLUSIONS

1. Fluorine in a–Si:H:F evolves at 120°C and at about 750°C in the form SiF4. 2. The moderate evolution at 120°C may be related to the adsorption of water in the air. 3. $\equiv SiF$ and $=SiF_2$ in the film change to SiF4, contributing to an abrupt evolution at about 750°C.

ACKNOWLEDGEMENTS

The authors would like to thank Mr. K. Kajiwara for making the EPMA measurements and Dr. N. Watanabe, Mr. J. Mizuguchi and Mr. M. Ikeda for useful discussions.

REFERENCES

1. A. Madan, S. R. Ovshinsky and E. Benn, Phil. Mag. B40, 259 (1979).
2. C. J. Fang, L. Ley, K. J. Gruntz, H. R. Shanks and M. Cardona, Phys. Rev. B22 6140 (1980).
3. T. Shimada, Y. Katayama and S. Horigome, Jpn. J. App. Phys. 19 (1980) L265.
4. G. Lucovsky, to be published in Proc. Kyoto Summer Inst. 1980.
5. H. Matsumura, private communication.

ON THE STRUCTURE OF FLUORINE DEFECTS IN AMORPHOUS AND CRYSTALLINE SILICON STUDIED BY HYPERFINE INTERACTION AND CHANNELING METHODS

K. Bonde Nielsen, S. Damgaard, J.W. Peterson, W. Schou
I. Stensgaard, and G. Weyer, Institute of Physics, University
of Aarhus, DK 8000 Aarhus C, Denmark

ABSTRACT

DPAD results on a-Si:F reveal a unique, amorphous, fluorine site stemming from 48% of the fluorine recoils. This component is also observed in crystalline Si:F with a population of 25% together with a second unique, "crystalline", component with a population of 40%. In a-Si:F the amorphous component is independent of temperature (80-900 K) whereas in crystalline Si:F it anneals at 700 K in favour of the crystalline component. Although the DPAD results indicate a unique orientation component of the F-orbitals in crystalline Si:F a specific lattice location could not be revealed in preliminary channeling experiments.

INTRODUCTION

It is of interest to gain insight in the microscopic nature of fluorinated amorphous silicon for a deeper understanding of its technologically important macroscopic properties. For this, the application of hyperfine interaction techniques offers an alternative to infrared spectroscopy[1]. The basic idea is to study the electronic structure, geometry and population of specific Si-F defects via the electric field gradient (EFG) at the fluorine nucleus and the electron density at its Si partner and, for crystalline material, to determine the position and symmetry of the fluorine atom in the Si lattice. Here we report on the first results which have been obtained for Ar-sputtered amorphous and fluorine-implanted crystalline silicon.

EXPERIMENTAL PRINCIPLES

The hyperfine interaction methods applied are perturbed angular correlation spectroscopy[2] (DPAD) and Mossbauer spectroscopy[3] (MS). The channeling technique[4] is adapted to the fluorine case. In combination with DPAD, it yields information on lattice location of fluorine.

1. The application of DPAD

In a classical picture the nuclear quadrupole moment of an (impurity) atom in a solid respond to the EFG of the environment by precessing the nuclear spin. In DPAD the impurities are implanted into the host material as recoil nuclei from nuclear reactions. A fraction of these recoils are left in an isomeric state for subsequent γ-decay. The precession is then reflected in a modulation of the γ-decay intensity, when recorded at a fixed angle with respect to the beam axis and time-correlated to the initiating reaction. The latter is achieved by the application of a pulsed beam and synchronizing the γ-detection to the beam frequency. The direct experimental output is a perturbation factor $G_2(t)$[5] or, if more than one "site" is populated, a superposition of such functions. The $G_2(t)$ contains the quadrupole interaction frequency $h\nu_Q = e^2Qq$, where eQ denotes the nuclear quadrupole moment. The EFG is a tensor, and is completely described by one parameter $eq = eq_{zz}$ in the case of axial symmetry. In the general case $G_2(t)$ depends on an asymmetry parameter $\eta = (eq_{xx} - eq_{yy})/eq_{zz}$. For single crystals the $G_2(t)$ depends on a further quantity, the orientation of the EFG tensor with respect to the lattice.

The $^{19}F(p,p')^{19}F^*$ reaction is technically very easy to deal with in DPAD. It populates a $\tau \sim 129$ nsec, I = 5/2 state at 197 keV. Furthermore, it turns out that $\nu_Q^{-1} \sim \tau$ for a typical F-compound, thus $G_2(t)$ can be followed over several periods of precession. This is important if more than one site is populated. The application of DPAD is therefore particularly attractive for fluorine and unique for EFG studies because nuclear quadrupole resonance spectroscopy (NQR) does not work for the spin½ ground state of the stable fluorine isotope.

2. The application of MS

In MS[3] the electron density at the Mossbauer probe nucleus can be extracted from the measured isomer shift. Unfortunately, neither Si nor F is a Mossbauer nucleus. However, a close similarity between Si and the isoelectronic element Sn offers alternativ approaches using the 24-keV Mossbauer transition of ^{119}Sn. Substituted Sn atoms on Si sites inherit the electronic structure of the host Si atoms[6]. By comparing Mossbauer data for fluorinated and non-fluorinated amorphous Si, the influence of fluorine on the electron density of Sn (and therefore Si) is deduced.

3. The application of channeling

For lattice location by channeling[4], the yields of backscattered particles or nuclear-reaction particles of γ-rays are recorded as a function of crystal orientation. Previously[7], the channeling technique has been applied for localization of deuterium in silicon using the $^2D(^3He,p)^4He$ reaction. In the case of fluorine in silicon, none of the above mentioned channeling methods work due to lack of sensitivity. However, the fact that the 129 nsec state of ^{19}F is populated strongly in a broad proton resonance at 2 MeV can be taken advantage of in the pulsed beam mode of operation. Here the delayed γ-ray of fluorine can be separated from the prompt Si-signal thus avoiding ruining background.

RESULTS

A typical DPAD spectrum obtained for an Ar sputtered a-Si:F target is shown in fig. 1. It reveals a unique fluorine site which is characterized by a quadrupole frequency of $\nu_Q = 23.1$ MHz and a damping of $\delta\nu_Q/\nu_Q \sim 3\%$. It is populated by $\sim 48\%$ of the fluorine recoils. The DPAD parameters for this site do not depend on fluorine concentration (range 0 - 20%) or target temperature

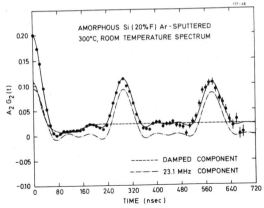

Fig.1
The non-normalized pre-cession amplitude $A_2 \times G_2$ (t) measured at room temperature for Ar-sput-tered a-Si:20%F. The dotted curves indicate the two components in the least-squares fit.

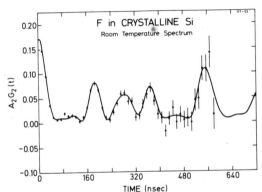

Fig.2
Typical DPAD spectrum for fluorine in crystalline silicon. The least-squares analysis includes a damped component and two components of $\nu_Q =$ 34 MHz and $\nu_Q = 23$ MHz. The probe atoms were re-implanted at a proton energy of 2 MeV from a layer ($\sim 5 \times 10^{17}$ cm^{-2}) produced by 100 keV implantation of BF_2^+.

(80 - 900 K). The remaining F-recoils in all cases are described by one, strongly damped component (cf. fig. 1) with $\delta\nu_Q/\nu_Q \sim$ 50% which reflects a distribution of sites. Figure 2 shows the corres-ponding spectrum for crystalline Si:F. One observes a unique site characterized by $\nu_Q =$ 34 MHz with a population of $\sim$40%, the "amor-phous" component ($\nu_Q \sim$ 23 MHz) with a population of $\sim$25% and a strongly damped component responsible for $\sim$ 35% of the fluorine recoils. The population dependence is shown in fig. 3. It is seen that the "amorphous" component anneals at 700K in favour of an increase in population of the high-frequency, "crystalline" site. A detailed analysis shows that the G_2(t) of the latter site is correlated with the orientation of the crystal; reflecting a unique orientation of the F-orbitals. The channeling data (so far obtained at a $\sim$ 5% level of accuracy) fail to reveal a unique position. For instance, the <100> scan (fig. 4) shows no dip in yield as was found for D in Si[7]). Work is in progress to perform channeling measure-ments at the 0.5% level and to obtain precise DPAD spectra as a function of crystal orientation, in an attempt to explain the struc-ture of the crystalline site.

114

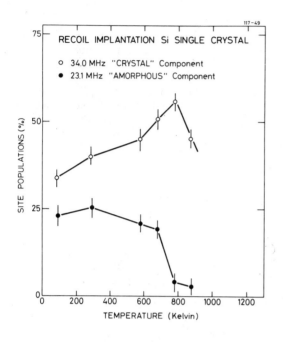

RECOIL IMPLANTATION Si SINGLE CRYSTAL

○ 34.0 MHz "CRYSTAL" Component
● 23.1 MHz "AMORPHOUS" Component

117-49

Fig.3

The site population of re-implanted fluorine in crystalline Si as a function of temperature.

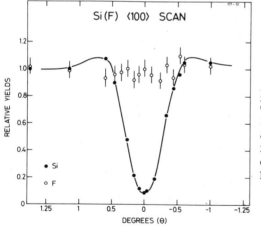

Si(F) ⟨100⟩ SCAN

117-51

● Si
○ F

Fig.4

Channeling spectrum for fluorine in silicon, ⟨100⟩ angular scan. The fluorine content was $5 \times 10^{15}/cm^2$ obtained by 100 keV BF_2^+ implantation at 500°C.

An example of the Mossbauer data obtained for Ar-sputtered a-Si:F in which ^{119m}Sn isotopes have been incorporated substitutionally at the Si sites is shown in fig. 5. It reveals a fluorine related component which has an exceptional large isomer shift of 4.5 mm/s relative to $CaSnO_3$.

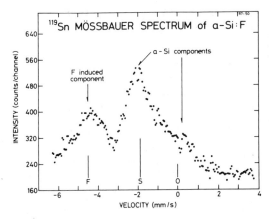

Fig.5
Mössbauer spectrum for substitutional Sn ($5 \cdot 10^{14}$ atoms/cm^2) in Ar-sputtered a-Si:7%F. The 4.5 mm/s line (F) is caused by the presence of fluorine. The components S and O are seen in a-Si alone.

DISCUSSION

The main conclusion from the DPAD data is the formation of two specific structures of F in Si by recoil implantation. The EFG value of the $\nu_Q = 23$ MHz, "amorphous" component points to a structure of large p-electron density at the fluorine atom. This combines favourably with the conclusion from the Mossbauer data that reveal a substitutional Sn-site which has delivered practically all of its valence 5p-electrons to presumably a neighbour F atom. Roughly estimated, the Sn configuration is changed from $5s^{1.6}5p^{2.4}$ to $5s^2 5p^{0.7}$. The large population of the "amorphous" component in a-Si:F strongly suggests it to be that responsible also for the dominating infrared absorption mode[1]. This has been assigned from chemical arguments to stem from the stretching mode of molecular-like $F-Si(Si_3)$ picturing dangling bond termination. Very little is known about quadrupole constants of fluorine but in a separate DPAD experiment[9] on a frozen SiF_4 target a dominating component of $\nu_Q = 37.5$ MHz has been found. The EFG of fluorine is dominated by the 2p-hole of the extremely electronegative fluorine atom[8], thus it should decrease with increasing bond ionicity. Consequently, the EFG is expected to be larger for SiF_4 than for a $F-Si(Si_3)$ structure. However, the difference in ν_Q between SiF_4 and the "amorphous" component is unexpectedly large[8]. Obviously, the molecular picture could underestimate the solid state influence on the electron flow towards fluorine.

The second, "crystalline" structure ($\nu_Q = 34$ MHz) has a significantly lower fluorine p-electron density. The above interpretation of the "amorphous" component implies a higher degree of covalency of the F-bonding in the "crystalline" component. This would be compatible with a structure similar to the one observed for deuterium in crystalline silicon by channeling. So far, however, the only conclusion from our channeling experiment with fluorine is that the F-position does not resemble that of deuterium. A key to a better understanding of the F-Si defects in general is the structure of the $\nu_Q = 34$ MHz component. The unique ν_Q, the influence of crystal orientation on $G_2(t)$, and the large site population does encourage further study.

The similarity in bulk properties which has been found for amorphous samples produced by ion-implantation and by other methods is reflected in the observation that the "amorphous" site is populated by recoil into crystalline silicon. This is interpreted as a result of correlated damage, i.e., damage created by the collision cascade of the probe nucleus itself. The finding that the site anneals at a lower temperature than that of recrystallisation indicates the increased stabilisation when the defect structures start to overlap.

ACKNOWLEDGEMENTS

We are grateful to Jacques Chevallier for the preparation of the amorphous samples.

This work has been supported by the Danish Natural Science Research Council.

REFERENCES

1. C. J. Fang, L. Ley, H. R. Shanks, K. J. Gruntz, and M. Cardona, Phys. Rev. B 22, 6140 (1980).
2. H. Haas. Physica Scripta 11, 221 (1975).
3. V. I. Goldanskii and R. H. Herber, "Chemical Applications of Mossbauer Spectroscopy" (Academic Press, New York 1968)
4. For instance, D. V. Morgan, "Channeling - Theory, Observation, and Application" (John Wiley & Sons, London 1973).
5. H. Fraunfelder and R. M. Steffen, in "Alpha-, beta- and gamma-ray spectroscopy" (North-Holland, 1965) vol. 2, p. 997.
6. G. Weyer, A. Nylandsted Larsen, B. I. Deutch, J. U. Andersen, and E. Antoncik, Hyp. Int. 1, 93 (1975).
7. S. T. Picraux and F. L. Vook, Phys. Rev. B 18, 2066 (1978).
8. E.A.C. Lucken, "Nuclear Quadrupole Constants" (Academic Press, London, 1969).
9. B. Toft and K. Bonde Nielsen, unpublished.

SMALL ANGLE SCATTERING OF 2 MICRON HYDROGENATED AMORPHOUS SILICON FILMS DEPOSITED AT 130°C AND 250°C

P. D'Antonio and J. H. Konnert
Laboratory for the Structure of Matter
Naval Research Laboratory, Washington, D. C.   20375

ABSTRACT

Small and intermediate angle x-ray diffraction data were collected on ~2μm device material films of a-Si:H grown in a dc proximity glow discharge system at ~130°C and ~250°C. The high temperature films, which are suitable for solar cells, produced no detectable small angle scattering. The error limits of the experiment were evaluated by placing the data on an absolute scale utilizing the a-Si peak in the intermediate angle data. Extensive small angle scattering was observed for the low temperature material which is not suitable for solar cells. A striking feature of this extensive scattering is that it arises primarily from very small regions of less than 10A in size.

INTRODUCTION

Small angle x-ray and neutron scattering studies of plama-deposited a-SiH films have been reported for films of 20μm and thicker.[1] These authors reported that some samples exhibited strong anisotropic scattering indicating rod-like microstructure normal to the film surface with a dominant rod diameter of ~60A. Other samples showed isotropic scattering with a similar dimension or no observable scattering. The objectives of the work reported here were to augment this earlier work in two ways: (1) data were collected on device material that was only ~2μm thick provided by Dr. David Carlson of RCA; (2) intermediate angle scattering data were collected so that the intensities could be placed on an absolute scale thereby allowing a quantitative evaluation of the low angle scattering.

DATA COLLECTION

Small and intermediate angle x-ray data were collected on films grown in a dc proximity glow discharge system at ~130°C (low T) and ~250°C (high T) with a SiH_4 pressure of 0.5 Torr and a flow rate of 50 sccm. Approximately 2μm films of a-SiH were deposited on 12μm Al foil upon which ~200A of Mo had been deposited. Small angle data were collected on four thicknesses of Al+Mo+a-Si:H film in the range $0.02 \leq s \leq 0.6A^{-1}$ with a Kratky small angle

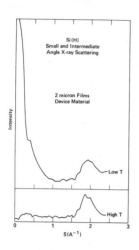

Fig. 1. Small and
intermediate angle
x-ray scattering for
2μm films of a-Si:H.

camera. Intermediate angle data in the range $0.1 \leq s \leq 2.5A^{-1}$ were collected with a diffractometer. The scattering parameter is $s=4\pi\sin\theta/\lambda$, where the angle between the incident and diffracted beam is 2θ, and λ is the wavelength. Background intensity data were collected with Al+Mo foils, and absorption measurements were made in order that the scaled background could be subtracted. The data sets were corrected for the aberrations associated with the different data collection geometries and scaled together. The diffraction patterns are illustrated in Fig. 1. These intensities may be approximately placed on an absolute scale by scaling the peaks at $\sim s=2A^{-1}$ to a value of 240 e.u. for an atomic scattering volume of $21.74A^3$. The values were determined through radial distribution analysis of high angle data obtained from bulk a-Si.

RESULTS AND DISCUSSION

The random errors associated with the inner region of the intensity curve for the high T material, indicate that the maximum possible intensity at $s=0.02^{-1}$ is approximately 1/6 of the peak at $\sim 2A^{-1}$. This maximum possible intensity of ~40 e.u. at $s=0.02A^{-1}$ can be used to estimate an upper limit on the fraction of the sample volume that could be composed of various sized voids. In the exponential approximation[2], the intensity for a polydispersed system of voids with radius of gyration R_O is

$$I(s) = M(R_O)V_a V(R_O)\rho^2 e^{-s^2 R_O^2/3} \tag{1}$$

where $M(R_O)$ is the volume fraction of voids, V_a is the atomic volume ($21.74A^3$) and ρ is the electron density ($14e/21.74A^3$). Setting $I(s)=40$ at $s=0.02A^{-1}$, one may solve for $M(R_O)$ in Eq. (1) for vaious R_O. Table I indicates the results of such a computation. It can be seen that the data are quite insensitive to regions with $R_O>350A$. The material appears to have a very uniform electron density with the hydrogen incorporated into the Si framework. If sufficient samples of a-Si:D could be prepared and high angle neutron diffraction data obtained, a radial distribution analysis should provide information on the atomic environment of the D atoms.

Table I. Maximum possible volume fractions for voids of radius of gyration R_o in a-Si:H films prepared at ~250°C.

R_o (A)	Maximum Void Volume Fraction
2.0	6.17×10^{-2}
2.5	3.16×10^{-2}
5.0	3.96×10^{-3}
10.0	5.00×10^{-4}
20.0	6.50×10^{-5}
40.0	9.54×10^{-6}
100.0	1.87×10^{-6}
200.0	1.27×10^{-5}
300.0	2.98×10^{-3}
350.0	1.43×10^{-1}

The intensity function for the low T material may be analyzed to obtain information on the size and number of voids (or regions of low electron density, x-rays are only weakly scattered by hydrogen atoms). This may be accomplished by integrating Eq.(1) over R_o.

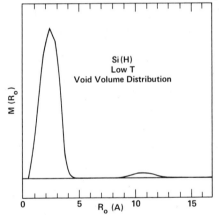

Si(H)
Low T
Void Volume Distribution

$M(R_o)$ has been expressed as an analytic, positive, flexible function defined by variables that may be adjusted in a least-squares fashion to reproduce as nearly as possible the observed intensity. The void volume function for the low T material is illustrated in Fig. 2. $M(R_o)$ indicates ~30% of the sample volume is occupied with voids having R_o=2.5A and 1% with voids of R_o=11A.

Fig. 2. Void volume distribution function for a-Si:H film prepared at ~130°C.

REFERENCES

1. A. J. Leadbetter, A. A. M. Rashid, R. M. Richardson, A. F. Wright and J. C. Knight, Solid State Comm. 33, 973 (1980).
2. A. Guinier and G. Fournet, Small Angle Scattering of X-rays (John Wiley and Sons, Inc., New York, 1955).

PHYSICOCHEMICAL EFFECT OF DOPING IN SPUTTERED a-Si : H

A.Deneuville, J.C.Bruyère
Groupe des Transitions de Phases, CNRS
B.P. 166, 38042 GRENOBLE CEDEX (France)

M.Toulemonde, J.J.Grob, P.Siffert
Groupe Phase, CNRS, Centre de Recherches Nucléaires
67037 STRASBOURG CEDEX (France)

ABSTRACT

The concentrations of As, B, H and Si versus depth of various combination of n^+, p^+, intrinsic sputtered a-Si : H are measured by helium Rutherford backscattering and nuclear reactions analysis. Excess and deficit of hydrogen by comparison with intrinsic a-Si : H H, are respectively found for As and B doping. Depending of the deposition rate this excess or deficit of hydrogen is directly correlated to the concentration of the dopants.

INTRODUCTION

One of the most studied problems of amorphous silicon materials is the role of hydrogen on the structure and on the electronic properties. If for intrinsic a-Si : H the situation begin to be lighted[1,2,3,4], scarce data are available when dopants are introduced. Only quantitative correlation between boron and hydrogen was determined[5,6] and a relative decrease of hydrogen from n layers to p layers was observed[7].

In the present work we shall follow the concentration of arsenic, boron, hydrogen and silicium using Rutherford backscattering (RBS) and nuclear reactions analysis (NRA).

ISSN:0094-243X/81/730120-05$1.50 Copyright 1981 American Institute of Physics

EXPERIMENTAL

The samples used in this study were prepared at 190° C by rf cathodic sputtering of a silicon target with different combinations of three reactive gaz mixtures at a total pressure of 9 x 10^{-3} torr (a) 20 % H_2 + 80 % Ar, (b) 19 % H_2 + 80 % Ar + 1 % AsH$_3$, (c) 19 % H_2 + 80 % Ar + 1 % B_2H_6. The substrate target holder voltages were kept at values corresponding the deposition rate between 58 Å/mn and 150 Å/mn for the three reactive mixtures. Each sample was deposited on a 100 Ω-crystalline Si. Their thicknesses have been measured by interference fringes and Talysurf techniques.

The RBS spectra (fig.1) were carried out using the 4 MV Van de Graaff accelerator in Strasbourg with α particles of energy ranging between 3 to 4 MeV and a particle detector placed at 160° relatively to the beam direction. Taking into account stopping power and cross section, profile and concentration are deduced.

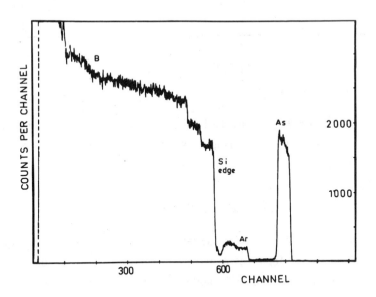

Fig.1 : The sample c-Si/a-Si : B : H (3500 Å)/a-Si : As : H (4000 Å) at a deposition rate of 80 Å/mn.

The hydrogen was extracted using the ^{15}N reaction which gives us a 40 Å depth resolution with a relatively high sensitivity[1,8] (fig.2). The boron concentration and profile were determined using the ^{11}B$(p,\alpha)^8$Be reaction[9] at proton energy of 168 keV. NB and B$_2$O$_3$ have been used as standards.

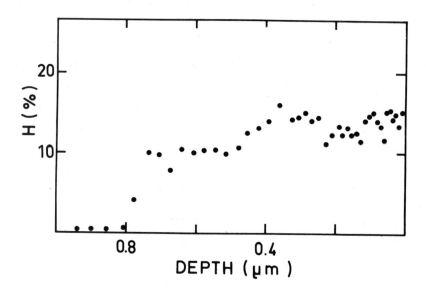

Fig.2 : The same sample as fig.1. Hydrogen profiling versus depth. The pourcentage of Hydrogen is related to the number of silicon.

RESULTS AND DISCUSSIONS

Two regimes have to be considered. The first one corresponding to low and medium deposition rate (fig.1,2,3), the second one to high deposition rate. The frontier of these two regime is 95 Å/mn (ref.4).

The low and medium deposition rate samples are characteristic of very high doping concentrations. For example at 80 Å/mn the N_{AS}/N_{Si} is 16 % and N_B/N_{Si} is 40 % . Even in this alloy regime for boron, from Hydrogen profiling we can see that there is more hydrogen in presence of arsenic than in presence of boron (fig.2). This feature is in agreement with previous results on glow discharge a-Si : H [Ref.7] .

In the case of high deposition rate more information can be extracted. On fig.3 the results corresponding to a thin n layer under intrinsic a-Si : H is reported. It is clear that the excess of Hydrogen in the n layer is quantitatively linked with the number of Arsenic. This can explained that no ESR signals is observed at low concentration of Arsenic[10]. In case of a p-n junction the results are reported on the table 1. Similar results was obtained for a p-n layer prepared at 120 Å/mn. Within the experimental errors the lack or the excess of hydrogen can be another time associated with the dopant concentration.

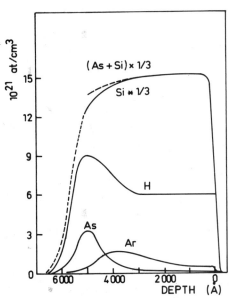

Fig.3 : At a deposition rate of 100 Å/mn the sample C-Si/a-Si:As:H(1000Å)/ a-Si : H.

Table 1 : As, B and H concentration (%) for the sample c-Si/a-Si H : As(1µ)/a-Si : H : B(1µ)deposited at 140 Å/mn.

	p-layer		n-layer
dopants	5		5
Hydrogen	4		13
H + B	9	H-As	8

In conclusion the doping of a sputtered a-Si : H presents similar behaviour for Hydrogen content than a glow discharge a-Si : H (ref.7). Moreover H seems to be linked quantitatively to the number of defective bonds left by the matrix including the dopants. This could explains the difficulties of doping sputtering a-Si : H since a significant part of "doping" atomes does not supply carriers.

References

1) M.H.Brodsky, M.A.Frish, J.F.Zeigler, and W.A.Lanford, Appl. Phys. Lett. 30, 561 (1977)

2) G.J.Clark, C.W.White, D.D.Allred, B.R.Appleton, F.B.Koch and C.W.Magee, Nucl. Instr. Meth. 149, 9 (1978)

3) J.Perrin, I.Solomon, B.Bourdon, J.Fontenille and E.Ligeon Thin Sol.films. 62, 327 (1979)

4) J.C.Bruyère, A.Deneuville, A.Mini, J.Fontenille and R.Danielou, J.Appl. Phys.51, 2199 (1980)

5) B.G.Bagley, D.E.Aspnès, R.E.Benenson, A.C.Adams, F.B.Alexander, and C.J.Mogab, BAPS 24, 399 (1979)

6) R.E.Benenson, L.C.Feldman and B.G.Bagley, Nucl. Instr. Meth. 168, 547 (1980)

7) G.Müller, F.Demond, S.Kalbitzer, H.Damjantschitsch, H.Mannsperger, W.E.Spear, P.G.Le Comber and R.A.Gibson, Phyl. mag.41B, 571, 1980.

8) M.Toulemonde, J.J.Grob, P.Siffert, A.Deneuville, J.C.Bruyère in "Nuclear Physics Methods in materials research" E.P.S. Meeting p.340 (1980)

9) E.Ligeon and A.Bontemps, J.of Rad.Chem. 12, 335 (1972)

10) R.J.Nemanich and J.C.Knights J. of Non.Cryst. Sol. 35 et 36, 243 (1980)

ATOMIC STRUCTURE AND SELF-CONSISTENT ELECTRONIC STRUCTURE
OF PERIODIC MODELS OF AMORPHOUS HYDROGENATED SILICON

C.-Y. Fong
Department of Physics
University of California, Davis, California 95616

Lester Guttman
Solid State Science Division
Argonne National Laboratory, 9700 South Cass Avenue
Argonne, Illinois 60439

ABSTRACT

Computer models of hydrogenated amorphous silicon have been constructed by adding hydrogen atoms to broken bonds in periodic random
network models of pure amorphous silicon. The average neutron scattering computed for 12 examples containing 10-13 at. % H is in good
agreement with recent diffraction data, supporting the assumption
that most of the hydrogen in this material is normally covalently
bonded to silicon. The one-electron wave-functions and associated
energies have been computed by the self-consistent pseudopotential
method for a number of these models. Soft core Si and H pseudopotentials are used. The occupied states associated with hydrogen are
identified from the electron density, and are found to lie in four
well-defined bands within the valence band region of the silicon network.

The material known as "amorphous silicon" has attracted much
attention, at first because it seemed to represent a simple class of
non-crystalline solids, and later because it offered a cheap road to
practical photovoltaic devices. It has turned out that the product
of silane decomposition contains much hydrogen and that its structure
and properties are strongly dependent on the conditions of preparation. The present work treats an idealized model of amorphous hydrogenated silicon in which each atom has its normal covalency, and no
defects are present.

THE MODEL

A systematic method of computer construction of random network
models of covalent glasses has been described previously.[1] Given
any example of such a model, which has no free surfaces and in which
every network node is perfectly four-coordinated, dangling bonds can
be made in pairs, and hydrogen atoms attached to them. From 6 to 8
H atoms were thus added to models containing 54 Si atoms in the re-
peating unit, giving 10-13 at. % H. The sites were chosen to avoid

ISSN:0094-243X/81/730125-05$1.50 Copyright 1981 American Institute of Physics

putting H atoms very close together, and additional modifications of the bond pattern were made to reduce the elastic strain. No Si atom was bonded to more than a single H atom, hence the models contained only "monohydride." Each example was relaxed to the minimum of a Keating-type potential to which was added a repulsive term of the form r_{Si-H}^{-6} for every pair of H and Si atoms not bonded directly. The strength of the repulsive force was that which was needed to prevent non-bonded pairs from approaching closer than 1.5 times the normal bonded distance (1.48 Å). Twelve examples were made in all.

Neutron diffraction measurements have been carried out on sputtered samples of a-Si and its hydride and deuteride.[2] From these data, it is possible to estimate separately the contributions to the coherent scattering from Si-Si pairs and from Si-H or Si-D pairs. A comparison is made in Fig. 1 between the latter, as derived from the difference between the hydride and deuteride, and the average Si-H structure factor computed for the models. Although there are differences, especially at the larger scattering angles, the main features of the patterns agree well. It may thus be claimed that the principles underlying the model have been verified, namely, that the hydrogen atoms are covalently bound to an otherwise random Si network. Further details of the model construction and comparison with experiment have been published elsewhere.[3]

ELECTRONIC STRUCTURE

The electronic structures of several of the examples described above, as well as those of a few with less hydrogen, have been computed by the self-consistent pseudopotential method, which is well-known for its successes in applications to true crystals. Because the present models are of a crystal with a large unit cell, the only difficulties are those connected with the unusually large numbers of atoms contained therein.

The valence electron eigenfunctions are taken to be Bloch functions made up of linear combinations of plane waves. An initial function is computed using an empirical pseudopotential. In the next iteration the charge density of this function is used to compute the Coulomb and exchange contributions which are added to an ionic pseudopotential to give a total potential, and the eigenvalue problem is solved again. The procedure is again iterated, the total potential at each step being taken as a linear combination of the potential used in the preceding step and that computed using the output eigenfunction from that step. When the two potentials are close enough to equal, the procedure is assumed to have converged to self-consistency.

The ionic pseudopotentials of Si^{4+} and H^+ which we used were first obtained by Ho et al.[4] In Fourier space, they are of the form

$$V(q) = a_1 q^{-2} (\cos a_2 q + a_3) \exp (a_4 q^4) \qquad (1)$$

where the coefficients $a_1, \ldots, a_4$ have the values in Table I. The

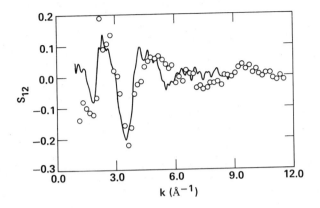

Fig. 1. Experimental intensity, a-(Si,D) minus a-(Si,H), (curve) and simulation (points).

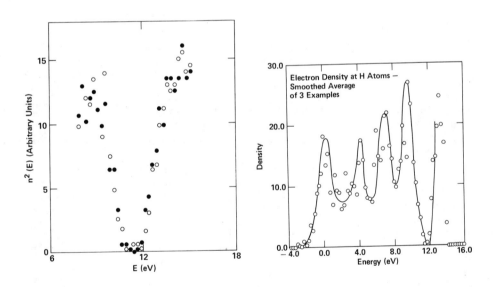

Fig. 2. Squared total density of states near Fermi energy, 2 examples, 10 at. % H.

Fig. 3. Average electron density at H atoms, 20 H

units of the a_i ($i>1$) and of the momentum q are atomic units (a.u.), and a_1 is determined by a normalization condition based on the unit cell volume of crystalline Si. The potential was cut off at $q = 4.0$ a.u. to match its inverse Fourier transform to the known real space pseudopotential. The iterations were started at the Γ point (000) of the zone, and the plane waves were limited at first to those within a sphere of squared-radius $E_1 = 16$ (in units of $q^2a^2/4\pi^2$, a being the unit cell edge). This sphere encloses 257 plane waves; about 300 more were included via the Löwdin perturbation scheme.[5] When the differences between the Fourier coefficients of the input and output potentials were all less than 0.001 a.u., the iterations were stopped. At this point, the eigenvalues of all the occupied states and of the lower unoccupied states had ceased to vary more than a few meV. The final potential was then used, without further iteration, to sample the eigenvalues only (not eigenfunctions) at 14 more points in the zone, namely, at (1/2 1/2 1/2), (1/4 1/4 1/4), and points of the form (1/2 0 0), (1/2 1/2 0), (1/4 0 0), (1/4 1/4 0) and their cyclic permutations. With some success, an accelerated iterative scheme has been used, following a method attributed to D. R. Hamann (Bell Telephone Laboratories) and communicated to us verbally by T. Jarlborg (Northwestern University).

By increasing E_1 to 20, the basis set was enlarged to 390 plane waves. Iterations to self-consistency at Γ then gave eigenvalues differing generally from those using the smaller basis by about 40 meV.

The total density of states of any example resembles that of pure a-Si found by the same method or by the OLCAO method,[6] as expected, since the hydrogen valence electrons amount to only 4% of the total for 13 at. % H. A region of low state density (see Fig. 2) near the Fermi level, as delimited by the intercepts of the sharply rising densities above and below it, is generally wider than we have found in our models of a-Si itself, and we believe this is due to the general reduction of strain when H replaces Si. We conjecture also that this gap would be entirely empty if the models had even smaller geometric distortions.

The states associated with hydrogen can be identified in at least three ways, which we have found in one case to give nearly identical results: (a) By calculating the s projection of the electron density on a sphere surrounding the H sites; (b) By calculating the average density inside such a sphere; (c) By evaluating the density at points along the line joining an H atom and its Si ligand. Using the second recipe for three examples, whose unit cells held 8, 6 and 6 H atoms, the histogram of Fig. 3 was compiled. Because there were only 20 atoms of hydrogen in the sample, and the electron density was computed only at Γ, the fluctuations were large, and it was helpful further to smooth the average by shifting the center of the histogram interval (0.25 eV) up and down by half its value.

The existence in the occupied region of at least four sub-bands of states having large amplitudes near the H atoms is evident in Fig. 3. Whether more structure is present, and what physical factors underlie these sub-bands cannot be answered at this stage.

Similar results have been reported[7,8] on the basis of computations that were much less extensive than our own, and comparisons have been made between them and electron photoemission spectra. Our experience shows that the data in Fig. 2 are barely adequate for location of the hydrogen sub-bands, let alone identification with features in the spectra, which are themselves subject to some uncertainty.

We are in the process of increasing the precision of these computations by using more examples and more points in the zone, and are intending to construct dihydride ($=SiH_2$) models. We intend also to improve the basis set by inclusion of atomic-like functions.

It is a pleasure to thank D. D. Koelling for his advice on computational techniques. This work was made possible by funding from the Department of Energy Photovoltaic Branch through the Solar Energy Research Institute.

Table I. Parameters of the ionic pseudopotential of Si^{4+} and H^+

	Si^{4+}	H^+
a_1	-77.545	23.327
a_2	0.791	0.280
a_3	- 0.352	- 1.538
a_4	- 0.018	- 0.007

REFERENCES

1. L. Guttman, A.I.P. Conf. Proc. 20, 244 (1974); 31, 268 (1976).
2. T. A. Postol, C. M. Falco, R. T. Kampwirth, I. K. Schuller and W. B. Yelon, Phys. Rev. Letters 45, 648 (1980).
3. L. Guttman, Phys. Rev. B 23, (February 15, 1981).
4. K. M. Ho, M. L. Cohen and M. Schlüter, Phys. Rev. B15, 3888 (1977).
5. D. Brust, Phys. Rev. 134A, 1337 (1964).
6. W. Y. Ching, C. C. Lin and L. Guttman, Phys. Rev. B16, 5488 (1977).
7. W. Y. Ching, D. J. Lam and C. C. Lin, Phys. Rev. Letters 42, 805 (1979); Phys. Rev. B21, 2378 (1980).
8. D. C. Allan and J. D. Joannopoulos, Phys. Rev. Letters 44, 43 (1980).

Electronic Densities of States in α-Si:H

D.A. Papaconstantopoulos.
Naval Research Laboratory, Washington, DC 20375

E.N. Economou
Department of Physics, University of Athens, Greece

ABSTRACT

We have used the coherent potential approximation to calculate the electronic densities of states for a model of hydrogenated amorphous silicon. The results are in good agreement with photo-emission, optical, photoconductivity and photoluminescence data.

Recent experimental work in α-Si:H has shown that hydrogen reduces the density of states (DOS) in the band gap by several orders of magnitude,[1] and also widens the optical gap.[2,3] In addition, other experiments have shown that hydrogen modifies both the valence[4] and conduction bands.[5]

For the purpose of understanding these experiments several theoretical models and calculations have been proposed.[6] We present here a brief account of our calculations[7] which we believe provide satisfactory explanations of the above mentioned measurements.

Our model assumes an effective lattice whose sites may have probability c of being vacant, and probability 1-c of having a Si atom. In addition, we have assumed that hydrogen atoms may be located along the lines connecting a vacant site with its nearest neighbors. Thus we have included in our model, at random, Si sites, vacancy sites, and sites that have one, two, three, or four hydrogen atoms. Using this model of disorder, we have used a tight-binding form of the coherent-potential approximation (CPA) to perform detailed calculations of the electronic DOS. Since we have not allowed for reconstruction, we believe that the most stable configuration to be compared with experiment is that in which a vacancy is replaced by a complex of four hydrogen atoms. This configuration is shown in two dimensions in Fig. 1.

The starting point of this calculation is a Slater-Koster (SK) Hamiltonian fit to the pseudopotential band structure of crystalline Si.[8] The basis is orthonormal with four orbitals (one s-like and three p-like) per atom. We have used 20 Si-Si matrix elements (three-center interactions) that include first, second, and

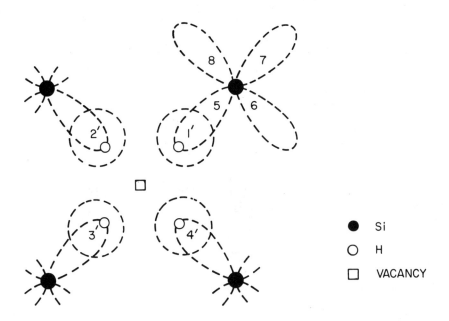

Figure 1.   Two-dimensional view of the atom configuration used in the present calculations.

third nearest neighbors. We have determined the H-H, and H-Si matrix elements from the SiH_4 molecule on an sp^3 basis, and then converted them to our SK basis.

The CPA effective Hamiltonian H_e has off-diagonal matrix elements which for the first nearest neighbors are a virtual crystal average (VCA) of the Si-Si and H-Si values. The off-diagonal second and third nearest neighbor interactions were assumed to have the Si-Si values. The diagonal matrix elements Σ_s and Σ_p form a diagonal 4x4 matrix (since each site is associated with four orbitals):

$$\tilde{\Sigma} = \begin{pmatrix} \Sigma_s & 0 & 0 & 0 \\ 0 & \Sigma_p & 0 & 0 \\ 0 & 0 & \Sigma_p & 0 \\ 0 & 0 & 0 & \Sigma_p \end{pmatrix} \tag{1}$$

and they are determined from the CPA condition:

$$\sum_j P_j \tilde{t}_j = 0 \tag{2}$$

where P_j is the probability for each configuration j, and

$$\tilde{t}_j = \tilde{U}_j [1 - \tilde{G}_e \tilde{U}_j]^{-1} \tag{3}$$

where $\tilde{G}_e$ is a 4x4 site diagonal Green's function corresponding to the effective Hamiltonian $\tilde{H}_e$, and

$$\tilde{U}_j = \tilde{E}_j(000) - \tilde{\Sigma} \tag{4}$$

where $\tilde{E}_j(000)$ is a 4x4, in general non-diagonal, matrix which contains the on-site SK parameters. Having determined Σ_s, Σ_p, and thus $\tilde{G}_e$ from the above equations we can calculate the DOS from the standard expression:

$$\rho(E) = - \frac{1}{\pi} \text{ImTr} \tilde{G}_e \tag{5}$$

Our calculated DOS are shown in Fig. 2 for the case of 5% vacancies which are all saturated by hydrogen resulting in a hydrogen concentration of 20%. From Fig. 2 we note first a bandgap $E_g=1.4eV$ that is wider by 0.4eV than the corresponding $E_g=1.0eV$ which our tight-binding Hamiltonian gives for the non-hydrogenated case.[8] This widening of the gap is due to a narrowing of the third peak of the DOS at the top of the valence band which we have identified to be a result of a decrease of the ppπ interaction due to hydrogenation.[7] This recession of the valence band by 0.4eV is in excellent agreement with the photoemission measurements of von Roedern et al.[4] Figure 2 also shows a site decomposition of the DOS. Concentrating on the H site DOS, we have identified hydrogen induced peaks at approximately 5.2 eV, 7.6 eV, and 13.5 eV below the Fermi level. This is also in good agreement with the photoemission data.[4]

We have further demonstrated the widening of the band gap by performing a joint DOS calculation and presenting our results in the same manner as that followed in the analysis of the measurements of the optical absorption coefficient α.[9] The calculated square root of the joint DOS is assumed to be proportional to the quantity $(\alpha E)^{1/2}$, and has been normalized to the experimental value[3] at E=4eV. A comparison with the measurements of Cody et al[3] is shown in Fig. 3. Although the experimental graph corresponds to a smaller hydrogen content (16%) than the calculated one, the agreement is good with the only discrepancy being that the theory predicts a smaller gap.

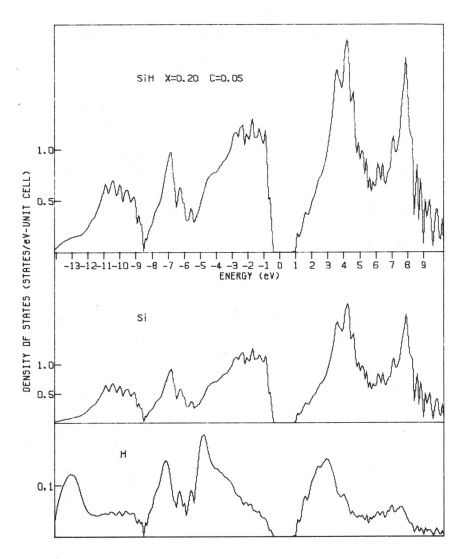

Figure 2. Total and site decomposed densities of states for SiH$_x$ with x=0.20. Note that the Si and H DOS have been multiplied by 1-c and c respectively (c=0.05). The Fermi level is located in the middle of the gap.

Figure 4 shows the variation of the band gap as a function of the hydrogen content. In all cases shown in this graph we are dealing with vacancies fully saturated by hydrogen. We note a monotonic increase of the band gap with increasing hydrogen concentration. This is in qualitative agreement with the experiments of

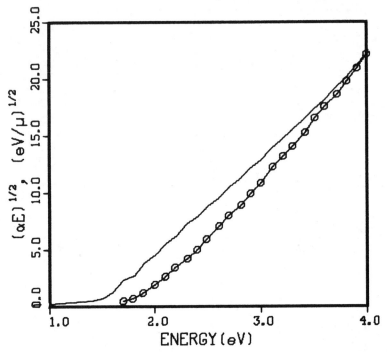

Figure 3. Plot of the square root of the joint density states versus energy. The open circles are the experimental values of the quantity $(\alpha E)^{1/2}$ (Ref. 3).

Moustakas et al[2] who have studied the dependence of the optical gap on hydrogen content for sputtered hydrogenated α-Si.

We should mention here that in addition to the hydrogen-saturated vacancy case we have also considered configurations where one, two, or three hydrogen atoms are present, leaving three, two, or one dangling bonds respectively. The results demonstrate the appearance of dangling bond states in the gap.[7]

Turning now to the conduction band, we have found from the site-decomposed DOS of Fig. 2 that the bottom of the conduction band has strong hydrogen character. This supports the notion that photoluminescence data[5] suggest the formation of Si-H antibonding states at the bottom of the conduction band.

We wish to acknowledge discussions with W.E. Pickett, T.D. Moustakas, L.L. Boyer, B.M. Klein, and G.D. Cody. We are also grateful to T.D. Moustakas for providing his unpublished data shown in Fig. 4. This work was supported in part by the Solar Energy Research Institute via an interagency agreement with the US Department of Energy.

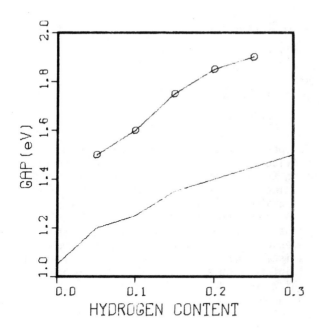

Figure 4.

Plot of band gap versus hydrogen content. The open circles are the measurements of Ref.2.

REFERENCES

1. W.E. Spear and P.G. LeComber, Solid State Commun. 17, 1193 (1975); D.E. Carlson and C.R. Wronski, Appl. Phys. Lett. 28, 671 (1976).

2. T.D. Moustakas, C.R. Wronski, and D.L. Morel, J. Non-Cryst. Solids 35 and 36, 719 (1980); T.D. Moustakas and W. Lanford, to be published.

3. G.D. Cody, C.R. Wronski, B. Abeles, R.B. Stephens, and B. Brooks, Solar Cells publ. by Elsevier Sequois-Lausanne (1981).

4. B. von Roedern, L. Ley, and M. Cardona, Phys. Rev. Lett. 39, 1576 (1977).

5. T.D. Moustakas, D.A. Anderson, and W. Paul, Solid State Commun. 23, 155 (1977).

6. W.Y. Ching, D.J. Lam, and C.C. Lin, Phys. Rev. Lett. 42, 805 (1979); D.C. Allan and J.D. Joannopoulos, Phys. Rev. Lett. 44, 43 (1980); K.J. Johnson, H.J. Kolari, J.P. deNeufville, and D.L. Morel, Phys. Rev. B21, 643 (1980); W.E. Pickett, Phys. Rev. (1981).

7. E.N. Economou and D.A. Papaconstantopoulos, Phys. Rev. B23, 2042 (1981).

8. D.A. Papaconstantopoulos and E.N. Economou, Phys. Rev. B22, 2903 (1980).

9. J. Tauc, R. Grigorovici, and A. Vancu, Phys. Stat. Sol. 15, 627 (1966).

ELECTRONIC STRUCTURE AS A PROBE OF BONDING IN
HYDROGENATED AMORPHOUS SILICON

Douglas C. Allan and J.D. Joannopoulos
13-2049 Department of Physics
Massachusetts Institute of Technology
Cambridge, Massachusetts 02139

ABSTRACT

We have recently developed a new approach to cluster Bethe lattice calculations which provides a practical scheme for incorporating n^{th} neighbor interactions in the tight-binding Hamiltonian used. We have used this scheme to include second-neighbor interactions in a realistic Hamiltonian, to examine the effects of "bulklike" and "surfacelike" surroundings on the electronic structure of a variety of Si-H bonding conformations in a-Si:H. We have found that the monohydride density of states depends markedly on its environment, which suggests that photoemission probes of the density of states may be used to gain structural information about a-Si:H. We propose a photoemission experiment which could distinguish between a microcrystalline form and a continuous random network form of a-Si:H. Implications for the doping mechanism of a-Si:H are discussed.

INTRODUCTION

Since the surprising discovery that hydrogenated amorphous silicon (a-Si:H) can be doped,[1] the body of experimental literature on this material has grown rapidly.[2-4] Owing to the difficulty in performing calculations for amorphous systems, realistic calculations for this system are just beginning.[4] Two related questions to be addressed by theory and experiment are (1) What kind of bonding structure is present in these films and (2) How does hydrogenation permit doping? The possibility of making devices(e.g. solar cells) of lower cost from a-Si:H by controlling its electronic properties spurs us to investigate the role of hydrogen in enabling doping. In this paper we will show the intimate relation between bonding structure and electronic structure for the high-substrate-temperature (low gap state density) modification[5] of a-Si:H. Two aspects of doping will be discussed in light of existing and proposed photoemission experiments. If substitutional impurities can be formed in the bulk of a-Si, then it is Fermi level pinning by a high concentration of gap states which prevents doping. It is well known that hydrogenation reduces the density of gap states, so that with P, As, or B fourfold coordinated in the bulk of the material, the Fermi level can be shifted.[1] It is possible, on the other hand, that the steric freedom of a-Si permits impurities to have arbitrary coordination, as suggested by Mott.[6] Since substitutional impurities do exist in hydrogenated samples, perhaps they are possible as a result of a structural relaxation which forms microcrystalline regions. Together with the reduction in gap states, the formation of microcrystalline regions with hydrogenation would provide a mechanism for doping. We will investigate possible structural relaxation by addressing yet a third question in this work, (3) What is the effect of bulklike and surfacelike environments on electronic excitations? By comparison with theoretical calculations, experimental probes of electronic structure may provide information about the spatial structure of a-Si and a-Si:H needed to answer questions (1) and (2) about structure and doping.

The paper is organized as follows. In section II we discuss the photoemission experiment[5] with which to compare our calculations, with mention of other interpretations of its features. In section III we sketch the theoretical method, which is explained in more detail elsewhere.[7-11] In section IV we discuss our results for a variety of Si-H bonding conformations, and make our conclusion.

II.   EXPERIMENTAL OBSERVATIONS

In Fig. 1(a) we show the ultraviolet photoemission spectra (UPS) for a-Si (dashed line) and a-Si:H. We attribute the featureless appearence of the a-Si spectrum to an averaging over a variety of local bonding topologies, i.e. a random distribution of rings of bonds.[10] Structure in the density of states (DOS) of a system of atoms arises from boundary conditions on the wavefunction in traversing rings of bonds. A system with many different ring sizes will have peaks in the DOS randomly shifted, hence the DOS will appear smooth.[9] The smooth a-Si spectrum indicates that a-Si is apparently not composed of microcrystalline regions. The effects of sixfold rings of bonds as in crystalline Si (c-Si), shown in Fig. 2(a), will be discussed in section IV. Notice that a-Si:H prepared by glow discharge decompostion of silane onto a substrate held at a temperature $\lesssim 350°C$, or by annealing films deposited at lower temperatures, or by a few other methods,[5] has the characteristic electronic structure seen in the solid curve of Fig. 1(a). This form of a-Si:H is apparently dominated by monohydride bonding,[5] and the C and D peaks were originally compared[5] with similar peaks seen in Si(111):H calculations[12] and experiments and in continuous random network (CRN) model calculations.[13] In section IV we will show that this comparison overlooks important topological and SiH-SiH interaction effects.

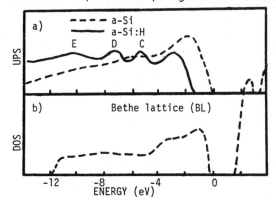

Fig. 1.
a) Ultraviolet photo-
   emission experiment
b) Bethe lattice
   density of states

III.   THEORETICAL METHOD

We use the cluster Bethe lattice method[7] to calculate the local
DOS of various H bonding conformations in a-Si:H. Each atom in the
tetrahedral Bethe lattice (BL) has its nearest neighbors tetrahedrally
oriented, but rings of bonds are analytically removed. We use an
empirical tight-binding Hamiltonian developed and applied successfully
by Pandey[12] to the study of Si(111):H. This uses an sp^3 basis per Si
atom, an s orbital per H, and includes all first neighbor interactions
and the second neighbor Si-Si interactions $pp\sigma 2$ and $pp\pi 2$. In the
BL the Green function can be solved for exactly,[7,11] and the resulting
DOS (Fig. 1(b)) has the same smooth appearence as the a-Si UPS.
When the local DOS is calculated for a cluster of atoms embedded in a
BL, structure in the DOS is an intrinsic property of the cluster and
not of the BL. This allows us to replace certain aspects of the
real local topology and interactions which are artificially removed
in the BL, to see their effects separately.

IV.   RESULTS

Having mentioned the connection between rings of bonds and DOS
peaks, let us consider the signature of a sixfold ring. Fig. 2(a)
compares the results of two calculations using the same Hamiltonian.
The dashed line is the calculation by Pandey[12] for the DOS of c-Si.
The solid line is our cluster BL calculation of the local DOS of an
atom participating in six sixfold rings of bonds, embedded as usual
in a BL. The three major peaks line up perfectly, showing that the
general features of the crystalline spectrum can be understood based
on topology alone. The lowest peak at the valence band minimum in
the BL DOS is a spurious artifact of the unphysical long range order
of the BL and should be ignored.[9] Now consider the local DOS shown
in Fig 2(b) for H on the Si(111) surface (dashed) and H bonded to the
Si atom with six sixfold rings in the cluster embedded in a BL.
These curves are again similar, as expected. Note in particular,
however, that the two lower peaks in the H DOS follow the peaks in
the underlying Si spectrum. Only the peak near -4.8 eV is intrin-
sically characteristic of the Si-H bond, as we domonstrate by considering Fig. 2(c). Here we have the DOS of a single SiH in a BL, all
rings of bonds removed. The single peak present is truly the signature of monohydride bonding, having removed local topological and
SiH-SiH interaction effects. With this in mind, the comparison of
UPS peaks for a-Si:H with DOS calculations for Si(111):H and SiH in
a CRN is ambigous unless the local environment of the SiH can in each
case be compared with that found in a-Si:H. If a-Si:H developes
microcrystalline regions, for example, then the hydrogenation of
internal surfaces would give rise to an environment similar to
Si(111):H and could be consistent with the observed UPS data.
Having considered the effects of sixfold rings of bonds, we now
investigate the effects of various kinds of interactions on the DOS.
We can model the interacting aspects of a surface without the
associated bonding topology by creating locally a "surface cluster"

to embed in a BL. We have considered in Fig. 3 the local DOS on a H atom and its underlying Si (a) surrounded by dangling bonds at second neighbors and (b) surrounded by SiH's at second neighbors, as in a partially and a fully hydrogenated surface but in the bulk of the material (as on the surface of a void). For comparison we show in (c) the DOS of two SiH's at nearest neighbors. This latter is a hydrogenated dimer, as might be found on a Si(100):H surface or possibly in bulk a-Si:H.[10] In every curve the characteristic Si-H peak near -4.8eV is seen. The structure arising from surfacelike environments

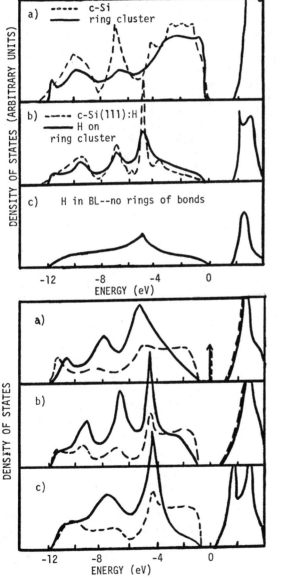

Fig. 2

a) DOS of bulk Si (dashed) and of a cluster containing six sixfold rings (solid).

b) DOS of H on c-Si(111) (dashed) and of H bonded to a sixfold ring cluster.

c) DOS of H bonded to Si in a BL, all rings removed.

Fig. 3

a) SiH surrounded by dangling bonds at second neighbors,

b) SiH surrounded by SiH's at second neighbors, and

c) a pair of nearest-neighbor SiH's. In each case the solid line is the local H DOS while the dashed line is the local DOS of the underlying Si atom.

(a) and (b), which arises solely from interaction effects, is in reasonable agreement with the UPS result shown in Fig. 1(a). The DOS of strongly interacting SiH's (Fig. 3(c)), with the underlying Si considered, is also consistent. What is not consistent is the isolated SiH in a topologically disordered Si environment (Fig. 2(c)).

These results have the following interpretation. It is possible that a-Si undergoes a structural relaxation upon hydrogenation, with the formation of large numbers of sixfold rings of bonds in microcrystalline regions. Hydrogen bonding to these Si atoms will have the signature seen in Fig. 2(b), which looks something like the UPS result. Another possibility is that no recrystallization occurs, but that H atoms bond proximally on the internal surfaces of voids believed to be present in the material[14], and create structure in the DOS by interactions as seen in Fig. 3. These two possibilities might be distinguished by taking an X-ray photoemission spectrum (XPS) on a-Si:H. Since XPS is not sensitive to H, a resulting spectrum with structure would indicate the presence of sixfold rings of Si bonds (i.e. recrystallization), while a smooth spectrum would indicate that H interactions are responsible for the structure seen in a-Si:H UPS. Partial recrystallization would explain the doping mechanism on the one hand, while H bonding to dangling bonds without recrystallization would lend credence to the view that substitutional impurities do form in a-Si (contrary to Mott's hypothesis[6]) and the reduction of gap states is all that is needed to move the Fermi level.

REFERENCES

1. W.E. Spear and P.G. LeComber, Solid State Comm. 17, 1193 (1975), and Philos. Mag. 33, 935 (1976).
2. J. Non-Cryst. Solids 35 and 36 (1980) and references therein.
3. M.H. Brodsky, ed., Amorphous Semiconductors (Springer-Verlag, New York, 1979).
4. Proceedings of this conference.
5. B. von Roedern, L. Ley, M. Cardona, and F.W. Smith, Philos. Mag. B 40, 433 (1979).
6. N.F. Mott and E.A. Davis, Electronic Processes in Non-Crystalline Materials, 2nd Ed. (Clarendon Press, Oxford, 1979), p. 44.
7. J.D. Joannopoulos and F. Yndurain, Phys. Rev. B 10, 5164 (1974).
8. J.D. Joannopoulos, Phys. Rev. B 16, 2764 (1977).
9. J.D. Joannopoulos and M.L. Cohen, Solid State Physics 31, 71 (1976).
10. D. C. Allan and J.D. Joannopoulos, Phys. Rev. Lett. 44, 43 (1980).
11. Generalization for nth neighbors: D. C. Allan and J. D. Joannopoulos, submitted to Phys. Rev. B.
12. K. C. Pandey, Phys. Rev. B 14, 1557 (1976).
13. W. Y. Ching, D. J. Lam, C. C. Lin, Phys. Rev. B 21, 2378 (1980).
14. T. A. Postal, C. M. Falco, R. T. Kampwirth, I. K. Schuller, and W. B. Yelon, Phys. Rev. Lett. 45, 638 (1980).

This work was supported in part by the National Science Foundation, Contract No. DMR-79-80895.

TOWARD A THEORY OF IMPURITIES IN AMORPHOUS SEMICONDUCTORS

John D. Dow and Otto F. Sankey
Loomis Laboratory of Physics and Materials Research Laboratory
University of Illinois at Urbana-Champaign, Urbana, IL. 61801

ABSTRACT

By drawing parallels with the theories of point and paired defects in crystalline materials, one can estimate which impurities are likely to form shallow dopants, deep traps, or suitable modifiers in amorphous semiconductors. It is suggested that Sb might behave differently from P and As in amorphous Si.

INTRODUCTION

The emergence of amorphous Si as a potentially viable material for large area photovoltaic cells astounded many physicists. Until a few years ago, it was widely believed that most amorphous semiconductors "could not be doped." This did not mean that impurities could not be inserted into the amorphous matrix, but rather that the impurities, once inserted, were not "electrically active" and did not form shallow impurity states. The introduction of "modifiers" such as hydrogen or halogens led to major improvements in a-Si as an electronic material; the modifiers "cleaned up the gap" by removing the deep trap states associated with dangling bonds. Clearly, impurities and defects play a major role in determining the viability of amorphous and crystalline semiconductors as optoelectronic materials, either adding electrically active shallow impurity states, producing deep-trap states, or modifying deep states by driving them out of the gap.

The purpose of this paper is to point out that there has been considerable progress recently in the theory of impurities in crystalline semiconductors: It is now possible to predict a priori (i) which impurities in a specific host are likely to produce "electrically active" shallow levels and which yield deep traps [1], and (ii) how a second "modifier" impurity will affect the energy levels of the defect it replaces or modifies [1][2].

PREDICTIONS FOR DEFECTS IN CRYSTALS

To illustrate these points, we display in Fig. 1 the predictions [2] for (spectator,oxygen) pairs in GaP, in comparison with data. The oxygen substitutes for P, and the various "spectators" are impurities on a nearest-neighbor Ga site. The theory is very simple, requiring as input only the electronic structure of the GaP host and a table of atomic energies; the model employs a nearest-neighbor, tight-binding Hamiltonian whose matrix elements are determined empirically [1][3]. The theory successfully

ISSN:0094-243X/81/730141-05$1.50 Copyright 1981 American Institute of Physics

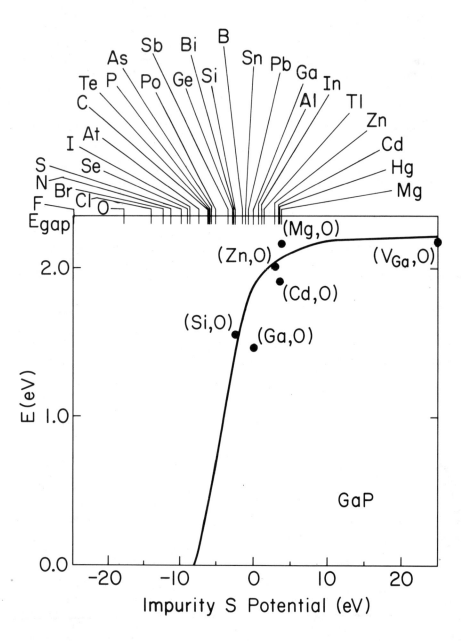

Fig. 1. Trends in the energy levels for nearest-neighbor paired complexes of a spectator impurity on a Ga site and an O defect on a P site in GaP. The dots are data, and the spectator atoms label the abscissa. Isolated O is the (Ga,O) pair.

reproduces the major chemical trends in the (spectator,0) pair data of GaP, and illustrates how the oxygen deep level (i.e., (Ga,0) pair) can be altered by a suitable spectator. In principle, by pairing oxygen with a spectator to the left of I in Fig. 1, the oxygen level can be driven out of the gap into the valence band; however, in practice, most of the spectator impurities capable of doing so are unlikely to occur naturally in significant concentration on Ga sites or else produce their own deep levels in the gap. Note that no spectator can drive the 0 level into the conduction band.

Corresponding predictions for substitutional point defects [1] and for (spectator,vacancy) pairs in crystalline Si are given in Fig. 2. The theory treats only the central-cell potentials of the defects, and neglects the long-ranged 1/r Coulomb potential. Thus shallow impurities, in this model, have zero binding energy and do not produce states within the gap; only the deep impurity levels lie within the gap (and within the figure). If no deep state is predicted to lie within the gap, then the central-cell potential creates a resonance in the band, and the impurity can produce a shallow level by virtue of the Coulomb potential outside the central cell. For example, in bulk Si, only F, 0, P and the impurities to the right of P (including As and Sb) are predicted to be capable [4] of forming shallow dopants (Fig. 2, dashed line). The impurities between Cl and C are predicted to yield deep levels.

A crude simulation of unmodified amorphous Si is achieved by introducing vacancies into the theoretical model for crystalline Si. In this model, the isolated vacancy's p-like dangling-bond levels lie near the middle of the gap. An impurity adjacent to a vacancy forms a pair of a1 (sigma-like) molecular orbitals whose energies are shown in Fig. 2. The right-most solid curve in Fig. 2 corresponds to a state with most of its wavefunction on the impurity's dangling bond, while the left-most curve corresponds to a wavefunction concentrated on the impurity's back-bonds. Impurities to the left of Se and between Po and Ga on the figure are predicted to produce deep levels in the gap. In particular, notice that for P (or As) the P dangling-bond-like level has been removed from the gap into the valence band (extrapolate the curve to the abscissa point of P). However this is not true for Sb. The Sb dangling-bond-like state is a deep level in the gap. Thus it is possible that in a-Si the dopants P and As may have characteristics different from those of Sb, if the dopant's environment is significantly non-tetrahedral.

The role of a modifier in this picture is both to saturate the dangling bonds of the vacancy and to drive the mid-gap dangling-bond level out of the gap. The first function has been widely appreciated for a-Si. However the possibility that the modified level might remain within the gap, but have altered occupancy, deserves more recognition. According to the dashed curve of Fig. 2,

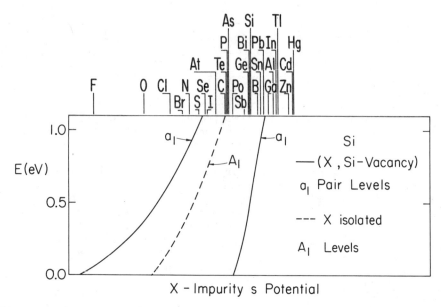

X - Impurity s Potential

Fig. 2. Predicted energies of substitutional deep impurity levels in crystalline Si for impurities X (on abscissa) on a Si site. Dashed line: A1-symmetric (s-like) levels of isolated X impurities; solid lines: a1 (sigma-like) levels of (X,vacancy) pairs. The zero of energy is the valence band maximum. A T2 (p-like) or e (pi-like) dangling-bond (vacancy) level is predicted at 0.5eV, and a branch of the curve for T2 and e levels rises from the valence band to the right of Hg, but is not shown.

F, O, and possibly Cl will drive the level into the valence band. A cluster of four hydrogen atoms, because their s energies approximate that of Si [5], will likely also drive the vacancy out of the gap. However H is not shown on the figures, because the model has limitations for Column I impurities [5].

DISCUSSION

The theory gives a global view of impurity levels in semiconductors, and can be useful for imagining novel doping schemes. However the theory is greatly simplified; it neglects lattice relaxation and the charge state splittings that result from different occupation of the levels by electrons. Moreover, the assumption that the impurities in Si occupy substitutional sites may be invalid. As a result of these numerous approximations, there is an uncertainty of several hundred meV in the model's predictions. The overall shape of the theoretical curve is reliable, but the theory is sufficiently simplified that some displacements and distortion of the predicted curves are necessary to allow for the approximate nature of the model. For example, the T2 isolated defect levels that emerge from the valence band for impurities more electropositive than Hg may be responsible for the In deep trap lying slightly above the valence band [6], even though the model predicts a resonance slightly below the band maximum. A complete discussion of the point defect levels in crystalline Si will be given by Hjalmarson et al. [7].

The theory has not yet been applied to amorphous Si, but we expect its predictions to be altered somewhat from the crystalline predictions on account of the disorder and the topological defects. There are no insurmountable impediments to the theory's application to amorphous semiconductors, provided a model of the amorphous structure is available [8].

Meanwhile, it might be worthwhile to test some of the predictions implicit in the general structure of the theory: For example, P and As should behave similarly as dopants, but Sb may behave differently.

ACKNOWLEDGEMENTS

We acknowledge stimulating conversations with R. E. Allen, H. P. Hjalmarson, W. Y. Hsu, and D. J. Wolford, and the support of this work by the Office of Naval Research (N00014-77-C-0537) and the Department of Energy (DE-ACO2-76-ER01198).

REFERENCES

[1] H. P. Hjalmarson, P. Vogl, D. J. Wolford, and J. D. Dow, Phys. Rev. Letters 44, 810 (1980), and references to earlier literature therein. Many of the ideas of this work are derived from an earlier phenomenolgical theory: W. Y. Hsu, J. D. Dow, D. J. Wolford, and B. G. Streetman, Phys. Rev. B 16, 1597 (1977).
[2] O. F. Sankey, H. P. Hjalmarson, J. D. Dow, D. J. Wolford, and B. G. Streetman, Phys. Rev. Letters 45, '1656 (1980).
[3] P. Vogl et al., to be published.
[4] A specific impurity produces a shallow dopant depending on the impurity-host valence difference and on the number of lower energy impurity states within the host band.
[5] H. P. Hjalmarson, Ph.D. thesis, University of Illinois, 1979.
[6] A. G. Milnes, Deep Impurities in Semiconductors, (Wiley, New York, 1973), p. 12.
[7] H. P. Hjalmarson et al., to be published.
[8] L. Guttman, Phys. Rev. B 23, 1877 (1981).

ELECTRONIC STRUCTURE OF AMORPHOUS SILICON ALLOYS

David Adler and Robert C. Frye*
Massachusetts Institute of Technology, Cambridge, MA 02139

ABSTRACT

A general discussion of the possible defect centers in primarily tetrahedrally bonded amorphous semiconductors is presented. Several different types of defects are likely to be present in such films. Because these defects do not have coordination numbers which differ by an even number (as in chalcogenides), an effective one-electron density-of-states approximation is invalid and can be very misleading. A much more complicated analysis is necessary. Although the two-fold-coordinated silicon defect almost certainly is characterized by a positive effective correlation energy, U_{eff}, tight-binding estimates suggest that the dangling bond may have a negative U_{eff} in amorphous silicon alloys. However, because of a rather large potential barrier between the lower-energy sp^3-coordinated and the higher-energy p^3-coordinated neutral dangling bonding, the former can be metastable at room temperature for very long times. It is suggested that these metastable states rather than optically induced defects, are responsible for the Staebler-Wronski effect in a-Si:H. Other experimental consequences of negatively correlated defects are discussed.

INTRODUCTION

Our understanding of the electronic structure of amorphous semiconductors has increased dramatically in recent years after the realization that well-defined defect centers are present in these materials.[1,2] The nature of these defects depends primarily on the chemistry of the constituent atoms, and tetrahedrally bonded amorphous solids differ considerably from chalcogenide and pnictide glasses.[3] In this paper, we discuss the probable nature of the major defects in a-Si alloys, analyze the sign of the effective correlation energy, consider the effects of these defects on the ground-state properties of the material, and examine the behavior under non-equilibrium conditions such as photoexcitation.

DEFECTS IN AMORPHOUS SILICON-BASED ALLOYS

Since tetrahedral coordination yields the maximum covalent-bond density involving s and p orbitals only, valence alternation is impossible and no low-energy negatively correlated defects exist in a-Si alloys. Nevertheless, strains during deposition can lead to significant densities of high-energy defects and some of these can be characterized by negative values of U_{eff}. The most likely such defect is the dangling bond, T_3^0 in the notation of Kastner et al.[2]

*Now at Bell Laboratories, Murray Hill, NJ 07974.

However, several other relatively low-energy defects are also possible and should not be overlooked. These include two-fold coordinated centers (T_2^0),[3] strained bonds,[4] or three-center bonds with bridging hydrogen atoms.[5] Strained bonds undoubtedly exist in a-Si alloys. However, it is unlikely that a large fraction of these bonds are sufficiently similar throughout the solid to contribute any sharp structure to the density of states. Rather, we would expect a continuum of energies to result, the bonding states merely forming the valence-band tail and the antibonding states the conduction-band tail. There is no evidence from silane chemistry for the existence of any three-center bonds, as is the case with boron-hydrogen molecules. Thus, it is probably that such a bond is unstable towards a conventional two-center bond and a dangling bond. On the other hand, there is a great deal of chemical evidence for two-fold-coordinated silicon, and we would thus expect T_2^0 centers to exist in a-Si alloys.

Tight-binding estimates[3] show that the effective correlation energy, U_{eff}, for two-fold-coordinated silicon centers is always positive. Consequently, these centers behave like conventional defects in semiconductors. The situation for the three-fold center is much less clear at present. Similar estimates[3] suggest that the reaction,

$$2T_3^0 \rightarrow T_3^+ + T_3^- \; ,$$

is exothermic, although more sophisticated calculations[6] have thus far not provided quantitative support for this conclusion. If indeed U_{eff} is negative for this defect center, it is due to the fact that T_3^+ is the lowest-energy configuration of an atom with three electrons in its valence shell and T_3^- is the lowest-energy configuration of an atom with five electrons in its valence shell. Although both charged centers have the same three-fold coordination, the bond angles are very different: T_3^+ most likely exhibits a resonance between sp^2 and sp^3 bonding and thus a bond angle between 109.5^0 and 120^0, while T_3^- would be expected to exhibit predominantly p bonding with a bond angle in the 90^0-100^0 range. Consequently, a T_3^0 center with a p-like configuration acts like an acceptor, whereas one with a hybridized sp-like configuration acts like a donor. The two neutral defects can interconvert by a local rearrangement, but since it is extremely likely that they are both at local minima, a potential barrier must be overcome to achieve this interconversion.

One possible objection to a negative U_{eff} in a-Si alloys in the existence of unpaired spins in the material. However, it is important to note that if the magnitude of U_{eff} is not too large, some T_3^0 centers are present at thermal equilibrium. In fact, there is a great deal of experimental evidence for the existence of large concentrations of spinless defects in a-Si alloys. The observed spin density appears to be several orders of magnitude lower than the density of localized states in the gap.[7] When atomic hydrogen is introduced into pure a-Si films, approximately 100 times as much H enters than the unpaired-spin density suggests.[8] Similarly, when a-Si:H films are heated, about 100 times as much H is given off than unpaired spins are created.[9] These spinless defects could be strained bonds, T_2^0 centers, or $T_3^+ - T_3^-$ pairs. When hydrogen effuses from an Si atom bonded to two H atoms, a T_2^0 center almost certainly results. Because of the dehybridization upon creation of a T_2^0 center, the process of effusing an H_2 molecule from a single Si center may well be exothermic. There is some evidence that this process occurs in the 320-350°C range,[7] where little or no increase in spin density is observed. In the 400-600°C range, hydrogen appears to effuse from sites at which only a single H is bonded, initially creating T_3^0 sites. These dangling bonds can reconstruct or become $T_3^+ - T_3^-$ pairs via charge transfer. Evidently only about 1% remain T_3^0 centers. It would appear to be unlikely that 99% of the dangling bond sites could reconstruct sufficiently in a primarily tetrahedral network to remove the unpaired spins. Thus, these results provide further evidence for the assertion that the dangling bond in a-Si alloys is negatively correlated. If we assume that the unpaired spin density in undoped a-Si films is due predominantly to the T_3^0 center, then we can estimate the magnitude of U_{eff} from the observation[4] that the incorporation of about 3% hydrogen passivates about 0.1% unpaired spins. This yields $U_{eff} \simeq -0.2eV$, a reasonable value.

It has been clear for many years that a-Si alloys are qualitatively different from chalcogenide glasses in most respects.[1,2] The view presented here attributes these differences not to the absence of negatively correlated defects in a-Si alloys, bur rather to the larger creation energy of these defects and the smaller magnitude of U_{eff}. Because of the larger creation energy, large densities are not necessarily present and the Fermi energy can be unpinned (e.g. by incorporation of H or F in the alloys); because of the smaller magnitude of U_{eff}, unpaired spins exist at thermal equilibrium. Another important consequence of the latter is the possibility of variable-range hopping conduction. If there are a sufficient number of T_3^0 defects (as is the case in pure a-Si films), hopping of electrons from T_3^- to T_3^0 centers can occur.

Several cautions should be noted. It is important to recognize that T_3^0 and T_2^0 centers cannot interconvert. When more than one independent strongly correlated center is present in any solid, there is no simple method for retaining an effective one-electron representation.[3] Consequently, it is incorrect to analyze trapping kinetics using fixed energy levels for the defect centers. Instead all quasi-particle excitation energies must be calculated explicitly and each should be used only to analyze the results of experiments which involve those particular excitations. A second caution is appropriate for any system with negatively correlated defects.[10] If, as suggested previously, a potential barrier exists between the two neutral defects, the equilibration kinetics could be extremely slow. In such a case, the effective density of states appears to be a function of time. In particular, the Fermi energy could be unpinned at short times but strongly pinned at long times. We shall return to this point later.

PHOTOCONDUCTIVITY

When negatively correlated defects are present and a potential
barrier exists between the two neutral centers, the equilibration
kinetics are controlled by a time constant exponentially lengthened
by the presence of the barrier.[10] The photoresponse depends sensitively on the relative separations in energy of the neutral donor
and acceptor from the Fermi energy. For an n-type semiconductor, if
the donor level is closer to E_F than the acceptor, electrons are
trapped more strongly than holes. The eventual release of these
trapped electrons yields a long tail in the photoresponse. The resulting increase in carrier concentration causes the quasi-Fermi
energy for electrons to increase, thus reducing the activation energy for conduction. Alternatively, if the acceptor level is closer
to E_F, holes are trapped more strongly than electrons. Their eventual release then suppresses the carrier concentration due to rapid
direct recombination. The quasi-Fermi energy is shifted away from
the conduction band, thus _increasing_ the activation energy for conduction.

Staebler and Wronski[11] observed an increase in activation energy by about 0.3eV following the exposure of a-Si:H films to light,
the recovery kinetics being controlled by a time constant which exponentially increases with an activation energy of about 1.5eV. These
results have a natural explanation in terms of negatively correlated
defects in which the acceptors are closer to E_F than the donors in
undoped samples. The 1.5eV activation energy then represents a large
barrier retarding acceptor-to-donor interconversion and suppressing
equilibration for very long times. With such a large barrier, the
metastable state created after absorption of the light pulse persists
for over 1000 years at room temperature.

The model presented here makes several predictions that can be
tested. For example, there should be an increase in the unpaired-
spin density due to the trapping of photogenerated electrons by the
T_3^+ centers. Such an increase has recently been observed.[7] In addition, the activation energy change induced by the light should be
extremely sensitive to the position of the Fermi energy at equilibrium. For example, as E_F is decreased by p-type doping, two additional effects occur. The donor density at equilibrium increases
relative to the acceptor density and shallow acceptors are introduced near the valence band. Both effects reduce the efficiency of
hole traps relative to that of electron traps, an occurrence which
could lead to an increase in the quasi-Fermi energy after absorption of light and thus a "negative" Staebler-Wronski effect. However, with continued doping, the material eventually becomes p-type,
at which point the increase in quasi-Fermi energy once again leads
to an increase in activation energy. At very high doping levels of
either type, the negatively correlated defects are saturated and the
entire effect must vanish. All of these effects have recently been
reported[7], providing strong evidence for the model presented here.
The model is also consistent with the observation of Staebler and
Wronski[11] that the recombination kinetics transform from bimolecular
to monomolecular after the photoexcitation. We feel that the major recombination centers are the T_2^0 defects discussed previously. If E_F

is   initially located just above these states, they are neutral at equilibrium and bimolecular recombination predominates. However, after illumination, the Fermi energy decreases, thus converting some of these states to T_2^+ centers and the recombination kinetics to monomolecular. This analysis suggests that lightly p-type samples should undergo the reverse type of transformation in recombination kinetics. No such experiment has yet been reported, however.

FIELD EFFECT

When negatively correlated defects are present, transient effects also complicate the analysis of field-effect measurements.[10] Again, the kinetics are controlled by the barrier between the two neutral defects. The effective density-of-states appears to be time dependent, although this is just an artifact of the negative correlation energy and the kinetics. A careful analysis of the time and temperature dependence of the field effect can be used to determine both the energy and the density of the negatively correlated defects.

CONCLUSIONS

We have proposed a model for a-Si alloys in which the dangling bond is characterized by a negative U_{eff} of magnitude about 0.2eV and the two configurations for the neutral dangling bond are separated by a 1.5eV barrier. This barrier explains the apparent photostructural changes observed in a-Si:H. The model is also consistent with many other previously puzzling observations in a-Si alloys.

ACKNOWLEDGMENT

This work was supported by the National Science Foundation-Materials Research under Grant DMR 78-24185.

REFERENCES

1. N. F. Mott, E. A. Davis, and R. A. Street, Philos. Mag. 32, 961 (1975).
2. M. Kastner, D. Adler, and H. Fritzsche, Phys. Rev. Lett. 37, 1504 (1976).
3. D. Adler, Solar Cells 2, 199 (1980).
4. D. Kaplan, Inst. Phys. Conf. Ser. 43, 1129 (1979).
5. R. Fisch and D. Licciardello, Phys. Rev. Lett. 41, 889 (1978).
6. D. C. Allan and J. D. Joannopoulos, Phys. Rev. Lett. 44, 43 (1980).
7. H. Fritzsche, Solar Energy Mat. 3, 447 (1980).
8. N. Sol, D. Kaplan, D. Dieumegard, and D. Dubreuil, J. Non-Crystall. Solids 35-36, 291 (1980).
9. D. Biegelsen, R. A. Street, C. C. Tsai, and J. C. Knights, Phys. Rev. B 20, 4839 (1979).
10. R. C. Frye and D. Adler, to be published.
11. D. L. Staebler and C. R. Wronski, J. Appl. Phys. 51, 32 (1980).

ELECTRONIC STATES OF AN ISOLATED PHOSPHORUS
ATOM IN AN AMORPHOUS SILICON MATRIX*

W. Y. Ching,
Department of Physics, University of Missouri, Kansas City, Mo. 64110

Chun C. Lin,
Department of Physics, University of Wisconsin, Madison, WI. 53706

ABSTRACT

We study the electronic states of an isolated P atom in an amorphous silicon matrix in several possible bonding configurations. Cluster type of electronic structure calculations are performed on local bonding structures of PSi_5, PSi_3 and PSi_4 embedded in a random network of a-Si. The local density of states of P and nearby Si atoms are extracted. For PSi_3, we find a dominating P peak about 4 eV below the valence band edge which is consistent with photoemission experiment. The PSi_5 results show more structures and differ significantly from the photoemission data. The results for PSi_4 are qualitatively similar to those for PSi_3.

INTRODUCTION

The successful doping of hydrogenated amorphous silicon (H-a-Si) with either n-type or p-type of dopants[1] rendered H-a-Si a leading candidate for low-cost photovoltaic solar cell material. In recent years, there has been an ever increasing amount of research work done on this material; however, up to this moment, thin-film H-a-Si photovoltaic solar cells have an efficiency of no more than 6 percent.[2] A serious limitation lies in the fact that H-a-Si still contains a large amount of defects in the gap which act as recombination centers for the charge carriers, resulting in the small diffusion length for the carriers generated by the photocurrent. In order to understand these defects and be able to increase the efficiency, numerous experimental investigation has been performed to study the nature and properties of these defect centers;[3] concurrently, various theoretical models[4,5] have been advanced to explain the origins of these centers. Although, it is apparent that these defect centers can be very complicated because of the various possible sources and atomic configurations, some progress has been made in identifying some of these defect centers.[6] Most of these studies concentrate on the defect models of dangling bonds, Si-H bonds and their interactions, and impurity atoms such as oxygen O, fluorine or other types of defect configurations. Little attention was paid to the bonding configuration of the dopant atoms themselves. Unlike the crystalline case, in which a pentavalent substitution impurity atom such as P gives up an electron as a negative charge carrier, the role of a P atom in a

*Supported in part by DOE Contract DE AC02 79ER10462 and in part by NSF.

non-crystalline a-Si is less apparent. The P atom can have a three-
or five-coordination (PSi$_3$ and PSi$_5$) in addition to a tetrahedrally
bonded PSi$_4$ configuration, since the non-periodic nature of a-Si network offers more flexibility to accommodate various bonding configurations.

In this paper, we report some preliminary results on a theoretical investigation of electronic states of an isolated P atom in an
amorphous Si matrix. Our approach is similar to our previous studies on hydrogenated,[5] flourinated[7] and oxygenated a-Si.[8] We build
clusters of tetrahedral network models of about 200 Si atoms, and
introduce at the center of each cluster, the specific type of bonding for the P atom. We studied the following three cases of isolated P atoms in a-Si with: (1) PSi$_5$, (2) PSi$_3$, and (3) PSi$_4$ type
of bonding configuration.

The electronic states are calculated using the first-principles
orthogonalized LCAO method as applied to cluster type of calculation which have been described in the literature.[9] The atomic-
orbital basis functions are centered at a cluster of about 40 central
atoms (including the P atom). The potential is constructed as a
superposition of atomic potentials of all the atoms in the cluster
network, with a Slater-type local exchange. From the resulting
eigenvalues and eigenvectors, we can extract the local density of
states (LDOS) of the P atom and of those Si atoms that are bonded to
the P atom (designated as Si*). The LDOS of Si* is useful in understanding the nature of P-Si bonds involved in each case. In conjunction with the available experimental information, the calculated
LDOS of the P atom in various bonding configurations in an a-Si
matrix provides a basis toward identifying the important configurations.

RESULTS

(a) PSi$_5$

As a starting point the geometry of the PSi$_5$ unit is taken to
be of the trigonal bipyramid form similar to the PF$_5$ molecule.[10]
To fully allow for pentavalent bonding we include in the basis set
3d orbitals of P in addition to 3s and 3p. In Fig. 1 (a) and 1 (b)
are shown respectively the LDOS of P and of Si* calculated by choos-
ing an equatorial P-Si distance of 2.25 Å and an axial P-Si distance
of 2.55 Å. The shaded area corresponds to the s orbital and the dark
area corresponds to the d orbitals. There are numerous structures
in the valence band (VB) region. The major ones are at -17.6 eV
(s-like) and -8.6 eV (p-like). The zero of energy is set at the VB
edge of bulk a-Si. There is a peak (1.4 eV) in the gap region. The
VB structures are insensitive to whether d orbitals are included in
the calculation. The photoemission spectrum observed by Ley[11] shows
only one peak (-4 eV) attributed to P atoms over the VB region of 0
to -9 eV. Other experimental evidence[3] indicates P inpurity states
near the CB edge which corresponds to 2-2.5 eV in the energy scale

of Fig. 1. It appears therefore that the LDOS of the PSi₅ configuration as shown in Fig. 1 differs significantly from experimental data.

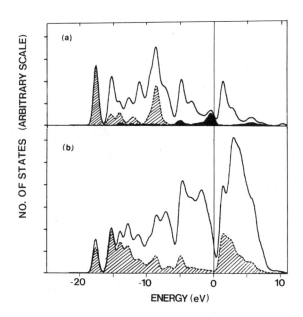

Fig. 1. The LDOS of (a) P atom, (b) Si* atoms in PSi₅ configuration. The zero of the energy is set at the top of VB of the bulk a-Si. The shaded area corresponds to the LDOS of the s orbitals and the dark area, the d orbitals.

(b) PSi₃

For the PSi₃ configuration we adopt a pyramid structure similar to PH₃ molecule[10] in an otherwise pure random network of a-Si. Figs. 2(a) and 2(b) show the calculated LDOS of P and of Si* respectively with a P-Si distance of 2.10 Å. In the VB region the structure is much clearer than the case of PSi₅. The major peaks occur at -17.6 eV (s-type), -14.1 eV (s-type), -13. eV (p-type), and -4. eV (p-type). The major peak at -4 eV is consistent with photoemission data.[11] In addition the peak at 1.9 eV corresponds to gap states close to the CB edge.

(c) PSi₄

The PSi₄ configuration is obtained by substituting a P atom for an Si atom in a random network model of a-Si such as the Polk model.[12] The P-Si distance is therefore about 2.35 Å. The LDOS of P and Si* in this four-coordination configuration are shown in Fig. 3. In the VB region the main structures include an s-like peak at -19.2 eV and a p-like peak at -4.9 eV. The gap-state peak at 2.1 eV is close to the CB edge resembling the shallow impurity levels of P impurity in crystalline Si. Both the LDOS peaks at -4.9 and 2.1 eV are consistent with experimental observations.

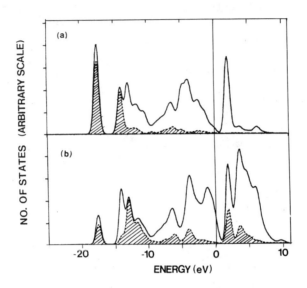

Fig. 2. The LDOS of (a) P atom and (b) Si* atom in PSi₃ configuration. Notation is the same as in Fig. 1.

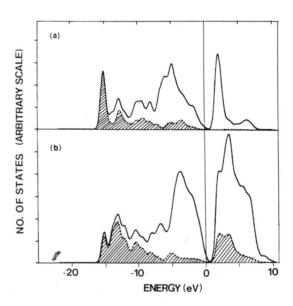

Fig. 3. The LDOS of (a) P atom and (b) Si* atom in PSi₄ configuration. Notation is the same as in Fig. 1.

CONCLUSION

Based on the results presented in the preceeding section, it appears that the PSi$_3$ and PSi$_4$ configurations are consistent with experiments but significant discrepancy is found for the PSi$_5$ configuration. However, before reaching a definitive conclusion, a systematic study of the variation of the calculated LDOS with respect to geometric parameters (P-Si bond lengths and SiPSi angles) must be made, and in this respect, more experimental information on the electron states of P atoms in a-Si will be very helpful. Furthermore, the present calculation does not take into account   the H atoms that are inevitably present near the P centers in H-a-Si of reasonable H concentration. It is difficult to ascertain the role of H atoms in the bonding configuration of P. Should the H atoms simply tie up the singly charged dangling bonds to form Si-H bonds with little effect on P atoms, then our analysis should remain valid. However in case of higher H concentration, various possible H bonding configurations definitely will affect the bonding configuration of the dopant atoms. Therefore, further experimental and theoretical work is needed to understand this highly complicated situation. One could also extend the present calculation to include the p-type dopants of B atoms in a-Si. Only when the electronic states of the dopants themselves in H-a-Si is well understood can we have more confidence in identifying various defect centers in H-a-Si films which so far had hindered the performance of H-a-Si as an efficient solar photovoltaic material.

REFERENCES

1.   W. E. Spear and P. G. LeComber , Solid State Commun. 17, 1193 (1975); Philos. Mag. 33, 935 (1976).
2.   D. E. Carlson and C. R. Wronski, Appl. Phys. Lett. 28, 671 (1976); D. E. Carlson, IEEE Trans. Electron Devices ED-24, 449 (1977).
3.   R. A. Street, to be published and references contained therein.
4.   D. Adler, Phys. Rev. Lett. 41, 1755 (1978); R. Fisch and D. Licciardello, ibid 41, 889 (1978). S. R. Elliot, Philos. Mag. B 38, 325 (1978).
5.   W. Y. Ching, D. J. Lam, and Chun. C. Lin, Phys. Rev. Lett 42, 805 (1979); Phys. Rev. B 21, 2378 (1980).
6.   For example see: Proceedings of the Eighth International Conference on Amorphous and Liquid Semiconductors, Boston, Massachusetts, 1979, edited by W. Paul and M. Kastner (North-Holland, Amsterdam, 1980).
7.   W. Y. Ching, J. Non-crystl. Solids 35 and 36, 61 (1980).
8.   W. Y. Ching, Phys. Rev. B 22, 2816 (1980).
9.   W. Y. Ching, C. C. Lin and D. L. Huber, Phys. Rev. B 14, 620 (1976); W.Y. Ching, C.C. Lin and L. Guttman, ibid, 16,5488 (1977).
10. For example see: A. Rank, L. C. Allen and K. Mislow, J. of Amer. Chem. Society, 94:9, 3035 (1972); A. Strich and A. Veillard, ibid, 95:17, 5574 (1973); A. Schmiedekamp, S. Skaarup, P. Dulay and J. E. Boggs, J. of Chem. Phys. 66, 5769 (1977).
11. L. Ley, private communication.
12. D. E. Polk, J. Non-cryst. Solids 5, 365 (1971).

HOLE CONDUCTIVITY THROUGH NEIGHBORING
Si-H BONDS IN HYDROGENATED SILICON

D.P. DiVincenzo
University of Pennsylvania, Philadelphia, PA 19104

J. Bernholc
Exxon Research and Engineering, Linden, NJ 07036

M.H. Brodsky, N.O. Lipari and S.T. Pantelides
IBM T.J. Watson Research Center, Yorktown Heights, NY 10598

ABSTRACT

The spatially-resolved electronic states of a model representation of Si-H bonds on vacancies in hydrogenated amorphous silicon (a-Si:H) have been calculated using a Green's-function technique. We find no gap states in the host Si bandgap. In the vicinity of the defect, states near the valence-band edge and, to a lesser extent, near the conduction-band edge are removed. We relate our results to a model of the Si-H bond as a barrier to band edge carriers. Parameters are derived that pertain to localization due to randomly located hydrogenated defects.

INTRODUCTION

Several calculations of the electronic structure of Si-H bonds in model environments have recently been carried out.[1-3] Studies are also available using CPA and other effective-medium theories.[4] The role of H in hydrogenated amorphous Si (a-Si:H), however, is still not thoroughly understood. According to a recently proposed quantum well model[5] of a-Si:H, Si-H bonds act as barriers to electron and hole conduction, leading to localization. The purpose of this paper is to present the results of a theoretical study of the electronic structure of Si-H bonds in a model environment, aiming to elucidate the role of these bonds as conduction barriers.

CALCULATION AND RESULTS

Our model defect is an isolated monovacancy in an otherwise infinite and perfect Si crystal (x-Si), where each of the four broken Si-Si bonds is saturated by an H atom. We take the Si-H bond distance to be 1.48 Å, its value in silane and on the hydrogenated silicon surface. No relaxation of the surrounding lattice is permitted. In this configuration, H atoms are separated by 1.42 Å, which is about twice the bond distance in the H_2 molecule.

We have used the self-consistent Green's-function method[6] to solve Schrödinger's equation for this defect. We separate the Hamiltonian H of the total system into $H=H^0+U$, where H^0 is the hamiltonian of the perfect x-Si, and U is the potential change induced by the defect. From the Bloch wave

ISSN:0094-243X/81/730156-05$1.50 Copyright 1981 American Institute of Physics

solutions for H^0,

$$H^0 | nk > = E_{nk} | nk >, \tag{1}$$

the Green's-function operator can be constructed:

$$G^0(E^+) = \lim_{\varepsilon \to 0} \sum_{nk} \frac{|nk> <nk|}{E - E_{nk} + i\varepsilon}. \tag{2}$$

Matrix elements of this operator contain all the necessary information about the perfect crystal. From it we obtain the complex quantity

$$D(E) = \det \left[1 - G^0(E)U \right]. \tag{3}$$

If D (E) is written in polar form:

$$D(E) = |D(E)| e^{i\delta(E)}, \tag{4}$$

then the change in the density of electronic states induced by the defect can be shown to be[6]:

$$\Delta N(E) \equiv N(E) - N^0(E) = \frac{d\delta(E)}{dE}. \tag{5}$$

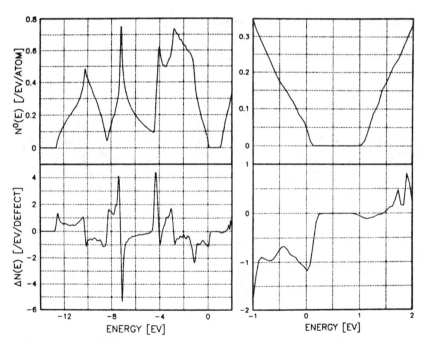

Fig.1 The host density of states $N^0(E)$ for pure x-Si and the change $\Delta N(E)$ due to the hydrogenated vacancy. The left panel shows the entire valence band and the conduction band up to 2 eV; the right panel expands the regions around the band gap.

In order to obtain $\Delta N(E)$ we must be able to evaluate Eqs. (2) and (3). In the present study, the Bloch states $|nk>$ were obtained from a fully-converged plane-wave pseudopotential band-structure calculation for x-Si. To find $D(E)$, the operator $1 - G^0(E)U$ must be evaluated in a complete set of functions. As reviewed in Ref. 6, only those functions for which U has non-zero matrix elements contribute to the determinant $D(E)$. We have chosen this basis set to be gaussian orbitals multiplied by spherical harmonics of $l=0, 1, 2$ and the xyz-like spherical harmonic of $l=3$. These orbitals were placed at the vacant Si site and at all first- and second-neighbor Si's of that site. We have used gaussians multiplied by spherical harmonics of $l=0$ and 1 on each of the four H sites. The defect potential U was taken to consist of a difference in ionic pseudopotentials[7] and a valence-electron contribution which was calculated self-consistently.

The change $\Delta N(E)$ in the density of states of pure x-Si induced by the hydrogenated monovacancy is shown in Fig. 1, along with the host Si density of states $N^0(E)$. $\Delta N(E)$ shows no bound states for the hydrogenated vacancy either in the bandgap or below the bottom of the valence band. Thus, the bound state of the dangling Si bonds is removed by the addition of hydrogens. The most prominent structures in $\Delta N(E)$ are associated with critical points in the density of states of x-Si.

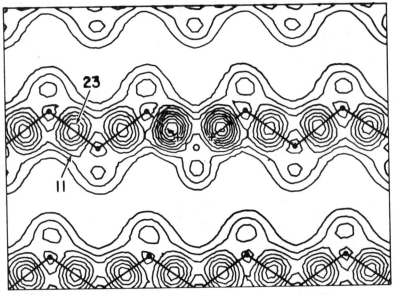

Fig.2   The total valence charge density is a (110) plane passing through the hydrogenated defect. The Si positions are indicated by solid circles, the H positions by crosses. Contours are given in electrons/Si unit cell.

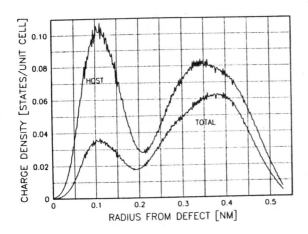

Fig.3 The spherically averaged charge density (TOTAL) for the energy range $-.25$ eV to 0 eV at the top of the valence band in the vicinity of a hydrogenated defect. The corresponding quantity for undisturbed x-Si (HOST) is shown for reference. The origin is at the vacant Si site with H atoms at $r=0.087$ nm, and Si's at $r=0.235$, 0.383, and 0.451 nm. The results are only accurate out to the second neighbor Si's.

The valence-charge density $\rho(r)$ in the vicinity of the hydrogenated defect is shown in Fig. 2. The Si-H bond charge is somewhat more concentrated and directional than the adjoining Si-Si bonds, which are essentially unchanged from pure x-Si. We can understand this gross similarity between the Si-H bond and the Si-Si bond by viewing the hydrogenated defect not as a Si vacancy with added hydrogen, but as x-Si with one Si nucleus split into four pieces to make the H nuclei (recall that a Si pseudoatom is equivalent to four protons). These pieces are then moved part of the way towards each of the nearest neighbors and are accompanied by only a slight shift of the electron cloud. However, an energy-resolved analysis of $\rho(r)$ reveals differences between the Si-H and the Si-Si bonds which are important in the vicinity of the band edges. As is shown in the FIg. 1, a large portion of the states near the valence-band edge is removed to lower energies. We quantify this effect in Fig. 3, which shows $\rho(r)$ for states within .25 eV of the band edge, spherically averaged about the vacant site. The corresponding quantity for the host perfect crystal $\rho^0(r)$ is shown for comparison. The Si-H bond charge in this energy region is reduced by 65% from the original Si-Si bond. This reduction is a consequence of the stronger Si-H bond, which causes a downward shift of the energy levels. Regions adjoining the defect are also affected: the nearest and next nearest Si-Si bonds have lost about 30% and 20% of their charge, respectively. There is a similar decrease in N(E) at the bottom of the conduction band (Fig. 1), but on a much smaller scale. The $\rho(r)$ plots for studies at the bottom of the conduction band are more complicated, with excess ρ on the Si-H bond and depleted ρ surrounding the defect. Also the energy range of the net depletion of N(E) is smaller for the conduction band than for the valence band.

DISCUSSION AND CONCLUSIONS

In order to assess the role of Si-H bonds, one would ideally like to know the properties of such bonds in various environments: isolated Si-H bonds, Si-H in multivacancies, Si-H on internal surfaces of larger voids, etc. Vacancies, including the model defect we have chosen, have some unique properties, such as the reestablishment of connectivity of the lattice. There are also general features of the results which are common to all Si-H bonds in a-Si:H. We now examine general implications of the results on the quantum well model[5] for a-Si:H. One of the main assumptions of that model is that Si-H bonds deplete the density of states at the top of the valence bands, causing localization of the Si eigenfunctions within 0.6 eV of the valence band edge. The model interprets the observed energies characteristic of transport and optical processes in terms of transitions between and activation from the localized levels. Using the results of our calculation, we can estimate the range of the disturbance to $\rho^0(r)$ emanating from the hydrogenated vacancy. We have approximately fitted the envelope of the charge disturbance in the top 0.25 ev of the valence-band as

$$\rho(r) = \rho^0(r)\left[1-e^{-r/a}\right] \tag{6}$$

with $a \approx 2.7$ Å. Classical percolation theory can be used to relate our results to the quantum well model; if more than 85% of the volume of the solid is disturbed by the defect, then percolation is cut off[8] and localized electronic states occur. If we assume that the hydrogenated defects are uniformly distributed throughout a-Si:H, then for reasonable defect concentrations of 5 to 15% the disturbance caused by the defect needs to have a range of 4.0 to 3.3 Å, respectively, for localization to occur according to the volume criterion. Of course, this estimate would be modified by quantum effects (cf. Anderson-Mott theory of localization) and by specific assumptions about the microstructure of a-Si:H. Still, this estimate is of the same order of magnitude as the 2.7 Å range which our calculation shows for the top 0.25 eV of the valence band. Although this cannot provide conclusive support for quantum wells, it shows that the disturbance caused by the Si-H bond is important for band edge electronic properties and transport in a-Si:H.

We thank S. Kirkpatrick and A.R. Williams for many useful discussions. This work is supported in part by the NSF on grant number DMR 76-80994, by the Solar Energy Research Institute under Subcontract No. ZZ-0-9319, and by ONR under contract N00014-80-C-0679.

REFERENCES

1. D.C. Allan and J.D. Joannopoulos, *Phys. Rev. Lett.* 44, 43 (1980).
2. W.Y. Ching, D.J. Lam, and C.C. Lin, *Phys. Rev. B* 21, 2378 (1980); K.H. Johnson, H.J. Kolari, J.P. de Neufville and D.L. Morel, *Phys. Rev. B* 21, 643 (1980).
3. W.E. Pickett (submitted to Phys. Rev. B)
4. E.N. Economou and D.A. Papaconstantopoulos, *Phys. Rev. B* 23, 2042 (1981).
5. M.H. Brodsky, *Solid State Communications*, 36, 55 (1980).
6. J. Bernholc, N.O. Lipari, and S.T. Pantelides, *Phys. Rev.* B 21, 3545 (1980).
7. Although the H atom has no core electrons we have obtained an ionic pseudopotential which accurately reproduces the atomic 1s eigenfunction and its energy. This amounts to smearing out the singularity of the potential at the origin.
8. R. Zallen and H. Scher, *Phys. Rev. B*, 4, 4471 (1971)

BONDING GEOMETRIES OF FLUORINE IN a-Si:F
A PHOTOEMISSION STUDY

L. Ley, K.J. Gruntz, R.L. Johnson
Max-Planck-Institut für Festkörperforschung
7000 Stuttgart, Federal Republic of Germany

ABSTRACT

The fluorine induced chemical shifts of the Si 2p lines in a-Si:F have been measured by photoemission. The shift per attached F atom is 1.15 eV. From an analysis of the spectra the distribution of F atoms among the different $Si-F_n$ (n=1...4) configurations have been determined as a function of the total F content. This distribution is in qualitative agreement with a distribution expected for a purely statistical incorporation of F in a-Si except for a marked surface enrichment of $Si-F_3$ units. Based on the information from the core level spectra the F 2p induced electronic structure has been obtained from the valence band spectra for each $Si-F_n$ configuration.

INTRODUCTION

Information about the way hydrogen or fluorine is bonded in a-Si has been obtained mainly from the analysis of the vibrational spectrum of the $Si-X_n$ (X=H,F) units as observed in infrared absorption spectra.[1-4] This analysis does not always lead to unambiguous identifications of certain absorption bands with a particular mode. Examples are the controversy over the 2100 cm^{-1} band in a-Si:H[5,6] and the 1010 cm^{-1} line in fluorinated a-Si (a-Si:F).[3,4]

Additional information about the bonding geometries of hydrogen in a-Si could be obtained from the analysis of the valence density of states (DOS) as measured in photoemission experiments.[7] Similar investigations on a-Si:F are expected to yield considerably more information since the highly electronegative F atom will induce measurable chemical shifts in the Si core levels that can be correlated with the number of F atoms attached to a given Si atom.

EXPERIMENTAL

The a-Si:F films were prepared by sputtering c-Si in an Argon-SiF_4 mixture onto Mo-substrates held at room temperature. Details of the preparation conditions are given in Ref.8. The sputtering chamber was attached to the photoemission spectrometer so that the specimens could be examined without exposure to air. We employed monochromatized Al K_α x-rays (hν = 1486.6 eV) for the excitation of the core level spectra (resolution 0.6 eV) and HeI (hν = 21.2 eV) and HeII (hν = 40.8 eV) radiation for the valence band spectra (resolution 0.3 eV). The spectra reported below were obtained on films containing only Si and F and no contamination.

ISSN:0094-243X/81/730161-05$1.50 Copyright 1981 American Institute of Physics

RESULTS AND DISCUSSION

Fig.1 shows the core level spectra of two films containing 14 at % and 37 at % fluorine, respectively.

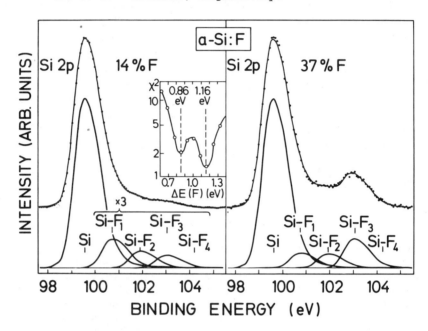

Fig.1. Si 2p core level spectra of two a-Si:F specimens (dots). The solid line is the result of a fit described in the text.

The main line at 99.6(1) eV binding energy corresponds to Si atoms bonded only to Si atoms. The intensity of the structure towards higher binding energies scales with the F concentration c_F and must therefore be due to chemically shifted Si 2p components. We were able to fit the spectra in Fig.1 to a sum of five lines corresponding to the five possible $Si_{4-n}-Si-F_n$ (n=0...4) units with the following restraints: (i) All lines have the same shape; (ii) the lines are equidistant. The last constraint requires that the charge transfer induced by the attachment of a F atom to a Si atom is independent of the number of F atoms already bound to it. This assumption has been tested for a series of chloromethylsilanes and was found to be true.[9] The fit obtained with a chemical shift ΔE_F of 1.16 eV per attached fluorine is also shown in Fig.1 as is the mean square deviation $X2$ between fit and data points as a function of ΔE_F. The average value of ΔE_F=1.15(2) obtained from 45 fits is compatible with the chemical shift between SiH_4 and SiF_4 assuming that the chemical shift induced by hydrogen is negligible.

The F 1s line has a binding energy of 686.2(2) eV. It is unaffected in shape or position by the fluorine concentration. We take that as evidence the F is bonded only in chemically equivalent positions in a-Si:F.

The results of the fitting procedure puts us in the position to calculate the F concentration due to each particular configuration $Si-F_n$ by multiplying the relative strength of the $Si-F_n$ component in the Si 2p spectrum with n, the number of F atoms in that configuration. In this way we obtain the data points of Fig.2a. The sum of all contributions in a given sample is, of course, the total F content denoted by c_F (Si 2p) in Fig.2.

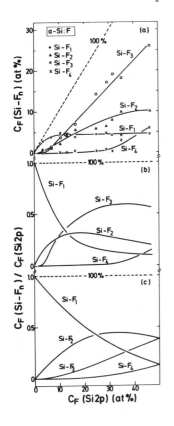

The implications of the results of Fig.2a become clearer when we consider the relative contribution of F atoms in each $Si-F_n$ configuration to the total F content as a function of c_F as shown in Fig.2b. These relative contributions must be compared with those of Fig.2c which have been calculated assuming a statistical distribution of F atoms in an ideal fourfold coordinated Si network. The statistical model predicts that the $Si-F_1$ units are dominant at low F concentrations and that the $Si-F_2$, $Si-F_3$ dominate at successively higher fluorine content at the expense of the lower coordinated $Si-F_n$ units.

The experimental fluorine distribution follows the statistical one only qualitatively. A notable quantitative deviation is the overemphasis of the $Si-F_3$ configuration which reach their maximum at much lower fluorine concentrations than expected statistically. The $Si-F_3$ units taken their weight initially from the $Si-F_1$ units which drop off faster than calculated and grow then at the expense of the $Si-F_2$ units. We could trace this deviation to a surface enrichment in fluorine. Depth profiling of c_F by the gradual removal of layers from the films through sputtering reveals a marked drop in the F content within a few Å from the surface. The spectral distribution of the Si 2p lines confirmed that the surface fluorine is bonded predominantly in $Si-F_3$ configurations. The extra fluorine concentration corresponds very nearly to three F atoms per Si surface atom.

Fig.2. The absolute (a) and relative (b) F concentrations in each $Si-F_n$ configuration as a function of the total F content c_F.
(c) The relative F contributions in $Si-F_n$ versus c_F based on a statistical distribution of F atoms in a-Si:F.

Fig. 3 shows He I and He II valence band spectra of three films with increasing amounts of fluorine. New, F induced features show up between 6 and 12 eV below the Fermi level E_F. They are predominantly F 2p derived. The F 2s states are at 31.3 eV

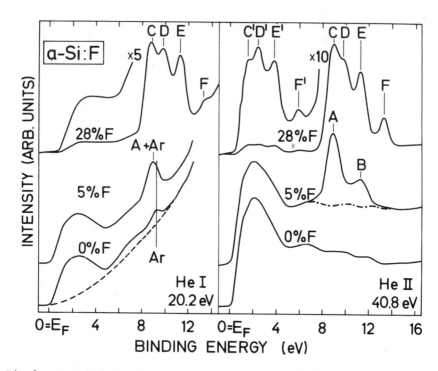

Fig.3. He I and He II valence band spectra of fluorinated and un-
fluorinated a-Si films. The features C', D', E' are due to He II
excitation.

below E_F. We have used numerous valence band spectra in conjunction
with the information from Si 2p core level spectra to obtain partial
F 2p DOS for each Si-F$_n$ (n=1...3) configuration. These partial densities compare very well with those calculated by Ching[10] for clusters of a-Si containing the various Si-F$_n$ units if we allow for a
rigid shift of 3 eV towards E_F of the latter (see Fig. 4). The number of peaks, their intensities and positions are well reproduced
except for the leading peak in the Si-F$_3$ spectrum. Here the calculation apparently underestimates the dispersion and gives only one peak
where we obtain two.

In closing, we mention that the addition of F to a-Si affects
the top of the valence bands in much the same way as does hydrogen.
The top of the valence bands recedes by as much as 0.7 eV when c_F
reaches ∿48 %. It should be remembered, however, that a large fraction of the fluorine is bonded near or more likely at the surface
in the form of Si-F$_3$. It is therefore unlikely that valence band
recession in the bulk reaches values as high as 0.7 eV.

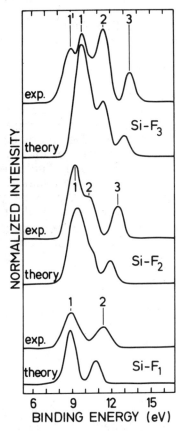

Fig.4. Experimental and theoretical F 2p partial densities of states for different Si-F$_n$ configurations.

REFERENCES

1. M.H. Brodsky, M. Cardona, and J.J. Cuomo, Phys. Rev. B16, 3556 (1977).
2. G. Lucovsky, R.J. Nemanich, J.C. Knights, Phys. Rev. B19, 2064 (1979).
3. C.J. Fang, L. Ley, H.R. Shanks, K.J. Gruntz, and M. Cardona, Phys. Rev. B22, 6140 (1980).
4. T. Shimada, Y. Katayama, J. Phys. Soc. Japan 49, Suppl. A, 1245 (1980).
5. S. Oguz, R.W. Collins, M.A. Paesler, W. Paul, J. Non-Cryst. Sol. 35+36, 231 (1980).
6. H. Shanks, C.J. Fang, L. Ley, M. Cardona, F.J. Demond, and S. Kalbitzer, Phys. Stat. Solidi (b) 100, 43 (1980).
7. B. von Roedern, L. Ley, M. Cardona, and F.W. Smith, Phil. Mag. B40, 433 (1979).
8. K.J. Gruntz, L. Ley, R.L. Johnson (to be published).
9. A.A. Bakke, H. Chen, W.L. Jolly, J. Electr. Spectr. 20, 333 (1980).
10. W.Y. Ching in: Amorphous and Liquid Semiconductors, W. Paul, M. Kastner editors (North-Holland, New York 1980), p. 61.

AUTOCOMPENSATION IN DOPED AMORPHOUS SILICON

D. K. Biegelsen, R. A. Street and J. C. Knights
Xerox Palo Alto Research Center, Palo Alto, CA 94304

ABSTRACT

Studies based predominantly on luminescence and electron spin resonance provide strong evidence for defect formation concomitant with doping of glow discharge produced a-Si:H. In samples doped with boron or phosphorus, the increase of non-radiative recombination observed in luminescence correlates with the increase of the dangling bond signal seen in light-induced ESR. This directly indicates an increase in the number of dangling-bond-like centers with doping. Compensation allows the Fermi level and dopant levels to be varied independently. In compensated samples with E_F near midgap, the number of dangling bond centers is reduced. An autocompensation mechanism is proposed to explain this Fermi level-dependent defect formation.

INTRODUCTION

For doped a-Si:H to be useful for electronic device applications the gap state density must be minimized. In this paper we present results which indicate that dangling-bond-type defects, which act as non-radiative recombination centers, are introduced in the process of dopant incorporation. An intrinsic process similar to autocompensation in crystalline semiconductors is shown to be consistent with the experimental results.

There is still uncertainty regarding the microscopic configurations giving rise to doping in a-Si:H. EXAFS measurements[1] of arsenic doped a-Si:H indicate that ~80% of dopant atoms are chemically accommodated in 3-fold coordinated sites, with corresponding bonding and anti-bonding energies lying respectively below and above the valence and conduction band edges. It is widely thought, though, that as in crystalline Si, the electrically active dopant is constrained during growth to bond in a 4-fold coordination. As in crystalline silicon, tetrahedral dopant incorporation is consistent with the "8 – N" rule in that, when E_F is below the dopant energy level, the dopant atom effectively has 4 valence electrons.

With the wide range of local constraints, allowing 3- and 4-fold bonding, it is not surprising that some 4-fold configured dopant sites could have associated distortion energies, such that bonding changes would be stabilized by change in electronic occupancy. Figure 1 is a schematic representation of the ground states of these hypothesized configurations as a function of E_F. E_n and E_p are demarcation levels separating the bonded, doping configuraton of a given site from the relaxed doubly three-fold coordinated configuration of opposite charge state. In this picture, then, when E_F is closer to the band edge than the demarcation level, it becomes energetically favorable to form an impurity-defect pair. It remains to be shown if these configurations are "frozen in" during deposition or can be altered dynamically (i.e., by shifting E_F). Because of the strong localization of the dangling bond electrons and the likelihood that the energy levels of the three-fold coordinated impurity are well outside the gap, the magnetic and optical properties of the autocompensated center can be expected to be very similar to those of isolated dangling bond defects in undoped material.

Fig. 1

Ground state configurations of auto-compensating dopants as a function of Fermi energy position. Double lines indicate a non-bonding lone pair; "clouds" indicate doubly occupied and empty dangling bond orbitals.

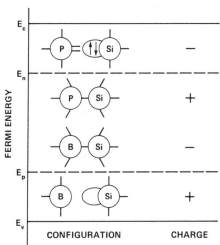

EXPERIMENT

In this section we present some of the experimental results which lead us to infer a Fermi energy-related mechanism of defect formation. (Much more data will be published elsewhere.[2]) It is well known that the intensity of luminescence in a-Si:H is quenched by doping.[3] The lower half of Fig. 2 shows the decrease of luminescence intensity and energy with doping. Also shown is the doping-dependent band at ~0.9eV which is also observed in undoped material having a high dangling bond defect density.[4] In these samples no electron spin resonance (ESR) is observed in the dark except at doping levels $\geq 10^{-3}$ [dopant]/[SiH$_4$]. The ESR and light-induced ESR (LESR) spectra have been shown to be decomposable into spectra of neutral dangling bonds, self-trapped band tail holes and band tail electrons.[5] In the upper half of Fig. 2 we plot only the dangling bond LESR as a function of doping. Because the strength of LESR depends on excitation intensity and lifetimes of the excited states, the measured spin densities are less than the total densities of such states. Nevertheless, Fig. 2 demonstrates that as doping increases, the defect densities increase strongly over that of the undoped material. This is complimentary to the luminescence results in showing that new (non-radiative recombination) dangling-bond-like centers are introduced by doping. It still remains to be shown if the defects are directly related to the position of E_F or explicitly tied to dopant incorporation.

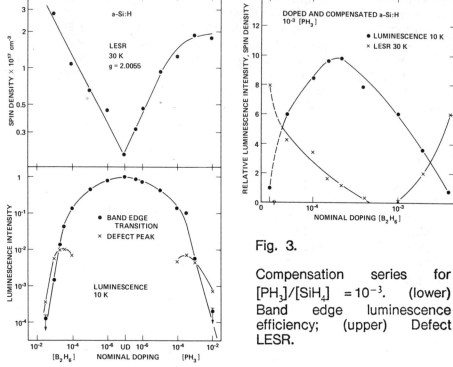

Fig. 3.

Compensation series for $[PH_3]/[SiH_4] = 10^{-3}$. (lower) Band edge luminescence efficiency; (upper) Defect LESR.

Fig. 2. (lower) Band edge and defect luminescence efficiencies versus dopant concentration;

(upper) Defect light-induced ESR versus doping.

Measurements of electrical conductivity and sample composition (by SIMS) show that compensation is effective in varying E_F independently of dopant concentration.[2] Compensation can thus be used to separate these two factors. The lower half of Fig. 3 shows the luminescence efficiency of band edge recombination for a representative double-doping sequence ($[PH_3]/[SiH_4]$ fixed at 10^{-3}). Although at these high doping levels the luminescence efficiency is much reduced from that in undoped material, the intensity does peak near nominal compensation and at a value ~10 times greater than the case of single-doping. This indicates that the density of non-radiative centers is reduced as E_F approaches midgap even though the total dopant level is high. In Fig. 3 we also plot the variation in defect-related LESR with compensatory doping for the same samples. From the disappearance of the dangling bond resonance in LESR (and its continued absence in ESR) at the nominal compensation composition (for which E_F is near midgap) we conclude that the dangling bond density is a function of position of E_F.

In undoped a-Si:H the dangling bond centers are neutral and paramagnetic so that the measured equilibrium spin density is a good measure of the electrically active defect density. In doped samples, the dangling bond centers are diamagnetic.[5] However, it is plausible to assume the same relationship between peak luminescence intensity and defect (non-radiative recombination center) density as in undoped samples.[6] In Fig. 4 we show the density of dangling bond sites estimated in this way as a function of single doping. Also plotted are the LESR spin densities. As mentioned above, the strength of LESR signals are underestimates of the total defect densities. The divergence at high doping reflects the effect on LESR of the recombination lifetimes, which are known to be reduced at high defect densities. These data show that doping (i.e., shift of E_F away from midgap) introduces a defect density ~1 – 10% of the doping concentration. It should also be noted that, at high doping levels, the defect density does not increase in direct proportion to the dopant concentration.

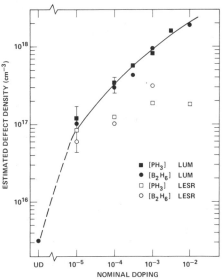

Fig. 4.

Estimates of dangling bond defect densities based on luminescence quenching; also plotted are defect LESR.

DISCUSSION

Experimentally we have found two qualitative regimes. For E_F within ~0.4eV of midgap, E_F is shifted readily by doping; whereas, on a relative scale, many dangling-bond-like defects are introduced. For E_F near or within the band tails, increase in dopant concentration has relatively little effect on E_F.[7] If the ineffectiveness of doping were due only to the sharply increasing band tail density of states, then the increase in defect concentration should be proportional to the increase in dopant concentration. To the contrary, though, the strongly sublinear relation (Fig. 4) indicates that another mechanism is operative. EXAFS measurements of arsenic-doped a-Si:H indicate that as the dopant concentration increases from the lowest value measured (~1%), the fraction of 3-fold coordinated dopant atoms incorporated into the silicon network is increased.[1] We therefore propose that the mechanism setting in at high concentrations is the topologically-allowed pairing of the 3-coordinated silicon atoms of two impurity-defect pairs. This results in two fewer defects, and two more 3-coordinated dopant atoms (which are electrically inactive). Said another way, at high dopant levels, the 4-fold constraints during deposition imposed by the silicon matrix are relaxed and 3-fold incorporation is much more likely. For the model presented here there should be a third regime corresponding to E_F lying between midgap and the demarcation levels. Here, doping should be efficient and a low ratio of defects to 4-fold dopants should exist. Experiments at very low doping are being carried out to access this regime.

CONCLUSIONS

We find that doping a-Si:H either n- or p-type introduces dangling-bond type defects. The results of compensation experiments indicate that a Fermi energy-dependent mechanism like autocompensation is operative.

ACKNOWLEDGEMENTS

We wish to thank R. Lujan for preparing and characterizing the many samples used in these studies. The work was supported in part by grant #XJ-0-9079-1 from the Solar Energy Research Institute.

REFERENCES

1. J. C. Knights, T. M. Hayes, and J. C. Mikkelsen, Jr., Phys. Rev. Letters 39, 712 (1977).

2. R. A. Street, D. K. Biegelsen, and J. C. Knights, Phys. Rev. B (to be published).

3. C. Tsang and R. A. Street, Phil. Mag. B37, 601 (1978); I. G. Austin, T. S. Nashashibi, T. M. Searle, P. G. LeComber, and W. E. Spear, J. Non-Cryst. Solids 32, 373 (1979); R. Fischer, W. Rehm, J. Stuke, and J. Voget-Grote, J. Non-Cryst. Solids 35 and 36, 687 (1980).

4. R. A. Street, Phys. Rev. B21, 5775 (1980).

5. R. A. Street and D. K. Biegelsen, Solid State Commun. 33, 1159 (1980).

6. R. A. Street, J. C. Knights, and D. K. Biegelsen, Phys. Rev. B18, 1880 (1978).

7. A. Madan, P. G. LeComber, and W. E. Spear, J. Non-Cryst. Solids 20, 239 (1976).

ESR AND IR STUDIES ON SPUTTERED AMORPHOUS Si-C-H, Si-Ge-H AND Ge-C-H

Tatsuo Shimizu, Minoru Kumeda and Yoshinari Kiriyama
Department of Electronics, Kanazawa University, Kanazawa 920, Japan

ABSTRACT

The change with annealing of the nature of dangling bonds and its relation to hydrogen content have been investigated in hydrogenated binary alloy systems of Si, Ge and C by means of ESR and IR absorption. In a-Si-Ge:H, the density of Ge dangling bonds is found to be larger than that of Si dangling bonds because of preferential attachment of hydrogen to Si. The increase in Ge dangling bonds by annealing is larger than that in Si dangling bonds. In a-Si-C:H and a-Ge-C:H, the density of dangling bonds increases by the detachment of hydrogen at higher temperature than in the case of pure Si and Ge, respectively.

1. INTRODUCTION

The nature of defects in alloy systems such as amorphous Si-C and Si-Ge is little known in spite of the growing interest in these alloys in the field of application. The purpose of the present work is to investigate the nature of defects in these amorphous systems and the variation of these defects by annealing. Questions are: (1) Which elements do dangling bonds originate from ? (2) What is the origin of the linewidth of the ESR due to dangling bonds ? (3) Which elements is hydrogen likely to bond with ? (4) At what temperature and from which elements is hydrogen detached by annealing ?
In order to answer these questions, we have carried out ESR and infrared (IR) measurements for hydrogenated amorphous Si-C, Si-Ge and Ge-C, and studied the change of the results of these measurements by annealing. The compositional dependence of the ESR for unhydrogenated samples have already been reported.[1]

2. EXPERIMENTAL

Samples were prepared by rf sputtering in a mixture of Ar and H_2. The total gas pressure was $1.1 \times 10^{-1} \sim 1.5 \times 10^{-1}$ Torr and the fraction of H_2 partial pressure was 40 %. The film composition was estimated from fractions of the target area occupied by the two component materials. Samples were deposited on crystalline Si wafers for IR measurements and on aluminium foils for ESR measurements. The aluminium substrates were removed by disolving in H_3PO_4. Isochronal annealing for 1 h was carried out in a vacuum of $\sim 10^{-5}$ Torr. The density of dangling bonds was measured by ESR at room temperature. The amounts of Si-H and Ge-H bonds were estimated from IR absorption peaks by using empirical factors obtained by Fang et al.[2] Inferring from the results by Guivarc'h et al.,[3] we estimated the amount of C-H bonds by assuming that the oscillator strength of stretching vibrations of C-H bonds is one sixth of that of Si-H.

3. RESULTS AND DISCUSSION

3 - 1. Si-Ge:H

Figure 1 shows an ESR spectrum for as deposited $Si_{0.5}Ge_{0.5}$:H. The lineshape and the intensity of the ESR signal change by annealing. We attempted to simulate these ESR signals by superimposing two signals. It is found that these spectra are not a single symmetric line nor a mere superposition of two signals. We assumed them to originate from two signals interacting strongly with each other, being deformed to tend to be a single line in the intermediate region. Therefore, the observed spectrum is fitted by two signals on both left and right sides as shown for example by dashed curve in Fig. 1. The changes of the spin densities for these two types of signals with annealing temperature are shown in Fig. 2 (a). The one type of signal has a g-value of 2.004 ∿ 2.006 and linewidth of 9 ∿ 13 G. The other type of signal has a g-value of 2.015 ∿ 2.019 and the linewidth of 28 ∿ 30 G. We identify the former narrow signal with the signal originating from Si dangling bonds and the latter broad signal from Ge dangling bonds by judging from the g-value and the linewidth (g = 2.0055 for Si and g = 2.020 for Ge). The spin densities for the broad lines (Ge) are always larger than those for the narrow lines (Si). Ge spin density increases by annealing at 300°C and Si spin density increases by annealing at 450°C.

Changes with annealing temperature of the concentrations of Si-H and Ge-H bonds are shown in Fig. 2 (b). These values were estimated from the intensities of IR absorption due to wagging modes of Si-H and Ge-H. Hydrogen is found to be detached from Ge-H at lower annealing temperature than from Si-H, which is consistent with the increase in Ge dangling bonds at lower temperature than Si dan-

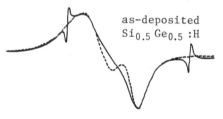

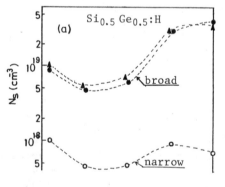

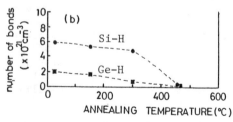

Fig. 1. An observed ESR spectrum and a superposition of two signals. Two sharp resonances at the left and right sides are ESR markers.

Fig. 2. Changes with annealing temperature of (a) the observed total spin density (triangles) and the spin densities for broad and narrow signals and (b) concentrations of Si-H and Ge-H bonds.

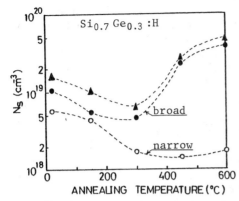

Fig. 3. Changes with annealing temperature of the observed total spin density and the spin densities for broad and narrow signals.

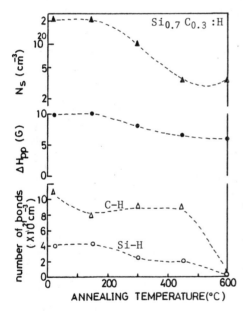

Fig. 4. Changes with annealing temperature of the spin density and the peak-to-peak linewidth of the ESR signal and the concentrations of Si-H and C-H bonds.

gling bonds. The quantity representing preferential hydrogen attachment to Si defined by[4]

$$\frac{\text{concentration of Si-H}}{\text{concentration of Ge-H}} \times \frac{\text{Ge content}}{\text{Si content}} \tag{1}$$

is $\sim$ 3 for as-deposited $Si_{0.5}Ge_{0.5}$:H.

The similar results for $Si_{0.7}Ge_{0.3}$:H are shown in Fig. 3. The ratio of the spin density for the narrow line to that for the broad line is larger for $Si_{0.7}Ge_{0.3}$:H than for $Si_{0.5}Ge_{0.5}$:H, because of the richer Si composition in the former than in the latter. This result also supports the present identification of the narrow and broad lines originating from Si and Ge dangling bonds. The quantity representing preferential hydrogen attachment to Si defined by eq. (1) is 1.4 for as-deposited $Si_{0.7}Ge_{0.3}$:H.

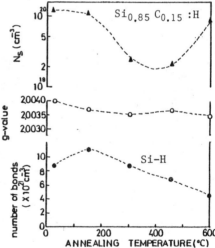

Fig. 5. Changes with annealing temperature of the spin density and the g-value of the ESR signal and the concentration of Si-H bonds from wagging modes.

3 - 2. Si-C:H

The ESR spectra in Si-C have a rather symmetric single line because of the close g-values for Si and C dangling bonds (g = 2.0055 for Si and g = 2.003 for C). Figure 4 shows the changes with annealing temperature of the spin density and the linewidth of the ESR signal and the amount of hydrogen estimated from IR stretching modes of Si-H and C-H for $Si_{0.7}C_{0.3}$:H. The spin density decreases up to 450°C probably due to thermal relaxation in amorphous structure. The linewidth decreases by annealing in a similar manner as the spin density because the linewidth of this alloy is mainly determined by dipolar interaction.[1] The g-value close to that for C dangling bonds does not appreciably change up to 600°C. Therefore, dangling bonds appear to be mainly those of C in this sample.

Concentrations of Si-H and C-H bonds largely decrease by annealing at 600°C. Hydrogen remains up to higher temperature in this case than in the case of Si-Ge system. Hydrogen detachment from Si and C is not so large up to higher temperature in comparison with the case of pure Si. Accordingly, the spin density does not increase by annealing below 600°C. The quantity representing preferential hydrogen attachment to C defined by the equation similar to eq. (1) is $\sim$ 6 for as deposited $Si_{0.7}C_{0.3}$:H. It is interesting that C dangling bonds predominate over Si dangling bonds in spite of the preferential attachment of hydrogen to C.

Figure 5 shows the results for $Si_{0.85}C_{0.15}$:H similar to Fig. 4. The spin density decreases up to 450°C and then increases. The g-value, which is closer to the value of Si than $Si_{0.7}C_{0.3}$:H, tends to decrease by annealing. The result indicates that Si dangling bonds decrease by thermal relaxation at lower temperature than C dangling bonds do. Although IR absorption due to C-H stretching vibrations is beyond the detection limit ($\le 5 \times 10^{21}$ cm^{-3}), the increase in the spin density by annealing at 600°C may be due to a dominant increase in C dangling bonds judging from the decrease of the g-value. The important point is that a-Si-C:H is more heat resistant than a-Si:H even in the sample with a small C content (15 at. %).

3 - 3. Ge-C:H

ESR results for $Ge_{0.7}C_{0.3}$:H are shown in Fig. 6. The g-value (g = 2.003) is close to that for C dangling bonds suggesting that dangling bonds are mainly those

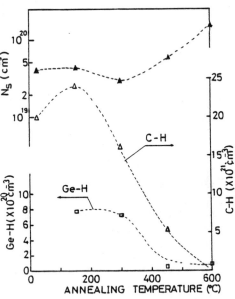

Fig. 6. Changes with annealing temperature of the spin density and the concentrations of Ge-H and C-H bonds.

of C. Concentrations of Ge-H and C-H bonds estimated from IR stretching modes are also shown in Fig. 6. The decrease in both concentrations are found to be appreciable at 450°C in accord with the increase of the spin density at that temperature. The results show that the incorporation of C into Ge makes a-Ge:H more heat resistant. The quantity representing preferential hydrogen attachment to C defined by the equation similar to eq. (1) is ~ 70 for $Ge_{0.7} C_{0.3}$:H annealed at 150°C. As in the case of Si-C, the density of C dangling bonds is larger than that of Ge dangling bonds in spite of preferential attachment of hydrogen to C.

4. CONCLUSIONS

(1) In the case of Si-Ge, the density of dangling bonds does not appreciably change up to 300°C by the balance of the small decrease by thermal relaxation and the small increase by the detachment of hydrogen from Ge and Si, and then increases largely by the rapid detachment of hydrogen. The rate of the increase is found to be larger for Ge dangling bonds than for Si dangling bonds. As expected by Paul et al.,[4] the density of Ge dangling bonds is found to be larger than that of Si dangling bonds because of preferential attachment of hydrogen to Si.

(2) In the cases of Si-C and Ge-C, the density of dangling bonds decreases by thermal relaxation and increases by the detachment of hydrogen at higher temperature than in the case of pure Si and Ge, respectively. The fact is in accord with IR results indicating that hydrogen is not detached from both Si and C in Si-C and both Ge and C in Ge-C up to higher temperature than in the case of pure Si and Ge, respectively. Accordingly, the incorporation of C is found to make a-Si:H and a-Ge:H more heat resistant. Hydrogen prefers to attach to C, but the density of C dangling bonds is larger than that of Si or Ge dangling bonds.

ACKNOWLEDGEMENTS

The authors wish to thank Mr. I. Kobayashi and Mr. T. Miura for their technical assistance. This work is supported by the Sunshine Project of Ministry of International Trade and Industry of Japan.

REFERENCES

1. T. Shimizu, M. Kumeda and Y. Kiriyama, Solid State Commun. (in press).
2. C. J. Fang, K. J. Gruntz, L. Ley, M. Cardona, F. J. Demond, G. Müller and S. Kalbitzer, J. Non-Cryst. Solids 35/36 (1980) 255.
3. A. Guivarc'h, J. Richard, M. LeContellec, E. Ligeon and J. Fontenille, J. Appl. Phys. 51 (1980) 2167.
4. D. K. Paul, B. von Roedern, S. Oguz, J. Blake and W. Paul, J. Phys. Soc. Jpn. 49 Suppl. A (1980) 1261.

CHANGES IN THE FIELD EFFECT DENSITY OF STATES OF a-Si:H WITH ANNEALING[*]

Nancy B. Goodman[†] and H. Fritzsche

The James Franck Institute and the Department of Physics
The University of Chicago, Chicago, Illinois 60637

ABSTRACT

The annealing dependence of the field effect density of states, $N_F(E)$, in plasma deposited hydrogenated amorphous silicon (a-Si:H) has been explored. Successive 50 minute vacuum anneals above the deposition temperature were made at increments of ~60°C on two samples. The sample made at $T_S = 280°C$ showed a smooth increase in $N_F(E)$ with each anneal from $\sim 10^{17} eV^{-1} cm^{-3}$ at midgap to $\sim 10^{18} eV^{-1} cm^{-3}$ after the final anneal. The sample made at $T_S = 160°C$ showed an even lower initial $N_F(E) \sim 3 \times 10^{16} eV^{-1} cm^{-3}$, a decrease in $N_F(E)$ after the first anneal at $T_A = 205°C$, followed by a systematically increasing $N_F(E)$ up to $\gtrsim 10^{18} eV^{-1} cm^{-3}$ after the final anneal at 505°C. This is much smaller than the density of hydrogen which is evolved during the anneals; it is comparable to the density of spins generated, but the relevant states are in different regions of the gap.

INTRODUCTION

When amorphous silicon films (a-Si:H) which are prepared by plasma deposition at temperatures T_S between 500-600K, are annealed at temperatures $T_A > 600K$, one finds that their concentration N_S of unpaired spins increases.[1-3] This increase in N_S is correlated with a decrease in the low temperature photoluminescence efficiency and a decrease in room temperature photoconductivity.[2-3] These annealing effects are accompanied by the effusion of hydrogen.[1-3] Since the concentration of spin centers generated by annealing is only a small fraction of the concentration of effused hydrogen, one conjectures that the majority of sites left behind by the effused hydrogen reconstruct and do not yield dangling Si bonds.

The paramagnetic dangling bond states are believed to lie in the lower half of the gap and the states for double occupancy in the upper half.[4] No measurements of changes of the density of states $N(E)$ near the gap center have yet been reported for high temperature anneals.

Madan et al.[5] have reported field effect measurements for a sample made at $T_S = 310K$ after anneals up to 485K. They showed a decrease in $N_F(E)$, which is consistent with the decrease in N_S and increase in photoluminescence reported by Biegelsen et al.[2] for similar samples after low temperature anneals.

This paper presents data on the field effect density of states $N_F(E)$ in a range spanning about 0.7eV around the gap center as a function of annealing. The highest annealing temperature $T_A \simeq 500°C$ lies above the temperature of the first peak in the hydrogen effusion rate.[3]

ISSN:0094-243X/81/730176-05$1.50 Copyright 1981 American Institute of Physics

RESULTS

Samples prepared at two substrate temperatures, T_S = 550K and 430K, were studied. They were ~0.7 µm thick and deposited onto 160 µm thick fused quartz plates from a (9:1) Ar-SiH$_4$ plasma gas mixture. Ohmic contacts were applied with evaporated nichrome on top of the films. The field effect was measured at (63±3)°C after heat drying the samples at 160°C in vacuum and in the dark. This removed the effects of light[6] and ambients[7] on the transport properties of the film. Fifty minute annealing treatments were carried out in a separate evacuated oven at increments of ~60°C.

Figure 1 shows the field effect conductance G of a T_S = 550K sample before and after various annealing steps. The abscissa shows the total charge per unit area applied by the transverse electric field. Our standard analysis[8] neglects the possible presence of interface states and assumes that the total applied charge resides in the space charge layer of the film. In order to keep note of this uncertainty and of the possibility that N(E) in the first 100-200 Å of the a-Si:H film differs from that in the bulk, we denote the field effect density of states by $N_F(E)$.

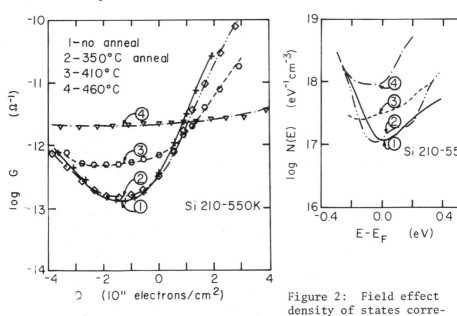

Figure 1: Field effect data for a sample deposited at T_S=550K after annealing at various temperatures.

Figure 2: Field effect density of states corresponding to curves through the data in Figure 1.

The lines through the data in Figure 1 are the results of computer fits. The corresponding $N_F(E)$ curves are shown in Figure 2.

The quality of the fits to the data demonstrates the self-consistency of the analysis. One notices first that the unannealed sample shows a conductance change of almost three orders of magnitude and that the field effect response is bipolar and asymmetric, indicating that the sample interface is slightly n-type.

There is only a minor change of $G(Q)$ and $N_F(E)$ with the first anneal at $T_A=350°C$, but a major increase in $N_F(E)$ at higher T_A. This increase is accompanied by a decrease of the conductivity activation energy from $E_a=1.0eV$ to $0.8eV$. As a consequence, a plot of $N_F(E)$ as a function of the energy away from the conduction band mobility edge, E_c, would look somewhat different since curves 3 and 4 would be shifted to the right by $\leq 0.2eV$. The magnitude of this shift is uncertain because of the decrease of the optical gap with hydrogen effusion[3] and also because of uncertainties in the measurement of E_a. The field effect analysis gives $N_F(E)$ as a function of $E-E_F$ directly.

Corresponding $G(Q)$ and $N_F(E)$ curves for a sample prepared at a lower substrate temperature $T_S = 430K$ are shown in Figures 3 and 4. Here again the $G(Q)$ curves in Figure 3 are computer fits to the experimental data. For curve 7 we could only obtain a lower limit of $N_F(E)>10^{18}eV^{-1}$ cm^{-3}, so no curve is shown in Figure 4. Also in this sample, a decrease in E_a from 1.0 to 0.8eV was observed near $T_A=400°C$.

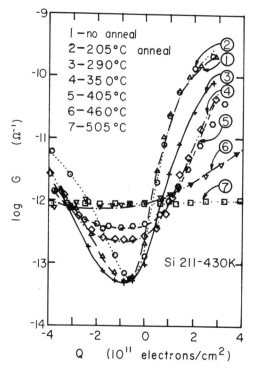

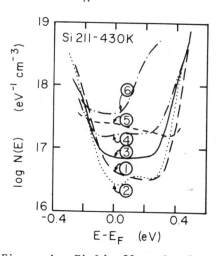

Figure 4: Field effect density of states corresponding to curves through the data in Fig. 3. For curve 7 we can only quote a lower limit of $N_F(E)$ $\gtrsim 10^{18}eV^{-1}cm^{-3}$.

Figure 3: Field effect data for a sample deposited at $T_S=430K$ after 50 minute anneals at various temperatures.

DISCUSSION

Both samples show an increase in the density of midgap states as hydrogen evolves during annealing. The increase in the number of localized states observed by the field effect method within the 0.7eV wide energy range around the gap center is about 10^{18} cm^{-3} after annealing at T_A =460°C. This number is more than three orders of magnitude smaller than the concentration of hydrogen atoms lost by effusion[3]. It is close to the concentration of spin defect centers observed by us[1] in similarly annealed samples. Since $N_F(E)$ gives an upper limit to the density of states $N(E)$ in the bulk[8], it is possible that one observes the overlapping tails of the distribution of singly occupied spin centers in the lower half of the gap and of the associated states for double occupancy in the upper half. Alternately, the midgap states which appear upon annealing may constitute stretched bonds or diamagnetic defects resulting from incomplete bond reconstruction during the annealing and hydrogen effusion process.

Since it is unlikely that the density of interface states increases with annealing, and increases of $N_F(E)$ by over an order of magnitude are observed, we conclude that the changes in $N_F(E)$ upon annealing as detected by field effect measurements are due primarily to gap states, as opposed to interface states.

The field effect response of the low T_S sample (Fig. 3) becomes sharper after the first anneal at 205°C leading to a lower $N_F(E)$ as shown by curve 2 in Figure 4. This decrease in density of states is expected for samples deposited at $T_S < 450K$. In such low T_S samples, N_S first decreases and only later increases with annealing temperature[1-3]. The fact that this behavior is also observed in $N_F(E)$ suggests that the interface density of states is smaller than 10^{11} cm^{-2}.

A comparison of the unannealed samples indicates that $N_F(E)$ is lower for the sample deposited at T_S=430°K than for the one made with T_S=550K. This is surprising because previously published work indicates that the reverse should be the case. We have measured many samples made at $T_S \sim 550K$, some of which have $N_F(E)$ lower than either of the samples discussed here; some higher. We only point out here that it is possible for a sample made at T_S=430K to have electronic transport properties as good as samples made at T_S=550K.

We wish to remark that the sharp increase in $N_F(E)$ for $E-E_F>0.4eV$ of the curves 1,2, and 3 in Figure 4 is probably caused partly by an uncertainty in the theoretical analysis. This sharp increase in $N_F(E)$ reflects the decrease in the slopes of the $G(Q)$ curves shown in Fig. 3 at large positive Q. We observed in other samples that the source-drain conductances become nonohmic in this range.[9] The true conductances are probably higher than those shown. The uncertainty in the analysis in this regime is associated with the following.[10] When one deals with a strong electron (or hole) accumulation layer, we have shown that 90 percent of the field effect current flows in a layer which is less than 50 Å thick. Under these circumstances the assumption that all states are shifted rigidly by the space charge potential without changing their conducting properties might no longer be valid. As a consequence, we believe that the $N_F(E)$ curves 1-3 in Fig. 4 increase less rapidly at large $E-E_F$. If our arguments are correct, the $N_F(E)$ curves 1-3 remain below the $N_F(E)$ curves 4-6 even after the latter are shifted towards the right by about 0.15eV needed to compare the density of states on a scale E_c-E which measures the energy separation from the conduction band mobility edge.

In conclusion, a smooth increase in $N_F(E)$ by about $10^{18}eV^{-1}cm^{-3}$ within a 0.7eV wide region around gap center after annealing at up to $460°C$ has been observed. This is the first explicit evidence for a change in the density of states near midgap due to annealing.

REFERENCES

* Supported by DOE and the Materials Research Laboratory program at The University of Chicago, funded by the NSF.
† Fannie and John Hertz Foundation Fellow.
1. H. Fritzsche, C.C. Tsai and P. Persans, Solid State Technology 21 (1978) 55.
2. D.K. Biegelsen, R.A. Street, C.C. Tsai and J.C. Knights,Phys. Rev. B20 (1979) 4839.
3. H. Fritzsche, Solar Energy Materials 3 (1980) 447.
4. R.A. Street and D.K. Biegelsen, Solid State Commun. 33 (1980) 1159.
5. A. Madan, P.G. LeComber and W.E. Spear, J. Non-Cryst. Solids 20 (1976) 239.
6. D.L. Staebler and C.R. Wronski, J. Appl. Phys. 51 (1980) 3262.
7. M.H. Tanielian, H. Fritzsche, C.C. Tsai and E. Symbalisty, Appl. Phys. Lett. 33 (1978) 353.
8. Nancy B. Goodman and H. Fritzsche, Phil. Mag. B42 (1980) 149.
9. Nancy B. Goodman, to be published.
10. Nancy B. Goodman, H. Fritzsche, and H. Ozaki, J. Non-Cryst. Solids 35/36 (1980) 599.

ANALYSIS OF CONDUCTIVITY AND THERMOELECTRIC POWER
MEASUREMENTS ON AMORPHOUS SEMICONDUCTORS

Paul Nielsen
University of Delaware, Institute of Energy Conversion
Newark, DE 19711

ABSTRACT

Döhler's method of analyzing the results of conductivity and thermopower of amorphous semiconductors is examined by applying it to $\sigma(T)$ and $S(T)$ calculated exactly from several models of the density of states $N(E)$ and mobility $\mu(E)$. The method works well in determining the Fermi level shift with temperature, but provides limited accuracy in reproducing the conductivity $\sigma(E)$. The reliability of the alternative two channel model for $\sigma(T)$ and $S(T)$ is examined by computerized least squares fitting of the seven parameters to data of Jones, et al. I find quite different parameter sets reproduce the data equally well.

METHODS

The conductivity $\sigma(T)$ and thermopower $S(T)$ in amorphous semiconductors can be described by the following expressions:[1,2,3]

$$\sigma(T;n) = \int_{-\infty}^{\infty} N(E)\mu(E,T)F(T;n)(1-F(T;n))dE \qquad (1)$$

$$S(T;n) = \int_{-\infty}^{\infty} N(E)\mu(E,T)((E-E_F)/kT)F(T;n)(1-F(T;n))dE/\sigma(T;n) \qquad (2)$$

where $F(T;n)$ is the Fermi function for doping level n and E_F is the Fermi energy at temperature T.

If conduction occurs in extended states above E_c, and in localized states at energy E_L with a hopping activation energy W, the two channel model[1,4] gives $\sigma \doteq \sigma_c + \sigma_L$ and $S=(S_c\sigma_c + S_L\sigma_L)/\sigma$ where:

$$\sigma_c = \sigma_{oc}\exp(-(E_c-E_F)_o/kT) \qquad (3)$$

$$\sigma_L = \sigma_{oL}\exp(-(E_L-E_F+W)_o/kT) \qquad (4)$$

$$S_c = -(k/e)(E_c-E_F)_o/kT + S_{oc} \qquad (5)$$

$$S_L = -(k/e)(E_L-E_F)_o/kT + S_{oL} \qquad (6)$$

To analyze experimental data requires the determination of the seven parameters defined above by a curve fitting procedure.

Döhler[5] has introduced a method of analyzing conductivity and thermoelectric power measurements which simultaneously uses both $\sigma(T)$ and $S(T)$ data to obtain values of the Fermi level shift with temperature and the differential conductivity $\sigma(E)$. The method is also useful in examining whether doping induced shifts of the Fermi level also produce changes in the conductivity $\sigma(E)$. Because the Fermi function is approximated by the Maxwell-Boltzman distribution and the statistical factor for the final state of the scattering process is set equal

ISSN:0094-243X/81/730181-05$1.50 Copyright 1981 American Institute of Physics

to 1, the approach is not applicable to situations in which the Fermi level lies within a region of high conductivity.[6]

The method relies upon specific relationship between functions $V(T)$ and $W(T)$ and the experimental values of $\sigma(T)$ and Peltier energy $\pi(T) = eS(T)T$, for various levels of doping n_D:

$$\sigma(T;n_D) = \sigma_o(T)\exp\{[E_o-E_F(T;n_D)]/kT\} \tag{7}$$

$$\sigma_o(T) = \sigma_{oo}\exp[-V(T)/kT] \tag{8}$$

$$-\pi(T) = W(T)+E_o-E_F(T;n_D) \tag{9}$$

where E_o is an arbitrary reference energy which should be independent of doping.

Equations (7), (8), (9) may be combined as

$$\ln\sigma(T)-eS(T)/k = \ln\sigma_{oo}+[W(T)-V(T)]/kT \tag{10}$$

Because $V(T)$ and $W(T)$ are defined to be doping independent, the quantity $\ln(\sigma(T)/\sigma_{oo})-eS(T)/k$ is independent of doping and hence independent of $E_F(0;n_D)$ if $\mu(E)$ and $N(E)$ do not change with doping level. A simple Laplace transform allows one to obtain $\sigma(E) = eN(E)\mu(E)$, if $W(T)-V(T) = nk(T-T_o)$.

In order to evaluate the reliability and accuracy of Döhler's method of analysis it is necessary to have a set of $\sigma(T;n_D)$ and $S(T;n_D)$ values applicable to known density of states $N(E)$, mobility μ, and $E_F(0)$ values. Such values were obtained for a number of $N(E)$ and $\mu(E)$ functions by accurate numerical integration of equations (1) and (2) as described in Ref. 6.

RESULTS AND DISCUSSION

Jones, et al.[4] have presented an analysis by the two channel model of a number of phosphorous doped amorphous silicon samples. Their experimental results are quite similar to the ones analyzed with success by Döhler[5] using a distributed conductivity. In order to evaluate the uniqueness of the parameters presented in (4), the S and σ points of their sample 8 were digitized and entered into a computer program which calculates the RMS deviations of S and of $\log_{10} \sigma$ from the calculated points at the same values of T.

Table I. Selected parameter sets, and RMS deviations for Sample 8 of Ref. 4. S_o values in mV/K, and RMS ΔS in μV/K, other energies in eV.

Set	σ_{oc}	E_c-E_F	σ_{oL}	E_L-E_F	W	S_{oc}	S_{oL}	RMS logσ	RMS ΔS
Jones	24	0.24	3	0.08	0.12	-0.56	-0.56	0.0178	26.17
1	23.2	0.24	3	0.08	0.12	-0.56	-0.56	0.0159	24.17
2	23.2	0.24	3	0.04	0.16	-0.5	-0.80	0.0159	24.40
3	23.2	0.24	3	0.00	0.20	-0.43	-1.035	0.0159	24.05

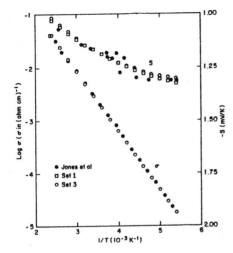

Fig. 1 S(T) and σ(T) and the two channel fits to the data.

It is evident from Table I that the choice of parameters made by Jones, et al is reasonable good. But by relaxing their essentially arbitrary requirements that S_{OC} = S_{OL} it is possible to vary $E_L - E_F$ from 0.08 to 0, while at the same time increasing W from 0.12 to 0.20, and changing S_{OC} and S_{OL}, to maintain or slightly improve the fit to the S data. Fig. 1 shows that the calculated values of S(T) for parameter sets 1 and 3 differ only slightly from each other. From this example I conclude that one cannot expect to get a unique set of two channel parameters if one allows $S_{OC} \neq S_{OL}$, as is physically reasonable.

Let us now consider the results of a Döhler analysis of calculated S(T) and σ(T) points. Two examples will be considered here. In both of them N(E) varies from 10^{17} to 10^{22} states eV^{-1} cm^{-3} according to:

$$\log N(E) = 17(g-h)+22(h-g+1) \tag{11}$$

with g = $[1+\exp(E/W)]^{-1}$, h = $[1+\exp[(E+Eg)/W]]^{-1}$, W = 0.15, and Eg = 1.4eV. However an additional peak centered at -0.2eV, with height of 0.699 in log N(E) and Lorentzian half width 0.05 is included in the second example. This peak has negligible effect on the results. μ(E) is given by:

$$[1+\exp [|40(0.2-E)|^{x}sign(0.2-E)]]^{-1} \tag{12}$$

where x is 1.4 for the second case (CS211) and 20 for the first case (CS209). Thus the second case has a gradual fall off in σ(E), as shown in Fig. 5, while the first case has a rapid decrease to zero, also shown in Fig. 5, and thus represents more closely the case of a crystalline semiconductor. Figs. 2 and 3 give the calculated σ(T) and S(T) for the second case. Also shown on the Figs. are the input values of E_F(0), activation energies in eV for different parts of the curves, and the values of A (=eS_0/k in Eqs. (5) or (6)). The results for the first case are generally similar to the higher T portion of these figures, with the activation energies remaining almost constant as the temperature is decreased.

The Döhler analysis for both cases are shown in Fig. 4, with the upper set of curves (for CS209) displaced vertically 100meV for clarity. In both cases the curves for W, V, and W-V for the different E_F(0) values from -0.5 to 0.0 lie atop one another, as Döhler predicted for an unchanging conduction mechanism. The variation of E_F with T cal-

184

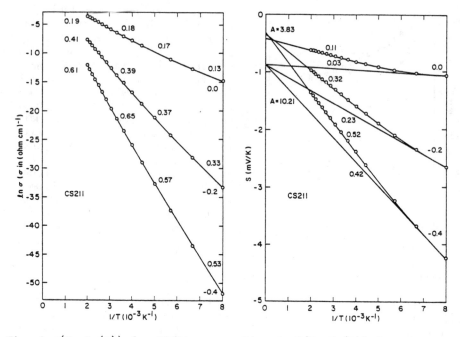

Fig. 2 $\sigma(T, E_F(0))$ for CS211   Fig. 3 $S(T, E_F(0))$ for CS211

culated from the Döhler analysis is within 10% of the variation calculated during the generation of $\sigma(T)$ and $S(T)$.

In order to apply the simple Laplace transform given by Döhler
in his Eq. 28 (in which the cosine factor should be $\cos[x(\tilde{\varepsilon} + n\ln|x-n|)]$),
W-V should be linear in T. This is the case for Model CS211.
Model CS209 gives a slightly curved W-V. The deviations from linearity is, however, relatively small and it is not clear that one would
necessarily decide that W-V was curved if the points also suffered
from experimental noise.

The insignificant deviations of W-V of CS211 from linearity produces deviations of $\sigma_T(E)$ from $\sigma(E)$ of less than a factor of 3 at
worst, and mostly less than 25%. However, the small deviation of W-V
from linearity in Model CS209 results in a factor of 10 error above
the mobility edge, and a very large error below it.

I consider that this method gives good results for the Fermi
level shift with temperature and a reasonable indication that the
transport mechanism is not changing with Fermi level. But it will
not determine $\sigma(E)$ to better than a factor of 3-10 if there is any
sharp structure in $\sigma(E)$, such as a sharp mobility edge, or narrow
peaks in $N(E)$ near the mobility edge.

ACKNOWLEDGMENTS

This work was supported by Contract # SERI-XG-0-9195-1.

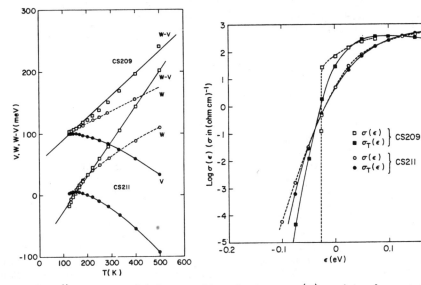

Fig. 4 Döhler analysis   Fig. 5 Input σ(E) and Laplace result
$\sigma_T(E)$

REFERENCES

1. N. F. Mott and E. A. Davis, <u>Electronics Processes in Non-Crystalline Materials</u>, 2nd Ed. (Oxford U. Press, Oxford, 1979) Chapters 2 and 7.

2. M. Cutler and N. F. Mott, Phys. Rev. <u>181</u>, 1336 (1969).

3. H. Fritzsche, Solid State Commun. <u>9</u>, 1813 (1971).

4. D. I. Jones, P. G. LeComber and W. E. Spear, Phil. Mag. <u>36</u>, 541-551 (1977).

5. G. H. Döhler, Phys. Rev. 8 <u>19</u>, 2083-2091 (1979).

6. P. Nielsen and V. L. Dalal, Appl. Phys. Lett. <u>37</u>, 1090-1092 (1980).

EVIDENCE FOR AN ADDITIONAL CONDUCTIVITY PATH IN P-DOPED a-Si:H
FROM SCHOTTKY BARRIER HEIGHT AND PHOTOCONDUCTIVITY
TEMPERATURE DEPENDENCE MEASUREMENTS*

P. Viktorovitch, G. Moddel and William Paul
Division of Applied Sciences, Harvard University
Cambridge, Massachusetts 02138

ABSTRACT

The results of conductivity and thermopower measurements in P-doped a-Si:H in the temperature range 200-400°K have been interpreted by some workers in terms of transport in the main conduction band and by others in terms of transport through a donor-impurity related band located 0.3 eV below the conduction band edge. In this report we present new and independent evidence, based on (i) the measurement of Schottky barrier heights (from both the activation energy of the saturation current and internal photoemission), (ii) the determination of the density of states distribution (from capacitance/conductance measurements) and (iii) the study of the photoconductivity temperature dependence on undoped and P-doped a-Si:H, confirming the second interpretation.

INTRODUCTION

Interpretations of experiments on conductivity (σ) and thermopower (S) in P-doped hydrogenated amorphous silicon (a-Si:H) proposed in the literature can be grouped into two categories: (a) transport above the main conduction band mobility edge (E_C) at temperatures larger than 200°K,[1] (b) transport in the conduction band above about 400°K changing to transport in a donor band located about 0.3 eV below E_C, at temperatures lower than 400°K.[2,3]

We present a study of transport and optical properties of Schottky devices on undoped and doped a-Si:H which provides additional evidence, essentially based on the measurement of the Schottky barrier height (ϕ_B), in favor of the second category of interpretations. We also determine the density of states (DOS) distribution in the material from capacitance/conductance measurements, using the Schottky device; we show that the only consistent way to reconcile the results of DOS and optical absorption measurements in the doped material is again to appeal to a second conductivity path. Finally, the results of photoconductivity temperature dependence measurements indicate that, unlike dark conductivity, the photoconductivity paths are the same in doped and undoped material.

EXPERIMENTAL

The sputtered a-Si:H was deposited onto substrates resting on a platform maintained at 275°C in an atmosphere of argon and hydrogen

*Supported by the Solar Energy Research Institute under Contract XW-0-9358-1.

with respective partial pressures of 5 and 1.6 mTorr. Doping was achieved by introducing phosphine in the sputtering gases. Schottky barriers were fabricated in Nichrome/a-Si:H/Pt sandwiches with the top surface Pt contact (5-7 nm thick) forming the barrier. The measurements of the spectral response of the Schottky devices and the absorption spectrum of the basic material, and the determination of the DOS distribution from the frequency (f) dependence of the zero-bias capacitance (C) and conductance (G) of the devices, have been described elsewhere.[4,5,6]

SCHOTTKY BARRIER HEIGHT MEASUREMENT

Activation Energy of the Saturation Current: The barrier heights (ϕ_B) of the Schottky devices on undoped and doped materials, corresponding to the activation energy of the saturation current density I_S of the diode, as derived from the temperature dependence of the extrapolation to zero voltage of the forward biased current-voltage characteristics, are given in the first column of Table I. The experimental error in ϕ_B is ±50 mV for all samples, except for the most heavily doped one, whose I_S does not show a well-defined activation energy. In the same table (2nd column) the pre-exponential factors I_0 of I_S divided by the surface field estimated from capacitance/conductance measurements are also shown. Given the error on ϕ_B, I_0/E_S is known within a factor of about 20. The transport of carriers across the junction being described by the diffusion theory,[7] I_0/E_S is an estimate of σ_0, the preexponential factor of the conductivity of the material, measured in the same range of temperature. The two last columns of the Table give the activation energy (E_σ),[8] and the preexponential factor (σ_0) of the conductivity of the different materials, as determined from conductivity measurements on codeposited samples in the coplanar configuration.

Table I Various transport parameters of the junctions and the material (see text)

	ϕ_B (eV)	I_0/E_S (cm$^{-1}\Omega^{-1}$)	σ_0 (cm$^{-1}\Omega^{-1}$)	E_σ (eV)
undoped a-Si:H	1.07 ±0.05	10^2-2×10^3	3-6×10^3	0.79 ± 0.01
P_{PH_3}=2×10^{-4}mT	0.8 ±0.05	0.8-15	10-20	0.29 ± 0.01
P_{PH_3}=6×10^{-4}mT	0.8 ±0.05	0.8-15	10-20	0.29 ± 0.01
P_{PH_3}=2×10^{-3}mT	0.6-0.8	-	10-20	0.29 ± 0.01

ϕ_B is found to be significantly smaller by about 0.3 eV (±0.05) in doped than in undoped material. The simplest way to explain this behavior is to appeal to an additional conductivity path located 0.3 eV below E_C, controlling the transport across the junction in doped material. It is notable that the reasonable agreement between σ_0

and I_0/E_s tends to confirm this analysis. Any important influence of the Schottky barrier lowering effect (ref. 9, p. 364) or of tunneling across the barrier, resulting in a lower barrier and likely to be relatively more important in the doped samples (because of their higher DOS, see last section, and hence higher surface field and thinner barrier), has been ruled out: the results of similar measurements on the same materials, but using Pd for the metal forming the barrier, and on other undoped samples with much higher DOS give similar differences between doped and undoped material.

Internal Photoemission. Internal photoemission was observed recently in Cr, Pd and Pt-a-Si:H barriers.[10] In order for photoemission to be used for determining the barrier height, its contribution to the total photocurrent must be significantly larger than that from carriers excited in the semiconductor. Figures 1a and b show the yield spectral response (η) (dashed line) of the Schottky devices on undoped material and on one of the doped materials ($P_{PH_3}=2\times10^{-4}$mTorr), respectively. We use the full line averaging through the interference fringes for the analysis of the data. On the same figure the normalized absorption coefficient (Y) (dotted line: the interference fringes have been suppressed for clarity) of the material, as determined from a combination of optical transmission and photoconductivity measurements,[5] is plotted versus hν in such a way as to make the two characteristics coincide at energies just below the band gap energy. In both cases there exists a range of photon excitation energy where a signal in excess, due to photoemission from the metal, is observed. It coincides with the presence of stronger interference fringes in η(hν),confirming the fact that the photocurrent originates from the very thin (5-7 nm) metal contact, where no spatial averaging of the fringes is possible.[10]

The internal photoemission is considerably larger in the doped sample and dominates the response over a significantly larger range of photon energy than in the undoped material, suggesting that the barrier height of the device is lower. We plot in fig. 2, $\sqrt{\eta}$ (circles) and $\sqrt{\eta-Y}$ (crosses) against the photon energy for both samples. The square root of the true internal photoemission signal follows an intermediate characteristic which clearly fits the standard linear form ($\propto A(h\nu - \phi_B)$: ref. 9, p. 404) for the doped samples. The fit is poorer for the undoped material, consistent with the relatively smaller contribution of the internal photoemission to η. The ϕ_B values are obtained from the intercepts of the straight lines in fig. 2 with the energy axis. Again we find that the barrier height in the undoped material is significantly larger than in the doped sample by about 0.25 eV, which is far beyond experimental error. This agrees with activation energy measurements. However, the ϕ_B optical values (1.02 and 1.28±0.05 eV) are systematically larger by about 0.2 eV than the ϕ_B activation energy values. This discrepancy may be due to the fact that the photoemitted electrons from the metal need an excess energy to escape the Coulombic attraction from the positive charge left in the metal. Such an effect is probably more important in a-Si:H than in crystalline semiconductors, given the lower mobility of electrons.

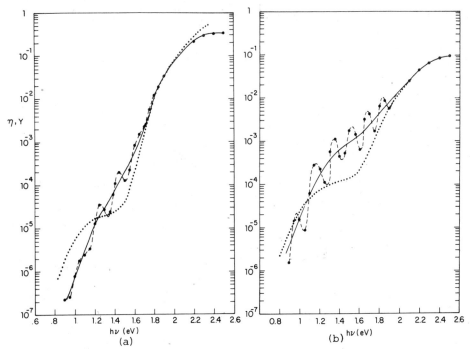

Fig. 1. Yield spectral response η (dashed line) of the Schottky devices and normalized absorption spectrum Y (dotted line) on undoped a-Si:H(a) and on one of the doped materials (b) $(P_{PH_3} = 2 \times 10^{-4}$ mT).

DENSITY OF STATES DISTRIBUTION

The D.O.S. distribution $N(E-E_F)$ spanning from (E_F) downwards approximately 0.3 eV, was determined from $C(f), G(f)$ measurements. In order to derive the exact position of the D.O.S. distribution with respect to E_c, we used the results of optical absorption measurements on the material (see fig. 1). The shoulder observed in the absorption data reveals the presence of an increase in the D.O.S. toward the valence band at an onset energy (E_{th}) which was found to be located around 0.8eV to 0.9 eV below E_c and to be approximately the same for doped and undoped samples[5]. This feature in the D.O.S. distribution has been identified also in $N(E-E_F)$ derived for $C(f)$, $G(f)$: however, such an identification requires us to appeal, in doped samples, to a second conductivity path located 0.25 to 0.35 eV below E_c, i.e., E_F is not located 0.29 eV below E_c as one might think from the value of E_σ (see Table I), but $E_\sigma + (0.25$ to 0.35 eV) = 0.55 to 0.65 eV below E_c. The Fermi level position is found to be the same in the three doped samples from both conductivity (same E_σ) and $C(f)$, $G(f)$ (similar E_F-E_{th}) measurements.

In fig. 3. the D.O.S. distributions of different materials are plotted versus the distance in energy below E_c. The Fermi level positions and the additional conducting path are shown also.

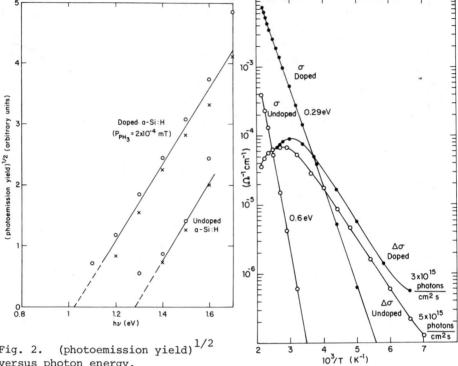

Fig. 2. (photoemission yield)$^{1/2}$ versus photon energy.

Fig. 4. Dark conductivity (σ) and photoconductivity ($\Delta\sigma$) for the shown photon fluxes at 1.96 eV versus 10^3/T for a doped and an undoped sample.

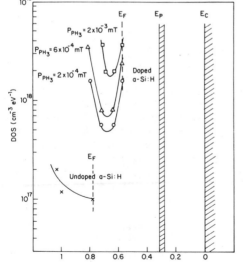

Fig. 3. Density of states D.O.S. distribution (error ±50%) for different materials versus energy referred to the conduction band edge E_C. The additional conductivity path E_P for doped a-Si:H and the Fermi level positions are shown also.

PHOTOCONDUCTIVITY

The temperature dependence of the photoconductivity ($\Delta\sigma$) of P-doped sputtered films exhibits qualitatively the same features as undoped films.[11,12] Its response time and deduced drift mobility are also similar, indicating that phototransport probably occurs at the same level in both cases. However, the relationship between the photoconductivity and dark conductivity (σ) temperature characteristics differ. In undoped films $\Delta\sigma$ is seen to peak at the temperature where its magnitude roughly coincides with that of σ,[13] whereas in doped films σ is far larger than $\Delta\sigma$ at the temperature where $\Delta\sigma$ peaks. This observation may be considered as corroborative evidence for additional dark transport at a level different from the conduction band edge. However, it should be treated with caution as we do not have, at the present time, a quantitative explanation for the high temperature behavior of the photoconductivity.

When the excess carrier density due to photo excitation is reduced below the equilibrium carrier density at a given level, any variation in the $\Delta\sigma$ response time (τ_R) with illumination intensity (F) is expected to cease.[14] In the doped film at $10^3/T = 2.7\text{K}^{-1}$ ($\sigma \sim 10 \times \Delta\sigma$) we find that $\tau_R \propto F^{-0.4}$. This again suggests that the σ (equilibrium) transport level is different from the $\Delta\sigma$ (excess) transport level.

REFERENCES

1. See for example, H. Overhof and W. Beyer, J. Non-Cryst. Solids, 35-36, 375 (1980).
2. See for example, D.G. Ast and M.H. Brodsky, Phil. Mag. B41, 273 (1980).
3. D. Anderson and William Paul (to be published).
4. P. Viktorovitch, G. Moddel, J. Blake and William Paul (to be published).
5. G. Moddel, D.A. Anderson and William Paul, Phys. Rev. B22, 1918 (1980).
6. P. Viktorovitch and G. Moddel, J. Appl. Phys. 51, 4847 (1980).
7. P. Viktorovitch, J. Appl. Phys. 52, to be published (1981).
8. For the rest of the paper E_σ will be considered as representing the energy difference between the conducting level and the Fermi level E_F. The correction which may be required to account for possible shifts in E_F with temperature is far less than the energy differences discussed here (see below).
9. S.M. Sze, Physics of Semiconductor Devices, Wiley-Interscience (1969).
10. C.R. Wronski, B. Abeles, G.D. Cody and T. Tiedje, Appl. Phys. Letters 37, 96 (1980).
11. T.D. Moustakas, J. of Electron. Mater. 8, 391 (1979).
12. G. Moddel, P. Viktorovitch and W. Paul (to be published).
13. W.E. Spear, R.J. Loveland and A.Al-Sharbaty, J. of Non-Cryst. Sol. 15, 410 (1974).
14. A. Rose, Concepts in Photoconductivity and Allied Problems, Interscience Publishers, p. 21 (1963).

HIGH-CONDUCTIVE AND WIDE OPTICAL-GAP BORON-DOPED Si:H FILMS

A.Matsuda, M.Matsumura, K.Nakagawa, T.Imura*, H.Yamamoto
S.Yamasaki, H.Okushi, S.Iizima and K.Tanaka
Electrotechnical Laboratory, 1-1-4 Umezono, Sakuramura, Niihari-gun,
Ibaragi 305, JAPAN

ABSTRACT

Doping of boron (B) into Si:H thin films by means of glow-discharge decomposition of SiH_4 and B_2H_6 mixed gas has been studied. A new deposition condition has been proposed for obtaining new p-type Si:H film which has a wide optical gap amounting to 1.8eV and dark conductivity exceeding $10^{-1}\Omega^{-1}cm^{-1}$. Optical and electrical properties of these B-doped Si:H films have been measured, and discussed in relation with the contents of bonded H and incorporated B atoms in the specimen. Annealing studies on the high conductive B-doped Si:H films have suggested that about 60-vol.% microcrystals (50A size) are embedded in amorphous network for this film.

INTRODUCTION

Phosphorus doping of hydrogenated silicon (Si:H) and fluorinated silicon (Si:F:H) has been done successfully by means of glow discharge decomposition of pre-mixed gas (PH_3 or PF_5 in SiH_4 or SiF_4 feed gas)[1-3]. However, as is well known, boron doping of hydrogenated silicon is generally accompanied with optical gap narrowing for the case of high doping which has been tentatively ascribed to a Si-B alloying effect[2,4,5].

In this report we present a new preparation condition for obtaining a high conductive B-doped Si:H films with a wide optical gap. We also show the origin of optical gap narrowing of highly B-doped Si:H films prepared by a conventional method through the measurements of optical absorption spectra, the concentration of incorporated B atoms and the content of bonded H.

EXPERIMENTAL

Two series of B-doped Si:H films were prepared by the RF-glow-discharge technique for two different deposition conditions using the capacitively-coupled chamber; one is conventional low-power and the other new high-power conditions. Detailed deposition conditions are listed in Table 1.

Dark conductivity (σ_d) and optical absorption spectrum (α-hν) were measured for each sample. Optical gap E_0 was graphically determined using the relation $\sqrt{\alpha h\nu} \propto (h\nu - E_0)$. Infra-red absorption and SIMS measurements were performed on all the specimen, from which the bonded H content and the concentration of incorporated B atoms in the specimens were determined. X-ray diffraction measurements were also carried out on the specimens for investigating their textures.

Table 1. Deposition conditions of B-doped Si:H films.

	Feed gas	Power	Pressure	Flow rate	T_s
low-power (conventional)	B_2H_6/SiH_4	5W	50mTorr	10SCCM	300°C
high-power (new)	B_2H_6/SiH_4+H_2 ($SiH_4/H_2=1/30$)	80W	1 Torr	10SCCM	300°C

[Electrode diameter; 80mmφ, Electrode distance; 40mm]

RESULTS AND DISCUSSION

Figure 1 shows the dark conductivity (σ_d) and the optical gap (E_O) of the two series of B-doped Si:H films plotted against the gaseous impurity ratio B_2H_6/SiH_4. E_O of the specimens deposited under conventional low-power condition decreases rapidly with an in-

crease in B_2H_6/SiH_4 ratio as in-dicated by the dashed line in the figure. On the other hand, E_O of the specimens deposited under the present high-power condition stays at a high value for all the doping region, and furthermore, σ_d exceeds $10^{-1}\Omega^{-1}cm^{-1}$ at the high doping region as shown by the solid line.

The activation energies (ΔE) of σ_d both of low- and high-power deposited specimens at high dop-ing level were 0.2eV and 0.03eV, respectively.

Figure 2 shows the concen-tration of incorporated B atoms in the specimens as a function of B_2H_6/SiH_4 ratio. As shown in the figure, B concentration incorpo-rated into the film increases with an increase in B_2H_6/SiH_4 ratio, and B concentration of the high-power sample is lower by one order of magnitude than that of the conventional low-power sample.

It is clear from Figs. 1 and 2 that "apparent doping effi-ciency" of high-power deposition condition is 10^4 times higher than that of conventional low-

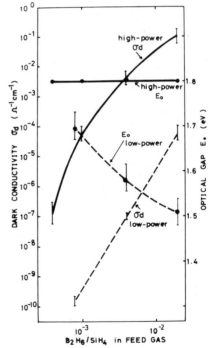

Fig.1. σ_d and E_O plotted against B_2H_6/SiH_4 ratio for low-power deposited films and new high-power deposited films.

194

power deposition condition.

It should be noted here that high-power deposited films have a mixed-phase structure, micro-crystals (50A) and amorphous network, while low-power deposited films stay amorphous, which has been checked both by X-ray diffraction and Raman scattering measurements[6]. Therefore, the apparent high B-doping efficiency of high-power deposited films should mainly be attributed to their crystalline nature, which is the same situation in high P-doping efficiency in high conductive n-type Si:H and Si:F:H films[3].

In order to investigate the nature of the microcrystals in the above two-phase structure, annealing study was carried out on this high-power deposited B-doped Si:H film. X-ray diffraction curve of the specimen was traced after each isochronal annealing (1hr, in flowing H_2), on which the peak intensity (I_p), the half width ($\Delta 2\theta$) and the peak angle (2θ) of Si (220) diffraction line from the microcrystals were determined.

Figure 3 shows I_p, $\Delta 2\theta$ and 2θ as functions of annealing temperature (T_a) for micro-crystals involved in high-power deposited film. As shown in the figure, I_p increases gradually up to T_a=550 °C, while $\Delta 2\theta$, a measure of the microcrystallite size, remains constant. For T_a>550 °C I_p increases rapidly and $\Delta 2\theta$ starts decreasing, indicating that the microcrystals grow up to larger sizes. More than 90% of bonded

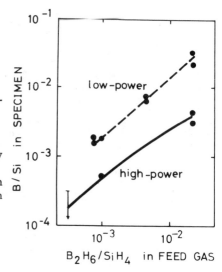

Fig.2. B/Si in the film plotted against B_2H_6/SiH_4 in feed gas.

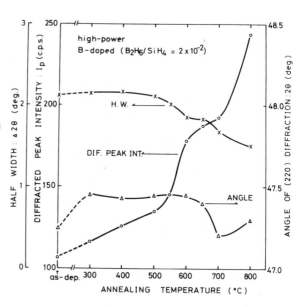

Fig.3. I_p, 2θ and $\Delta 2\theta$ of Si (220) diffraction line (Cu-Kα ray) from the microcrystals in the high-power B-doped Si:H film as functions of T_a.

H in the specimen was evolved out at $T_a=550°C$, which seems to be related with a rapid rise of I_p for $T_a>550°C$. At $T_a=800°C$, a whole volume of the specimen was crystallized. Assuming that a product of I_p and $\Delta 2\theta$ is proportional to a volume of the microcrystals in the two-phase structure of the specimen, we estimated the volume fraction of the micro-crystals in the as-deposited film. It has been turned out that microcrystals amounting to 60 vol.% are involved in amorphous network.

Figure 4 shows the $\sqrt{\alpha h\nu}$-$h\nu$ curves of two different B-doped Si:H films, high-power deposited sample (denoted by P) and conventional low-power deposited sample (denoted by A), respectively. The data for undoped a-Si:H (GD and SP) as well as Si crystal are also shown in the figure as refer-ences. As shown in the figure, the $\sqrt{\alpha h\nu}$-$h\nu$ curve is shifted to lower energy region with a

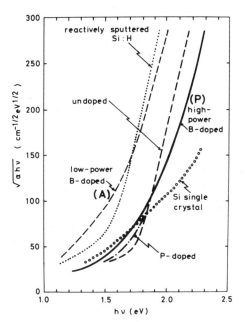

Fig.4. $\sqrt{\alpha h\nu}$-$h\nu$ curves of low-power B-doped film (A) and high-power B-doped film (P). The data for undoped film, crystal-line Si and reactively-sputtered Si:H are also shown.

simultaneous change of its slope when B is doped under the conven-tional low-power condition. But the characteristic curve of the B-doped Si:H deposited under high-power condition (curve P) lies almost at the same energy region as that of undoped Si:H although α-$h\nu$ relation does not precisely obey the square-root law due to its microcrystalline-amorphous mixed phase.

The content of bonded H in the film was determined by the ir absorption spectra in order to investigate the origin of optical-gap narrowing in the conventional low-power deposited p-type Si:H films.

Figure 5 shows the relationship between E_0 determined from $\sqrt{\alpha h\nu}$-$h\nu$ curve and the content of bonded H. The data points of re-actively-sputtered Si:H (SP) were taken from our earlier work[7]. It is clear from the results shown in the figure that optical gap E_0 is mainly affected by the bonded H content independent of whether the material is GD, SP, undoped or B- (or P-) doped film when the depo-sition temperature (T_s) is fixed. Namely, optical-gap narrowing in highly B-doped Si:H deposited under the conventional low-power con-dition should be mainly ascribed to a low content of bonded H in the film but not to the Si-B alloying effect[5]. The B-doped Si:H depo-sited under high-power condition shows a fairly large E_0 which orig-inates in a large amount of bonded H involved in the film, as is clear from Fig.5.

CONCLUSION

(1) New high-power deposition condition with low deposition rate produces a high conductive B-doped specimen ($>10^{-1}\Omega^{-1}cm^{-1}$) with large optical gap of around 1.8eV. The specimen contains around 60 vol.% of micro-crystals ($\sim$50A in size) in amorphous network.

(2) Optical-gap narrowing in conventional B-doped amorphous Si:H should be mainly attributed to a decrease in bonded H in the sample.

REFERENCES

1. W.E.Spear and P.G.LeComber; Philos. Mag. 33 (1976) 935.
2. A.Madan, S.R.Ovshinsky and E.Benn; Philos. Mag. 40 (1979) 259.
3. A.Matsuda, S.Yamasaki, K. Nakagawa, H.Okushi, K.Tanaka, S.Iizima, M.Matsumura and H.Yamamoto; Jpn. J. Appl. Phys. 19 (1980) L305.
4. D.E.Carlson; J. Non-Cryst. Solids; 35&36 (1980) 707.
5. C.C.Tsai; Phys. Rev. B19 (1979) 2041.
6. K.Tanaka, K.Nakagawa, A. Matsuda, M.Matsumura, H. Yamamoto, S.Yamasaki, H.Okushi and S.Iizima; Proc. 12th Conf. Solid State Devices (Tokyo, 1980) (in press).
7. S.Iizima, H.Okushi, A.Matsuda, S.Yamasaki, K.Nakagawa, M. Matsumura and K.Tanaka; Proc. 11th Conf. (3rd International) Solid State Devices (Tokyo, 1979); Jpn. J. Appl. Phys. 19 (1980) Suppl. 19-1, 521.

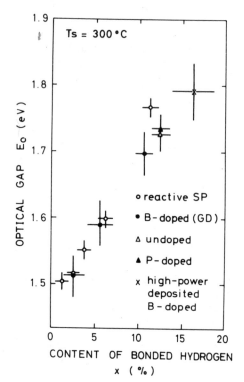

Fig.5. Relationship between content of bonded H and optical gap E_0 in low-power B-doped Si:H ($\bullet$), high-power B-doped Si:H ($\times$), reactively-sputtered Si:H ($\circ$), undoped GD-Si:H ($\triangle$) and P-doped Si:H ($\blacktriangle$).

* Osaka University, Yamada-kami, Suita-shi, Osaka 565, JAPAN

A PHYSICAL INTERPRETATION OF DISPERSIVE TRANSPORT
IN AMORPHOUS SILICON HYDRIDE

T. Tiedje, A. Rose and J. M. Cebulka
Corporate Research Laboratory
Exxon Research and Engineering Co.
Linden, NJ 07036

ABSTRACT

A physical interpretation of dispersive transport based on the progressive thermalization of electrons in an exponential distribution of traps, is used to explain the temperature dependence of the electron and hole drift mobilities in amorphous silicon hydride.

INTRODUCTION

The temperature dependence of the electron and hole drift mobilities in amorphous silicon hydride ($a-SiH_x$) is known to be exponential in $1/T$ with an activation energy in the 0.13-0.25 eV range for electrons and 0.26-0.54 eV for holes.[1] One explanation for the exponential temperature dependence is that the carriers interact with a distribution of localized states that has a sharp low energy cut-off.[2] The problem with this interpretation is that the physical reason for the sharp edge in the localized state distribution is not clear and there is no evidence from optical absorption measurements,[3] for example, that the density of states has the required form. In this paper we generalize the above-mentioned interpretation of the drift mobility to a continuous distribution of localized states with no sharp cut-off. We discuss the effect of this modification on the drift mobility in terms of a novel physical interpretation of the dispersive transport process,[4] and show that a simple exponential tailing of the density of states into the band-gap can explain the temperature dependence of the electron and hole drift mobility in $a-SiH_x$, as measured by the time-of-flight technique.

DISPERSIVE TRANSPORT MODEL

At the beginning of a time-of-flight experiment a packet of electrons is introduced at one end of a sample, by a flash of light. Within one trapping time ($\sim 10^{-11}$s) all of the carriers will be trapped with a distribution that runs parallel with the density of localized states, if all the states have the same capture crossections. By a detailed balance argument one can show that the thermal release time τ is an exponential function of the form,

$$\tau = \nu^{-1} \exp(\frac{\varepsilon}{kT}) \qquad (1)$$

of the trap depth ε, where ν is an attempt rate ($\sim 10^{12}$ s^{-1}) and T is the temperature.

A number of trapping times after the injection pulse the electrons that were initially trapped in the shallow states will have had a chance to be thermally emitted and retrapped many times and the population in the shallow traps will approach an equilibrium Boltzmann distribution. Similarly, there will be electrons in deep states that have remained frozen in the same traps since the initial injection. The energy $\varepsilon(t)$ that separates the equilibrium fraction from the frozen part sinks steadily deeper into the trap distribution with time, as the frozen part progressively thermalizes. This energy $\varepsilon(t)$ equals kT ln νt, namely the depth of the deepest trap from which an electron can be thermally emitted in the time t. If we postulate that the density of states decreases exponentially below the conduction band edges as $\exp(-\varepsilon/kTc)$, then after a large number of trapping times (ν^{-1}), the charge will be localized in energy around $\varepsilon(t)$, as shown in Fig. 1. The density of the equilibrated part of the charge above $\varepsilon(t)$ decreases towards the conduction band because of the Boltzmann factor (for $T_c>T$) and the density of charge in the frozen part below $\varepsilon(t)$ decreases towards the Fermi level because of the density of states.

This concentration of the injected charge at a well-defined energy, suggests that we treat the drift mobility as a single trap level problem where the depth of the level increases with time and the density of levels decreases with time. Taking into account the time dependence of both factors we find,

$$\underset{\sim}{\approx} \frac{\mu_0 \quad N_c kT}{N_t(\varepsilon(t))[kT_c + \frac{kT}{1-\alpha}]\exp(\frac{\varepsilon(t)}{kT}) + N_c kT} \tag{2}$$

where $\alpha = T/T_c$, μ_0 is the free carrier mobility, and N_c ($\sim 10^{21}$ cm^{-3} eV^{-1}) is the density of states at the conduction band mobility edge. Substituting kT ln νt for $\varepsilon(t)$ we find,

$$\mu_D = \mu_0(1 - \frac{T_c}{T}) \tag{3}$$

for $T \gtrsim 1.5 \ T_c$ and for $T \lesssim 0.8 \ T_c$

$$\mu_D(t) \underset{\sim}{\cong} \mu_0\alpha(1-\alpha)(\nu t)^{\alpha-1} \tag{4}$$

These equations demonstrate that the temperature T_c defines a transition from a time independent mobility at high temperatures where the transport is diffusive to a time dependent mobility at low temperatures where the transport is dispersive. A crucial assumption of our model is that there is a mobility edge which separates localized states with zero mobility from finite mobility band states.

In a time-of-flight experiment the drift mobility is usually defined in terms of a transit time which is approximately equal to the time t_T at which the center of gravity of the charge packet reaches the back contact or,

$$\int_0^{t_T} \mu_D(t)Edt = L \tag{5}$$

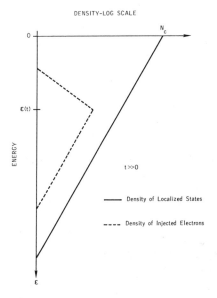

Fig. 1. Energy distribution of injected electrons.

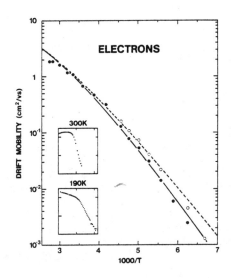

Fig. 2. Fit to electron drift mobility with $T_C = 312K$, $\mu_0 = 13$ cm^2/Vs and $\nu = 4.6 \times 10^{11}$ s^{-1}.

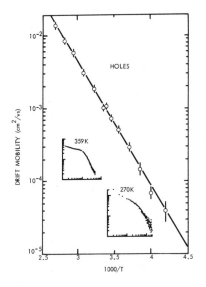

Fig. 3. Fit to hole drift mobility with $T_C = 500K$, $\mu_0 = 0.67$ cm^2/Vs and $\nu = 1.6 \times 10^{12}$ s^{-1}.

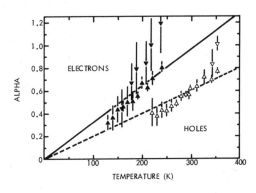

Fig. 4. Temperature dependence of dispersion parameter α.

where E is the electric field and L the sample thickness. This expression can be solved for the transit time in the low temperature limit ($T < T_c$) to give,

$$t_T \simeq \frac{1}{\nu} (\frac{\nu}{1-\alpha})^{1/\alpha} (\frac{L}{\mu_o E})^{1/\alpha} \qquad (6)$$

which has the field and sample thickness dependence expected for dispersive transport. [5]

The current up to the transit time was calculated from a drift mobility argument based on an effective trap level at $\varepsilon(t)$. After the transit time this approach is no longer applicable since an electron that is thermally emitted from a deep state will be collected before being retrapped below $\varepsilon(t)$. Thus the occupancy of the deep states stops increasing after the transit time. The current after t_T is a thermal emission limited current such that for each factor of two increase in time a slice of trapped electrons about kT wide at $\varepsilon(t)$ is thermally emitted and collected. This idea can be expressed mathematically as

$$I(t) = eLfN_t(\varepsilon(t))kT/t \qquad (7)$$

where $I(t)$ is the current density and f is the occupancy of the deep states at the transit time. By substituting for $\varepsilon(t)$ one can show that,

$$I(t) \propto (\nu t)^{-1-\alpha} \qquad (8)$$

This expression has the time dependence expected for the second branch of the current transient in dispersive transport. [5]

TIME-OF-FLIGHT-MEASUREMENTS

Now we compare the predictions of the model with time-of-flight measurements [7] of the carrier mobilities in a-SiH$_x$, as a function of temperature. The measurements were performed on 2mm^2 Pd/a-SiH$_x$/n$^+$a-SiH$_x$/Cr Schottky diode structures on glass substrates. The electron drift mobility was measured on a 3.9μm thick rf glow discharge deposited film and the hole drift mobility measurements were made on a 1.7μm thick d.c. glow discharge film doped with 1.7 ppm of boron. The photocurrent transients were excited with an 8ns dye laser pulse at 457nm. The electron photocurrent decay, following the light flash, is plotted on a log scale in the insets in Fig. 2 for two different temperatures. At low temperatures the photocurrent transients are dispersive (lower inset in Fig. 2) and at high temperatures the current decay has the abrupt fall-off at the transit time characteristic of conventional diffusion broadened transport (upper inset in Fig. 2). Thus the electron transport undergoes a transition from dispersive at low temperatures to non-dispersive at high temperatures.

Also plotted in Fig. 1 is the electron drift mobility, defined by the standard expression $\mu_D = L^2/(Vt_T)$ where V is the applied bias. The transit time, t_T was determined experimentally from the intersection of linear fits to the two branches of the current decay on the log plots. The temperature dependence of the hole drift mobility is shown in Fig. 3. Like the electrons the holes show more dispersion at low temperatures than at high temperatures, however, unlike the electrons the hole transport is dispersive over the entire range. The dispersion parameter α was determined from the slope of the current decays prior to the transit time and after the transit time. The experimentally determined values of α, are plotted in Fig. 4.

Based on the linear fit to the data shown in Fig. 4, the characteristic temperatures for the conduction and valence band tails are 312K and 500K respectively. Using these numbers we can determine μ_0 and ν by fitting the temperature dependence of the drift mobility with Eq. (6) at low temperatures and by a numerical solution of Eq. (2) near T_c and above. The best fits are shown as solid lines in Figs. 2 and 3. The open circles and broken line in Fig. 2 are experimental and calculated drift mobilities for a bias field twice as large (2×10^4 V/cm) as the other data.

The material parameters derived from the fitting procedure (see Figure Captions) are physically reasonable. For example, an electron free carrier mobility of 13 cm^2/Vs corresponds to a mean free path of about four nearest neighbor distances for an electron with thermal velocity 10^7 cm/s and effective mass unity. The smaller hole free carrier mobility of 0.67 cm^2/Vs may reflect a larger effective mass or strong hole lattice interactions.[7] The attempt rates ν can be related to capture cross-sections by detailed balance. The attempt rate (4.6×10^{11} s^{-1}) for the electron traps implies a capture cross-section of 1.5×10^{-15} cm^2 and the corresponding number for hole traps (1.6×10^{12} s^{-1}) implies a crosssection of 5×10^{-15} cm^2, for an assumed conduction band edge degeneracy of 3×10^{19} cm^{-3}. These capture cross-sections are of atomic dimensions as expected for neutral centers.

We thank G. D. Cody and C. R. Wronski for advice and assistance, and B. Abeles and D. L. Morel for supplying the samples.

REFERENCES

1. P. G. LeComber, A. Madan and W. E. Spear. J. Non-Cryst. Solids 11, 219 (1972); A. R. Moore, Appl. Phys. Lett. 31, 11 (1977); D. Allan, Phil. Mag. 38, 381 (1978); W. Fuhs, M. Milleville, and J. Stuke, Phys. Stat. Sol. (b) 89, 495 (1978); T. D. Moustakas, J. Elect. Mat. 8, 391 (1979).

2. W. E. Spear, D. Allan, P. LeComber and A. Ghaith, Phil. Mag. B41, 419 (1980).

3. B. Abeles, C. R. Wronski, T. Tiedje and G. D. Cody, Solid State Commun. 36, 537 (1980); R. S. Crandall, Phys. Rev. Lett. 44, 749 (1980).

4. T. Tiedje and A. Rose, Solid State Commun. (to be published).; J. Orenstein and M. Kastner (to be published).

5. G. Pfister and H. Scher, Adv. Phys. 27, 747 (1978).

6. T. Tiedje, C. R. Wronski, B. Abeles and J. M. Cebulka, Solar Cells, 2, 301 (1980).

7. C. Tsang and R. A. Street, Phys. Rev. B19, 3027 (1979).

Anomalous Carrier Drift in a-Si Alloys

T. Datta and M. Silver
Department of Physics and Astronomy
University of North Carolina, Chapel Hill, N. C. 27514

ABSTRACT

Transient pulse photocurrent measurements have been made on a-silicon alloys sandwiched between a metal blocking and an injecting contact. The detailed time response is anomalous and cannot be explained on the basis of dispersive drifting carriers.

EXPERIMENTAL RESULTS

Recently, interest in drift mobility results has heightened because of the large difference in results between the previously accepted values[1], $\mu_e \simeq 0.1$ cm^2/v-sec, and the newer figures obtained by T. Tiedje et al[2] of $\mu_e \simeq 1.0$ cm^2/v-sec. Transit time measurements have usually not shown such large discrepancy in crystalline substances unless there is also a large difference in the trap distribution between the materials. In amorphous specimens such as a-silicon alloys large differences in their electronic properties depending upon preparation, have been found. Consequently one might speculate that the discrepancy between the previously accepted values and the newer ones is also due to material preparation, in which, the higher mobility results from a narrower and shallower trap distributions at a low concentration.

In order to attempt to shed light on this field, at Chapel Hill we have been investigating a-Si;F:H alloys (prepared and characterized by A. Madan and his co-workers at Energy Conversion Devices) using the transit time technique. The films were sandwiched between a metal blocking and a semiconducting injecting contact. We used a N$_2$ nano-second dye laser to produce excess carriers. The details of the material can be found in the paper by Madan[3] et al and our experimental arrangement is given in a previous paper[4].

Most previous drift studies involved only reverse bias. Significant dispersive transport was observed[1,5]. In our experiments we have employed both forward and reverse biases. Our reverse bias data conforms with previous results and is suggestive of dispersive transport. Log i vs log t results are shown in figure 1. The typical power law response[6], was found; ie an initial $i \sim t^{(-1+\alpha)}$ followed by a region where $i \sim t^{(-1-\alpha)}$ is seen where $\alpha = 0.8$. The apparent dispersive transit time of around 250 nano seconds is clearly seen. It was surprising to see such a long transit time with such a large value of α because for dispersive transport the effective mobility at a given time depends only on the band mobility, the attempt to escape frequency, and α. As α approaches unity, dispersion should tend to disappear and transit time should be comparable to $L^2/\mu_o v$. Under our experimental conditions, this would be less than the laser pulse time, about 6 nano second. This was the first indication that the transit time response is not solely due to drift.

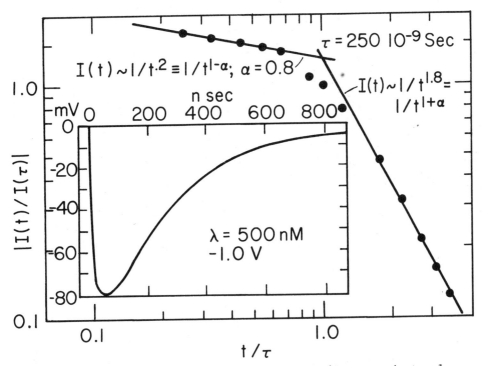

Fig. 1. Log I vs log t; insert, corresponding transient pulse.
The initial peak photo current was directly proportional to the photon
flux indicating that the excess charge was small compared with CV.

Our results on forward bias are much more definitive in demon-
strating that other factors besides drift determine the detailed
shape of the transient response. Figure 2 shows our transient
signal when a small forward bias is applied. One observes at first
a short time negative current followed by a reversal of the current
which persists for a very long time.

At first glance one may be tempted to interpret these results
in terms of drift. With a pulsed forward bias whose magnitude is
comparable to the built in potential, one would expect a potential
minimum between the electrodes. Thus, carriers generated on the
metal side of the minimum would give a negative current while
carriers on the other side would give a positive current.

A fast negative response compared with the slow positive one
would mean that the minimum is located near the metal contact. This
simple drift picture, fails however when one compares what happens as
a function of voltage and absorption depth of the light. Comparison
between the negative pulses at different voltages reveals that both
the time and the peak current do not scale with voltage. In fact the
negative peak current changes by 7 to 1 when the voltage changes by
only 1 to 1.5 The time for the negative current also doesn't scale
with voltage.

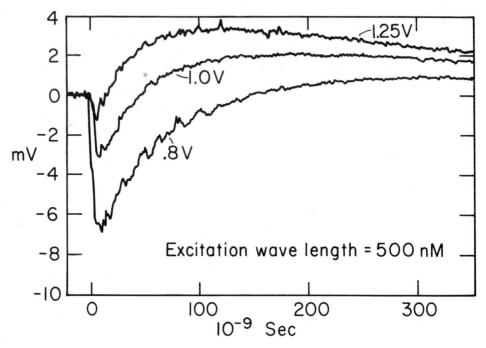

Fig. 2. Transient responses for three different forward biases

The accepted wisdom of a drift response, (even with such a distorted potential) appropriately scaling with applied field is grossly violated. Further the pulse shape is completely deformed and mutilated as the bias is varied. Even the peaks value for both the negative and positive currents do not scale.

The wave length dependence of the shape of the forward bias response is even more revealing, regarding the deficiency of a pure drift picture in explaining our results. Figure 3 shows the transient response for three different wave lengths. The peak negative current should have scaled with the reciprocal of the absorption coefficient. Further for very weakly absorbed light the initial positive peak should have been delayed because of the effect of carriers generated in front of the potential minimum. Finally, since the intensity was about the same for each wavelength, the total area under the current curves which should be proportional to the total excess charge, and independent of wavelength. As is obvious from figure 3, these expectations are not fulfilled.

In light of all the evidence, we believe that the "transit time" response is not only due to drifting carriers. We have previously proposed that there is space charge reorientation which distorts the signal thereby rendering them inappropriate for drift time determination. Hence, we suggest that the published values for the mobility in these materials are suspect. Further, we predict that the apparent mobility, defined by $\mathcal{M} = L^2/Vt_d$, should increase substantially with the thickness of the samples used. Recently reported results seem to bear out this prediction. We do not as yet have a quantitative picture for the space charge relaxation. We are continuing our studies in order to develop a self consistent picture.

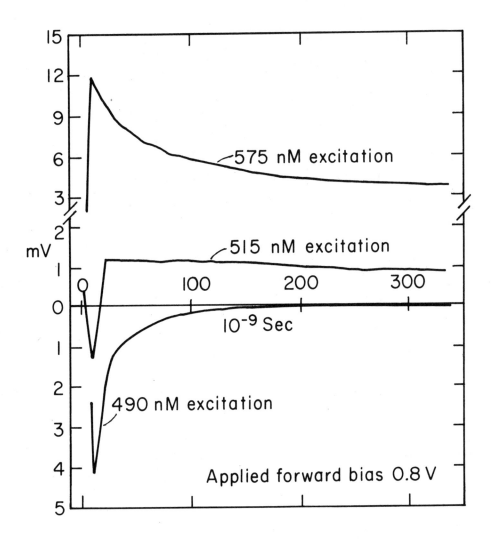

Fig. 3. The response as a function of excitation wave length. Notice the temporal coincidence of the peaks for all positive and all negative pulses (top and bottom curves).

ACKNOWLEDGEMENT

We would like to thank Prof. Mel Shaw of Wayne State University for some helpful discussion on the nature of the relaxation process, NSF for support of this research grant #DMR7920023 and the Army Research Office for use of equipment purchased under grant #DAA929-7750081.

REFERENCES

1. a) A. R. Moore, Appl. Phys. Letts. 31, 762 (1977)
   b) P. H. LeComber, A. Madam et al., J. Non Cryst. Sol. 11, 219 (1972).

2. T. Tiedje, B. Abeles, D. L. Morrel et al., Appl. Phys. Letts, 36, 695 (1980).

3. A. Madan et al., to appear in Appl. Phys. Lett., No. 1980.

4. T. Datta and M. Silver, to appear in Sol. St. Comm.

5. W. Fuhs, M. Milleville and J. Stuke, Phys. Stat. 501 (b) 89, 495 (1978).

6. H. Scher and E. W. Montroll, Phys. Rev. B, 16, 4466 (1977).

TIME-OF-FLIGHT STUDIES IN SPUTTERED a-Si:H

P.B. Kirby and William Paul
Gordon McKay Laboratory
Division of Applied Sciences
Harvard University
Cambridge, Massachusetts 02138

P. Jacques and J.L. Brebner
Departement de Physique
Université de Montréal
Montréal (Qué.), Canada H3C 3J7

ABSTRACT

This paper concentrates on electron drift signals observed in standard time-of-flight measurements on sputtered a-Si:H in the Schottky diode configuration. Values of mobility of 0.1 $cm^2s^{-1}v^{-1}$ at room temperature have been found in material that has good photoelectronic properties. The mobility is found to be activated in the range 250-350 K in a manner similar to previous results on glow-discharge produced material. Both highly dispersive and constant current transients are observed at room temperature independent of the density of states at the Fermi level. The effects of increased light intensity and bias relaxation on samples displaying constant current transients will be presented briefly. An attempt at an analysis of anomalous transients will be reviewed.

INTRODUCTION

Interest in time-of-flight measurements is two-fold. They serve as a means of obtaining values of mobilities for device operation and as a means of studying carrier propagation which in amorphous semiconductors is often controlled by non-Gaussian statistics. The first time-of-flight measurements on glow-discharge a-Si:H were based on an analysis of photocurrent transients where the carriers propagate as a Gaussian pulse.[1] Values of room-temperature mobilities in the range $0.01 - 0.1$ $cm^2s^{-1}v^{-1}$ and activation energies of $0.17 - 0.2$ eV were found.

Recently measurements by Tiedje et al.[2] on glow-discharge a-Si:H have clearly shown that it is possible to obtain either highly dispersive or non-dispersive electron transients dependent on the preparation conditions of the films. Very high trap-controlled mobilities ~ 0.8 $cm^2v^{-1}s^{-1}$ were found in films having non-dispersive behavior. Tiedje et al.[2] also made measurements on sputtered material that gave dispersive transport and considerably lower values of mobility than those found for glow-discharge a-Si:H. An interesting model to explain the different transient shapes has recently been put forward by Tiedje and Rose.[3] In this model the transient response prior to the transit time is determined by a time dependent drift mobility and at later times by a thermal emission current from traps.

ISSN:0094-243X/81/730207-05$1.50 Copyright 1981 American Institute of Physics

EXPERIMENTAL

Schottky barriers were formed with Nichrome/a-Si:H/Pt or Pd sandwiches. The 100-500 nm sputtered unhydrogenated a-Si layer creates an ohmic contact to the a-Si:H film. Films over a wide range of preparation conditions have been used, but for this study typical conditions are sputtering onto a substrate held at 250°C in an atmosphere of argon and hydrogen with partial pressures of 5 and 1.6 m Torr respectively.

Measurements were performed using a fraction of a 10 nanosecond pulse of wavelength 3371 Å from a nitrogen pumped dye laser incident on the front surface of the Schottky diode. Transient photocurrents were recorded in either single-shot mode on a storage oscilloscope or at 10 pulses/second with a boxcar averager. In the repetitive mode a frequency divider was available to help eliminate the effects of any build-up of trapped space-charge.[4] Except at the lowest temperatures no difference has been observed between the single-shot and repetitive mode of operation. Samples of thickness greater than one micron were preferred so that the varying electric field in the barrier region extends for only a small fraction of the sample's thickness.

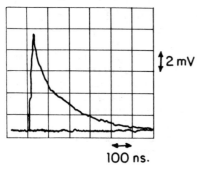

Fig. 1. Experimental single-shot photocurrent observed in a-Si:H at 280 K. The applied voltage is 10 volts and the thickness of the sample is 4.6 microns.

EXPERIMENTAL DATA AND DISCUSSION

Transient photocurrents have been observed in twelve films to date. No difference has been observed in the overall transient current shape between platinum and palladium used as the

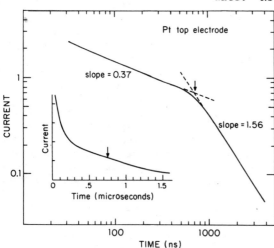

Fig. 2. Photocurrent for sample of Fig. 1 at 257 K in a $\log_{10}$ vs. $\log_{10}$ t representation and units of I vs. t (insert). The arrows mark the position of the transit time obtained from the intercept of the tangents in the main figure for a field of 2.8×10^4 V/cm applied across the specimen.

blocking front contact. The majority of transients observed have been of the dispersive type quite commonly observed in amorphous semiconductors.[5] Such a dispersive transient is shown in Fig. 1 which was recorded in the single-shot mode. In the usual analysis of such photocurrents the transit time is identified by a change of slope on a plot of log current versus log time. This is understood to arise from a distribution of event times with an algebraic tail[5] characterized by a dispersion parameter α.

Such a logarithmic plot for the sample of Fig. 1 is shown in Fig. 2. The algebraic dependence is well observed and the change of slope gives rise to a sharp fiduciary mark. Verification of this feature as the transit time for carriers reaching the back contact is made in Fig. 3 by plotting the reciprocal transit time versus applied voltage. In the low voltage regime a linear relationship holds and so the mobility is a good parameter. The mobility values obtained from the slopes in Fig. 3 are shown in the insert at various temperatures. An activation energy of 0.23 eV is obtained, a value that is somewhat higher than previous measurements on glow-discharge produced a-Si:H.[1] The slope of pre-transit current is found to depend on the applied field, maximum dispersion occurring at low voltages. Similar behavior was found in crystalline anthracene[6] and was interpreted as consistent with a multiple trapping model of transport. Multiple trapping should also be accompanied by a superlinear dependence of the reciprocal transit time on applied voltage.[5] Scher and Montroll predict that the reciprocal transit time should vary as $1/\alpha$ for highly dispersive transport. Figure 3 is clearly not in agreement with this prediction, superlinearity only setting in for fields greater than 6.0×10^4 V/cm.

The sample examined in Figs. 1 to 3 has been found to have 1×10^{16} cm^{-3}eV^{-1} states at the Fermi level from $C(\omega)$ measurements. The room temperature mobility is 0.1 cm^2/Vs, higher than the previous measurements on sputtered a-Si:H[2] but still significantly lower than the value of 0.8 cm^{2}V^{-1}s^{-1} reported on glow-discharge a-Si:H.[2] The film of Fig. 1 is 4.6 microns in thickness; identical values of mobility have been observed in 1 micron films which limits the possibility of a strong

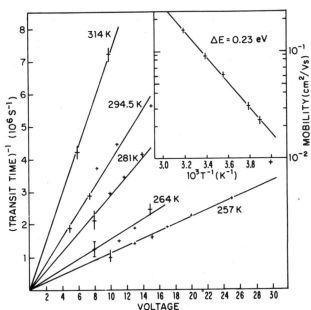

Fig. 3. Voltage dependence of the transit times for the dispersive transient of Fig. 1 and Fig. 2. The insert shows the temperature dependence of the mobility calculated in the linear low voltage region.

210

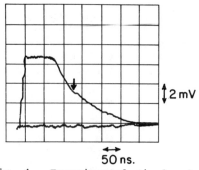

↕2 mV

←→
50 ns.

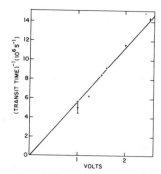

Fig. 4. Experimental single-shot photocurrent displaying a constant current regime (1.5 V across 1.35 μ).

Fig. 5. Voltage dependence of the transit times for the film in Fig. 4.

dependence of the measured mobility on the thickness of the sample.[7] Tiedje[2] found a stronger dependence of the mobility on applied field than is evident in Fig. 3, which we also observe in some films.

In a subset of samples we have observed constant current transients more typical of non-dispersive behavior. Such a transient recorded in the single-shot mode is shown in Fig. 4. It is characterized by carriers moving with a constant velocity before reaching the back electrode. The fall-off from the current maximum cannot be described in terms of diffusion alone so that the situation is similar to that of the trap-controlled Gaussian transport in amorphous selenium at high temperatures.[5] In that case it has been shown that the time for the current to reach 50% of its initial value is a good measure of the transit time.[8] This corresponds to the maximum of a Gaussian pulse of carriers reaching the back contact. Confirmation for this identification is shown in Fig. 5 by the linear relationship between the reciprocal transit time and the applied field. We have also studied the effects of field relaxation and light intensity on the photocurrents and find effects consistent with non-dispersive transport. When a DC bias is applied the constant current disappears and a rapid fall-off from an initial peak with a long slow tail results. The difference is due to the field now being dropped completely across the highly resistive Schottky barrier region. When the light intensity is increased so that the amount of injected charge introduced perturbs the applied field the transients displayed in Fig. 6 are observed. The transients are typical of space-charge limited currents commonly observed in materials with non-dispersive transport.[2,9] The effects of temperature, light intensity and applied voltage on the constant current transients have been studied in detail and will be presented in a future publication.[10] The mobility at room temperature for the film in Fig. 4 is ~0.2 cm^2/Vs, similar to the value found for the dispersive transient of Fig. 1. Thus it is apparent that both dispersive and non-dispersive transients can occur for films having a similar value for the carrier mobilities.

In some films it has not been possible to define a transit time by the standard methods of analysis. This is particularly observed in very thin films and ones having a large density of states at the Fermi level. A mild example of such a transient plotted in logarithmic

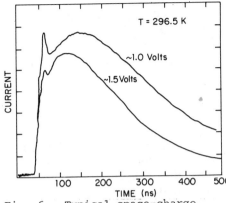

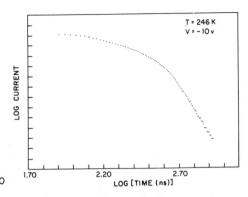

Fig. 6. Typical space-charge limited transients observed for films having a constant current region (incident intensity ~10^{12} photons/cm^2). Signal intensities refer to separate scales.

Fig. 7. Anomalous photocurrent observed in a thin film (< 1 micron).

units is shown in Fig. 7. It is difficult to draw two asymptotes on a log i - log t plot. In order to obtain a fiduciary mark corresponding to a transit time we have employed differentiation of the current transient to identify points of inflexion corresponding to a peaked distribution of carriers reaching the back contact. We are presently pursuing this method which might prove useful in the analysis of anomalous transients.[11]

CONCLUSIONS

On the short time scale of the present experiments (~ 300 nanoseconds) we have observed that the carriers propagate through the material in a manner dependent on the sample's preparation conditions. The relevant property of the films which controls the transport has yet to be identified. Another question is whether the propagation mechanism observed at these short times can be extrapolated to longer times and lower applied fields. Photoconductivity decay measurements would seem to be a promising method of testing this.

Research supported by the Department of Energy under Subcontract No. XW-0-9358-1 with Solar Energy Research Institute.

REFERENCES

1. P.G. Lecomber, A. Madan, and W.G. Spear, J. Non.-Cryst. Sol. 11, 219 (1972).
2. T. Tiedje, B. Abeles, D.L. Morel, T.D. Moustakas and C.R. Wronski, Appl. Phys. Letts. 36, 695 (1980).
3. T. Tiedje and A. Rose, to be published in Solid State Communications.
4. W. Spear, J. Non.-Cryst. Solids 1, 197 (1969).
5. G. Pfister and H. Scher, Adv. Phys. 27, 747 (1978).
6. J.B. Webb, D.F. Williams, J. Noolandi, Solid State Communications 31, 905 (1979).
7. T. Datta and M. Silver, to be published.
8. G. Juska, A. Matulionis and J. Viscakas, Phys. Status Solidi 33, 533 (1969).
9. L.B. Schein, R.W. Anderson, R.C. Enck and A.R. Mchie, J. Chem. Phys. 71, 3189 (1979).
10. P.B. Kirby, William Paul, to be published.
11. P. Jacques, J. Brebner, presented for publication.

212

ELECTRONIC DEFECT LEVELS IN PLASMA-DEPOSITED AMORPHOUS SILICON

N. M. Johnson, M. J. Thompson,* and R. A. Street
Xerox Palo Alto Research Centers, Palo Alto, California 94304

ABSTRACT

Defect levels in plasma-deposited amorphous silicon were investigated with deep-level transient spectroscopy. Both voltage-pulse excitation and photoexcitation were used to fill deep levels with charge carriers in Schottly-barrier diodes, and the current transient was monitored to detect trap emission. The results are analyzed with a conventional trap-limited emission model to deduce trapped-charge distributions in the bandgap of the amorphous silicon. Applicability of the model is critically evaluated.

INTRODUCTION

Compared to its crystalline counterpart amorphous silicon offers a unique challenge for the characterization of electronic defects by deep-level transient spectroscopy (DLTS). In crystalline semiconductors deep levels appear at discrete energies in the forbidden energy band and in well controlled material are usually present in low to moderate densities (i.e., $<10^{15}$ cm^{-3}). In amorphous silicon, on the other hand, the localized electronic levels are continuously distributed in energy and the densities generally exceed 10^{16} cm^{-3}. Continuous trap distributions have been measured by DLTS in the metal-insulator-semiconductor structure in which the defect levels are spatially localized at the insulator-semiconductor interface (1). The present study was directed toward an evaluation of current-transient techniques to characterize bulk defects in hydrogenated amorphous silicon. Similar techniques have previously been applied to studies of amorphous silicon (2,3). The present study includes a critical examination of the techniques and model-dependent results.

SAMPLE PREPARATION AND MEASUREMENT TECHNIQUES

Schottky-barrier diodes were fabricated on quartz substrates. Cr or Ni was deposited to form a bottom electrode followed by the deposition of a 50-nm layer of doped (phosphorus) n$^+$ a-Si:H and then a 0.6-μm layer of undoped a-Si:H. The amorphous silicon was deposited by the glow-discharge decomposition of silane as described elsewhere (4). Pd dots of 1-mm diameter and 4-10 nm in thickness were vacuum deposited on the undoped material to complete the test device. The n$^+$ layer

*On sabbatical leave from the Department of Electronic Engineering, University of Sheffield, England.

ISSN:0094-243X/81/730212-05$1.50 Copyright 1981 American Institute of Physics

provided an ohmic contact for dc current-voltage characterization and voltage-pulse transient-current measurements.

The basic technique used here for defect detection was deep-level transient spectroscopy (5). In the present study the measurement consisted of creating a non-steady-state distribution of trapped charge and then monitoring the transient current as the material relaxed to steady state. The Schottky-barrier structure provided blocking contacts under reverse bias, which is a necessary condition for trap-emission limited transient currents. Trap filling was accomplished by either forward biasing the diode with a voltage pulse to inject electrons into the amorphous silicon or pulse illuminating the material, with uniformly absorbed light (633-nm wavelength), through a semitransparent metal

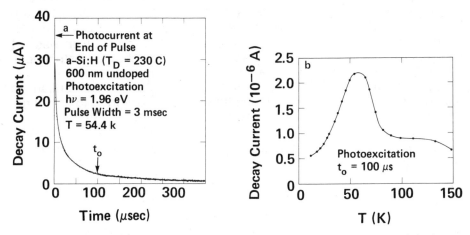

Fig. 1. Formation of DLTS Spectrum from Current Transient: (a) decay current after photoexcitation and (b) spectrum obtained from the temperature dependence of the decay current, which is monitored at a specific time t_0 after photoexcitation.

electrode to generate free carriers. For illustration a current transient after photoexcitation is shown in Fig. 1 (a). A DLTS spectrum is obtained by recording the decay current, measured at a fixed time t_0 after trap filling, over a range of temperatures, as shown in Fig. 1 (b). The time t_0 defines the emission rate window of the current-transient spectrometer.

CURRENT-TRANSIENT ANALYSIS

The amorphous silicon thin film is modeled as a homogeneous material with localized electronic levels continuously distributed in energy between the extended states of the conduction and valence bands. After trap filling, carriers are thermally emitted to the extended states with the emission time for electrons, τ_n, given by

214

$$1/\tau_n = \nu_n \exp(-E/kT), \tag{1}$$

where ν_n is the attempt-to-escape frequency, E is the trap depth below the conduction-band mobility edge, k is Boltzmann's constant, and T is the absolute temperature. If the current transient is limited by emission of trapped charge, the current i at time t after the trap filling event is (2,6)

$$i(t) = (qAlkT/2t)\, n_{t0}(E), \tag{2}$$

where $E = kT \ln(\nu t)$, q is electronic charge, A is the electrode area, and I is the film thickness; the factor of 2 in the denominator of Eq. (2) arises from the assumption that the trapped charge is distributed uniformly in the film. The quantity $n_{t0}(E)$ is the density of trapped charge at energy E at the end of the trap filling event (i.e., at t = 0). Only if the traps are fully occupied with electrons at t = 0 does n_{t0} yield the actual trap distribution in the bandgap. In the present study this condition was not in general met so that the measured trapped-charge distributions provided lower limits for the actual trap distributions.

From a DLTS spectrum, the trapped-charge distribution is computed from Eq. (2). The temperature scale is converted to an energy scale with the assumption of a constant attempt-to-escape frequency ν of 10^{11} sec^{-1} (2). From Eq. (2) it follows that the current at time t_0, divided by temperature, is proportional to the trapped-charge density at energy $E = kT \ln(\nu t_0)$.

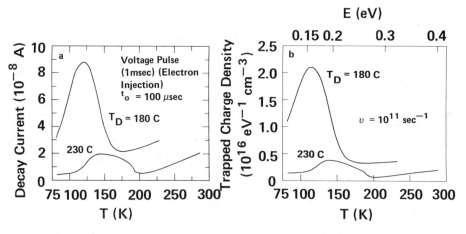

Fig. 2. DLTS Analysis of Voltage-Pulse Excited a-Si:H: (a) current-transient spectra for samples deposited at T_D = 180 and 230 C and (b) trapped-charge distributions for same.

RESULTS

Results for voltage-pulse excited diodes are presented in Fig. 2. In Fig. 2 (a) are shown DLTS spectra for amorphous silicon layers deposited at 180 and 230 C. The diodes contained the n^+ layer and were annealed after Pd deposition to achieve near ideal current-voltage characteristics (7). The emission spectra were recorded under identical experimental conditions so that the differences may be ascribed to variation in defect density with deposition temperature. In Fig. 2 (b) are shown the trapped-charge distributions obtained from the current-transient analysis. The distributions display broad peaks in the energy range of 0.15-0.2 eV, with densities of the order of 10^{16} eV^{-1} cm^{-3}. The distributions suggest a higher trap density in the 180-C than in the 230-C deposited material; defect densities measured by electron spin resonance show a similar trend. In addition, the features in the current-transient spectra are also observed in thermally stimulated current (TSC) spectra obtained after photoexcitation.

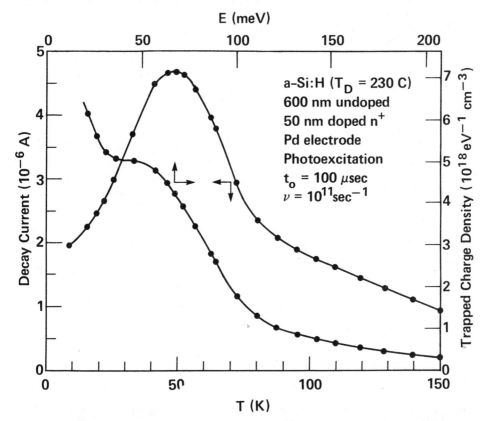

Fig. 3. Current-Transient Spectrum and Trapped-Charge Distribution for a Photoexcited Schottky Diode. The a-Si:H was deposited at 230 C.

Photoexcitation DLTS yielded results whicii differ significantly from those above. In Fig. 3 are shown both a spectrum and the trapped-charge distribution for a 230-C deposited sample. The spectrum was constructed from a series of fixed-temperature measurements. The trapped-charge density is of the order of 10^{18} eV^{-1} cm^{-2} and decreases with increasing energy.

DISCUSSION

The spectra and trapped-charge distributions obtained with voltage-pulse (Fig. 2) and optical (Fig. 3) excitation overlap sufficiently in temperature and energy to permit a comparison. Two striking differences are evident: peaks in the spectra appear at different temperatures, for the same t_0, and the scales of trapped-charge density differ by two orders of magnitude. These features reflect primarily the distinct forms of trap filling. In the case of voltage-pulse excitation, traps are populated by electron injection from the back contact, and carrier freeze-out at that contact can significantly reduce the amount of injected charge at low temperatures. In addition, the amount of trapped charge cannot exceed the initial capacitive charge on the electrodes since at this point the electric field at the injecting electrode vanishes. However, DLTS spectra from voltage-pulse excitation are qualitatively similar to photoexcited TSC spectra. Photoexcitation with uniformly absorbed light generates holes and electrons which are trapped at low temperatures. In this case the net charge can be much less than the electron density. The influence of bulk space charge on the current decay is not considered in the above analysis. A consequence of the above considerations is that the measured trapped-charge distributions are dependent on the experimental conditions as well as on defect properties. Thus, device and measurement parameters, such as film thickness and applied electric field, require further study to determine the influence of measurement conditions on deduced trapped-charge distributions.

One of the authors (NMJ) is pleased to acknowledge helpful discussions with R. S. Crandall. The authors also express their appreciation to R. Lujan and D. Moyer for technical assistance. The work was supported in part by Grant # XJ-0-9079-1 from the Solar Energy Research Institute.

REFERENCES

1. N. M. Johnson, Appl. Phys. Lett. <u>34</u>, 802 (1979).
2. R. S. Crandall, J. Electron. Mater. <u>9</u>, 713 (1980).
3. J. D. Cohen, D. V. Lang, and J. P. Harbison, Phys. Rev. Lett. <u>45</u>, 197 (1980).
4. R. A. Street, J. C. Knights, and D. K. Biegelsen, Phys. Rev. <u>B18</u>, 1880 (1978).
5. D. V. Lang, J. Appl. Phys. <u>45</u>, 3023 (1974).
6. T. G. Simmons and L. S. Wei, Solid-State Electron. <u>17</u>, 117 (1974).
7. R. J. Nemanich, C. C. Tsai, and M. J. Thompson, these proceedings.

DETAILED CALCULATION OF THE DENSITY OF GAP STATES OBTAINED
BY DLTS MEASUREMENTS OF DOPED a-Si:H SCHOTTKY BARRIER DIODES

J. D. Cohen, D. V. Lang and J. P. Harbison
Bell Laboratories
Murray Hill, New Jersey   07974

ABSTRACT

A full numerical analysis of the nonequilibrium response of a
Schottky-barrier space charge region for an arbitrary density of
states, g(E), has been developed. We apply these methods to our
measurements of Deep Level Transient Spectroscopy (DLTS) in n-type
a-Si:H. This gives a quantitative picture of g(E) extending, in
some cases, over 70% of the mobility gap. This analysis gives
qualitative agreement to our previous interpretation of similar
data but produces more reliable quantitative results and, in addition, discloses features in g(E) not apparant from our simpler
approach. In particular it identifies the correct value of the
thermal emission energy gap (near 2.0 eV).

We have made an extensive series of transient response measurements on the admittance of PH_3-doped a-Si:H Schottky barriers. These
include TSCAP, admittance vs. temperature and DLTS which are the
most useful techniques for the study of gap states in crystalline
semiconductors. A preliminary account of this work has been given;[1]
however, the earlier analysis was an extension of that for discrete
levels and is not fully justified in the limit of large concentrations of deep states. We report here a detailed numerical analysis
which correctly interprets thermally stimulated effects in junctions
with an arbitrary density of states, g(E), or spatial variation,
g(x,E).

As with earlier analyses of junction measurements[2-4] we start
with the integral-differential equation describing the band bending,
Ψ, in the space charge region in thermal equilibrium which is modified for the case of large applied bias to account for an occupation
in deep depletion determined by a quasi-Fermi energy, E_F^*, near
midgap. We solve this problem numerically using a modified Noumerov
technique[5] which converges very rapidly for this problem. Since
this method explicitly generates $\rho(x)$ rather than $\rho(\Psi)$, as favored
by others,[2-4] we may trivially include spatially nonuniformities.

The Noumerov method is especially crucial for an analysis of the
nonequilibrium response. In Fig. 1 we illustrate the approach to
equilibrium of a Schottky barrier in which a nonequilibrium gap
state occupation has been introduced by a sudden increase of reverse
bias voltage (at t=0). Initially (t=0+) the charge distribution is
unchanged, but at later times (t=t₁) there develop 3 fairly distinct
regions. Near the interface (region A) the material is depleted of
free carriers and the occupied states are too deep to have emitted
any electrons. Thus, the charge distribution is unchanged. In region
B, also depleted of free carriers, states have emptied down to an

ISSN:0094-243X/81/730217-05$1.50 Copyright 1981 American Institute of Physics

energy depth $E_1 = kT \, \ell n(\nu t_1)$ where ν is the prefactor for carrier emission.[6] The charge density is roughly constant. Finally, in region C, both emission and capture of free carriers are balanced for times t_1 so that the bulk Fermi level describes the gap state occupation.

For each time (or energy) increment the band bending is calculated. The complex admittance is also calculated for each increment using the very general equations developed by Losee.[7] This allows us to construct the DLTS and TSCAP spectra for any arbitrary $g(x,E)$. Since voltage pulse methods allow us to observe only states in the upper half gap, we employ a laser pulse to perturb states below midgap and observe hole emission as discussed previously.[1] The method for calculating the capacitance transient response is completely analogous to the voltage filling case.

Let us demonstrate the analysis with DLTS data taken on PH_3-doped a-Si:H. These

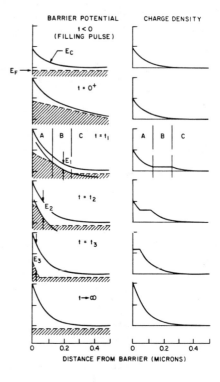

Fig. 1 Time evolution of space charge region following voltage pulse.

samples were prepared by the standard rf decomposition of SiH_4 as described elsewhere.[1] In Fig. 2 the DLTS voltage and laser pulse signals versus _temperature_ are closely related to the densities of states versus _energy_ measured down from E_C and up from E_V for states in the upper and lower half of the mobility gap, respectively. A negative signal indicates electron emission; a positive signal indicates a predominance of hole emission. The proportionality of the energy scale to the temperature scale is determined by recording spectra for several rate windows, $1/\tau_m$. Thus the deep minimum for voltage pulse data between 200 K and 250 K reflects a corresponding minimum in $g(E)$ in the upper half of the gap. The peak near 350 K is due to the midgap cutoff imposed by E_F^*.

This interpretation of the DLTS signal gives the first trial guess for $g(E)$ shown in Fig. 3. The overall scale is determined by requiring that the _integrated_ $g(E)$ over energy agree with TSCAP data. The laser signal is doubled in the diagram to compensate for a 50% _assumed_ filling fraction for laser excitation. Since the laser pulse spectrum is the _net_ hole _minus_ electron emissions, the voltage pulse spectrum is _added_ back to give the trial $g(E)$ in the lower half gap. From this trial $g(E)$ we numerically calculate the DLTS spectrum given by the solid line shown in Fig. 2. This is

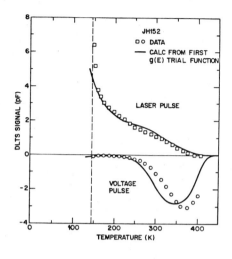

Fig. 2 Measured DLTS signal for τ_m = 100 ms (open symbols) compared to calculated signal (solid lines) from first trial g(E).

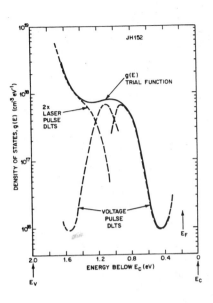

Fig. 3 Method for generating the first trial g(E) from the DLTS data. For this trial the gap energy, E_g, was taken to be 2.00 eV.

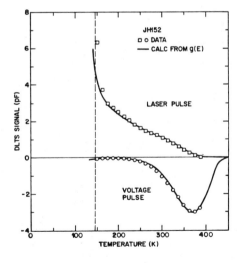

Fig. 4 Final fit to DLTS data calculated from g(E) shown in Fig. 5.

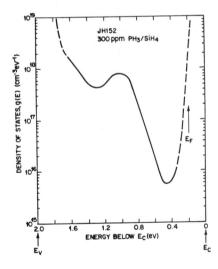

Fig. 5 Density of states obtained after several iterations. A value E_g=2.06 eV was found to give the best fit.

already reasonably close to the data. After a few iterations the final fit is shown in Figs. 4 and 5. Note, comparing Figs. 3 and 5, that relatively small changes in g(E) produce comparable changes in the predicted DLTS spectra. This sensitivity is to be contrasted with steady state capacitance methods to obtain g(E).[3,4]

In Fig. 6, a fit to DLTS data on a second PH_3 doped a-Si:H sample is shown. This second sample indicates that there is no universal g(E) for all a-Si:H samples although there are qualitative similarities. We also use data on this sample to illustrate two additional important points.

One test of the DLTS energy scale is the extent to which our model fits changes in the DLTS spectrum with rate window. We compare the calculated spectrum and actual data for two different rate windows in Fig. 7. The g(E) in Fig. 6 was obtained by fitting the τ_m = 100 ms DLTS data with a constant ν = 10^{13} sec^{-1}. Since the 20 ms data is also fit with the same ν and no adjustable parameters, this is strong evidence that this assumption is justified within the limits of experimental uncertainty.

The spatial variation of g(E) giving rise to the DLTS signal may be measured directly by using voltage pulses of varying amplitudes. Because of discrepancies among various g(E) models in the literature[1-4] it is important to show directly that our DLTS spectra related to the true bulk g(E). The amplitude of the 350 K maximum in the voltage pulse spectrum is plotted vs. filling pulse amplitude in Fig. 8 along with our calculated amplitude using the g(E) from Fig. 6. The fit to the data is remarkably good provided the filling pulse duration is adequately long. This proves conclusively the bulk origin of the DLTS measured signal. This is particularly important in view of surface and near surface anomalies indicated by previous measurements.[8,9]

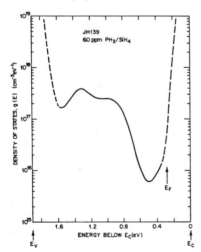

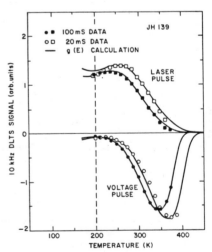

Fig. 6 Density of states obtained from fit to DLTS data shown in Fig. 7. Here E_g = 1.9 eV.

Fig. 7 Fit of DLTS data for 2 different rate windows calculated from g(E) of Fig. 6.

We wish to acknowledge the valuable assistance of A. J. Williams, A. Savage and A. M. Sergent in sample preparation and to thank V. Narayanamurti and G. A. Baraff for helpful discussions.

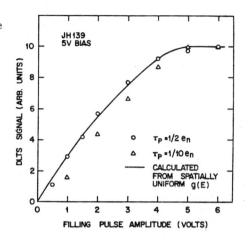

Fig. 8 Calculated and measured variation of 350 K electron emission peak with filling pulse amplitude.

REFERENCES

1. J. D. Cohen, D. V. Lang and J. P. Harbison, Phys. Rev. Lett. 45, 197 (1980).
2. W. E. Spear, P. G. LeComber and A. J. Snell, Phil. Mag. B38, 303 (1978).
3. A. J. Snell, K. D. MacKenzie, P. G. LeComber and W. E. Spear, Phil. Mag. B40, 1 (1979).
4. M. Hirose, T. Suzaki and G. H. Döhler, Appl. Phys. Lett. 24, 234 (1979).
5. See W. E. Milne, Numerical Calculus, (Princeton U. Press, Princeton, 1949), p. 140.
6. See D. V. Lang in Thermally Stimulated Relaxation in Solids ed. by P. Bräunlich (Topics in Applied Physics, vol. 37, Springer-Verlay, Berlin, 1979), p. 93.
7. D. L. Losee, J. Appl. Phys. 46, 2204 (1975).
8. I. Soloman, T. Dietl, and D. Kaplan, J. de Physique 39, 1241 (1978).
9. D. G. Ast and M. H. Brodsky, J. Non-Cryst. Sol. 35 and 36, 611 (1980).

MEASUREMENT OF MOBILITY IN AMORPHOUS
SILICON USING TRAVELING WAVES

D. Janes, S. Datta, R. Adler and B. J. Hunsinger

Coordinated Science Laboratory
University of Illinois
Urbana, IL 61801

ABSTRACT

We report a new method to measure low carrier mobilities in amorphous thin films using the acousto-electric effect. Mobilities as low as .08 cm^2/V-sec have been measured and we believe that still lower values down to .001 cm^2/V-sec can be measured. A traveling wave electric field is generated in the film by placing it close to a piezoelectric solid carrying surface acoustic waves. The charge carriers in the film are dragged along by the traveling wave and this effect is detected as a dc current in an external circuit. In our experiments, the external bucking voltage needed to null out this current is measured (thus eliminating contact resistance problems). This voltage is proportional to the carrier mobility, independent of the number of carriers. The mobility is thus calculated directly from the measured voltage. Our measurements were made using 20 MHz traveling waves with an inverse radian frequency of 8 ns. Traps slower than this do not affect the measurement. This technique should be a useful complement to the transient charge technique.

INTRODUCTION

A fundamental parameter in characterizing electronic transport is the mobility, μ, of the carriers. The Hall effect is widely used to measure μ in crystalline semiconductors; however, such measurements are difficult to interpret in disordered materials when the carrier mean free path is so reduced by disorder as to be comparable to the interatomic spacing.[1] In such materials, the transient charge technique (TCT) is used to perform a direct time-of-flight measurement of carrier mobility; the transit time of a pulse of injected carriers moving in an external dc field is observed giving a measure of the carrier drift mobility.[2,3] In this paper we will report a new method to measure low carrier mobilities in amorphous thin films, using a traveling wave excitation.

It has been pointed out in connection with TCT measurements that, due to trapping effects, there is often a significant differ-

ISSN:0094-243X/81/730222-05$1.50 Copyright 1981 American Institute of Physics

rence between the effective drift mobility, μ_D, of excess carriers and the free carrier drift mobility, μ_C. Under usual experimental conditions, the TCT measures μ_D. To our knowledge there is no experimental technique to measure μ_C. The measurement technique to be described here uses traveling wave electric fields produced by a surface acoustic wave in a neighboring piezoelectric medium; the effect of traps on the measured mobility depends on the traveling wave frequency used. At usual ultrasonic frequencies (we used 20 MHz) the inverse radian frequency is ~ 10 ns. The measured mobility is not affected by the slower traps.

TRAVELING WAVE MEASUREMENT TECHNIQUE

The traveling wave measurement technique that we propose to use is based on the acoustoelectric effect.[4] This effect is due to the drift of charge carriers caused by the traveling electric field associated with an acoustic wave. The essential feature of this technique is the traveling wave electric field rather than the acoustic wave. For this reason we call it the traveling wave technique rather than the acoustoelectric technique. Measurements of electronic properties in high mobility electronic semiconductors based on the acoustoelectric effect have been reported previously.[5-7] However, to our knowledge, such measurements in low mobility materials have not been performed before. The test film is placed in proximity with surface acoustic waves propagating on an insulating piezoelectric substrate (Fig. 1). The carrier drift is observed as a dc current in the external circuit, given by

$$J_{AE} = qn \frac{(\mu E)^2}{v_s} \tag{1}$$

where J_{AE} is the dc current density caused by the traveling wave
$\quad$ n $\quad$ is the carrier density
$\quad$ μ $\quad$ is the mobility of carriers
$\quad$ E $\quad$ is the rms. traveling wave electric field in the film
$\quad$ v_s $\quad$ is the velocity of the wave
and $\quad$ q $\quad$ is the electronic charge.

Diffusion effects are neglected.

Equation (1) may be derived from a rather simple argument. For simplicity, let us consider a traveling square (rather than sinusoidal) wave. The electron thus finds itself in an electric field E that periodically reverses polarity. The electron velocity is μE during the time it is in the positive field, and $-\mu E$ when it is in the negative field. This would seem to give it zero average velocity; however, it spends more time moving with the wave than moving against the wave. Quantitatively, it has a velocity μE for a length

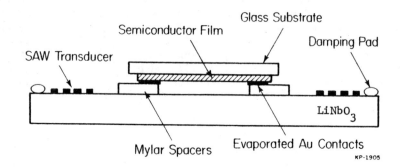

Figure 1: Experimental setup for acoustoelectric mobility measurement.

of time proportional to $1/(v_s - \mu E)$ and a velocity $-\mu E$ for a length of time proportional to $1/(v_s + \mu E)$. It thus has an average velocity $\langle v \rangle$ given by

$$\langle v \rangle = \mu E \cdot \frac{\dfrac{1}{v_s - \mu E} - \dfrac{1}{v_s + \mu E}}{\dfrac{1}{v_s - \mu E} + \dfrac{1}{v_s + \mu E}}$$

$$= (\mu E)^2 / v_s \tag{2}$$

This produces a dc current density $J_{AE} = (qn\langle v \rangle)$ in agreement with Eq. (1). A more rigorous analysis based on the bunching of carriers by a traveling electric field gives the same result.[4]

It will be noted that J_{AE} is proportional to $n\mu^2$ whereas the current due to dc fields is proportional to $n\mu$. It is thus possible to obtain μ from these two measurements. To avoid contact effects, we usually measure the bucking dc field E_{AE} needed to null out the current due to the traveling wave:

$$E_{AE} = J_{AE}/qn\mu = \mu \cdot \frac{E^2}{v_s} \tag{3}$$

Knowing E and v_s, we can obtain μ by measuring E_{AE}.

TRAPPING EFFECTS

Now we come to the interesting question of whether the measured mobility is μ_C or μ_D. The answer depends on the frequency of the traveling wave. At high frequencies the traps cannot participate and one measures the free carrier mobility μ_C. At low frequencies the traps can fully equilibrate with the mobile electrons and one measures the effective drift mobility μ_D. To put it quantitatively, let us consider a single trap level with a capture time τ_C (average time an electron remains free) and a release time τ_r (average time an electron remains trapped). It has been shown[8] that the measured mobility μ is given by

$$\mu = \mu_C \cdot \frac{f_o + \omega^2 \tau^2}{1 + \omega^2 \tau^2} \tag{4}$$

where ω is the radian frequency

$$\tau = \tau_C \tau_r / (\tau_C + \tau_r)$$
$$f_o = \mu_D / \mu_C = \tau_C / (\tau_C + \tau_r)$$

At low frequencies ($\omega\tau \ll f_o^{\frac{1}{2}}$),

$$\mu = \mu_D \tag{5a}$$

At high frequencies ($\omega\tau \gg 1$),

$$\mu = \mu_C \tag{5b}$$

At intermediate frequencies ($f_o^{\frac{1}{2}} < \omega\tau < 1$) the measured mobility increases with frequency. It will be noted that there is a close parallel with the TCT measurements, the role of the transit time being played by the inverse radian frequency $1/\omega$. However, while it is difficult to make measurements with short τ_t, it is fairly straightforward to use ultrasonic waves with frequencies in this range. In our first experiment we used a wave frequency of 20 MHz corresponding to $1/\omega \sim 8$ ns; so that the effects of all slower traps were excluded from the measurement.

MEASUREMENT SENSITIVITY

The acoustoelectric current (and hence the bucking d.c. field E_{AE}) reverses direction if the direction of wave propagation is reversed. This property can be used to separate it out from any spurious voltages due to thermal gradients or other causes.

Measuring the bucking d.c. field E_{AE} mentioned previously involves nulling the d.c. current. The accuracy of this measurement depends on how small a fraction of the short-circuit d.c. current can be detected. Therefore measurement sensitivity depends strongly on the magnitude of this current. It can be shown that

$$I \propto \frac{\mu}{R_\square}$$

where $R_\square$ is the sheet resistivity of the film.

Our experiments[9] were performed using 145 mW of acoustic power at a frequency of 20 MHz. The amorphous silicon samples were about 5 mm x 5 mm in size. A sample with $R_\square = 3.2 \times 10^9$ Ω/square produced a current of 38 pA; this yields a mobility of .5 cm^2/V-sec. The Hall mobility measured with similar samples at the RCA Laboratories is about .1 cm^2/V-sec. A second sample with $R_\square = 1.1 \times 10^8$ Ω/square produced a current of 177 pA, implying mobility of .08 cm^2/V-sec. The limit on how low a mobility can be measured depends on the sheet resistance. At 20 MHz with 400 mW of acoustic power, a mobility of .001 cm^2/V-sec in a material with 10^{10} Ω/square would give about 1 pA of current which can be measured with commercially available ammeters.

CONCLUSIONS

A traveling wave technique (TWT) for measuring low carrier mobilities in thin highly resistive amorphous films has been described. The traveling wave electric field is produced by ultrasonic waves generated in a nearby piezoelectric medium. The measurement is made under null current conditions so that contact effects are minimal.

REFERENCES

1. Record of a Meeting on the Hall Effect in Disordered Systems held at the Cavendish Laboratory, Cambridge, Phil. Mag. B 38, 463 (1978).
2. W. E. Spear, J. Non-cryst. Solids 1, 197 (1970).
3. M. Martini, J. W. Mayer and K. R. Zanio, Applied Solid State Science, Vol. 3, ed. Raymond Wolfe, Academic Press, New York and London 1972, p. 181.
4. N. I. Meyer and M. H. Jørgensen, Festkörperprobleme X, ed. O. Madeling, Pergamon Vieweg 1970, p. 21
5. A. Bers, J. H. Cafarella and B. E. Burke, Appl. Phys. Lett. 22, 399 (1973).
6. H. Gilboa and P. K. Das, IEEE Trans. ED-27, 461 (1980).
7. K. A. Ingebrigtsen, J. Appl. Phys. 41, 454 (1970).
8. A. R. Moore and R. W. Smith, Phys. Rev. 138, A1250 (1965).
9. R. Adler, D. Janes, B. J. Hunsinger and S. Datta, Appl. Phys. Lett. 38, 102 (1981).

STUDY OF GAP STATES IN a-Si:H ALLOYS BY MEASUREMENTS OF PHOTOCONDUCTIVITY AND SPECTRAL RESPONSE OF MIS SOLAR CELLS*

P. E. Vanier, A. E. Delahoy, and R. W. Griffith
Brookhaven National Laboratory
Upton, NY 11973

ABSTRACT

A picture of the density of gap states $n(E)$ in glow discharge a-Si:H is constructed using four different kinds of transport measurement on a large number of samples. The minimum in $n(E)$ lies 0.4 eV below E_c, rather than in the middle of the gap. A distribution of fast recombination centers lies at mid-gap, and two sets of hole traps lie between mid-gap and the valence band. Modifications in $n(E)$ have been studied by the effects of selected impurities on the conversion efficiency and spectral response of MIS and p-i-n solar cells.

INTRODUCTION

One underlying assumption of this paper is that, to the zeroth approximation, all our samples of a-Si:H have the same types of gap states, and that the transport properties observed in a given specimen are primarily determined by the position of the dark Fermi level, E_F. The sample preparation, measurement techniques and models used to explain the features seen in photoconductivity have been discussed elsewhere.[1-3] In addition to shifting E_F, impurities or conventional dopants added to the discharge can, of course, modify $n(E)$ and in fact are found to degrade solar cell performance. These effects have been investigated in MIS and p-i-n diagnostic devices using additives such as N_2, O_2, NO, air or PH_3 in the plasma.[4] Salient results are presented here.

DARK CONDUCTIVITY $\sigma_d(T)$

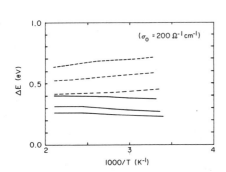

Fig. 1. Temperature dependence of effective activation energy.

Using measurements of $\sigma_d(T)$ we estimate $E_F(T)$ by a new simple method. Beyer et al.[5] have shown that kinks in curves of $\sigma_d(T)$ and thermopower $S(T)$ can be explained by shifts of E_F with temperature, and that if the effects of these shifts are cancelled out the data can be explained using a single conduction pathway. Such nonlinear statistical shifts affect the interpretation of the slope E_σ and intercept σ_0 of Arrhenius plots of σ_d. Therefore, we assume a fixed value

*Work performed under the auspices of the U.S. Department of Energy under Contract No. DE-AC02-76CH00016.

228

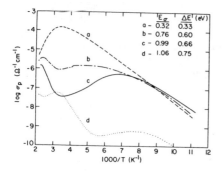

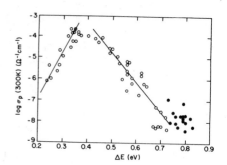

Fig. 2. Temperature dependence
of σ_p for samples with different
activation energies. Flux f =
= 10^{14} photons cm^{-2} s^{-1}; λ = 600 nm.

Fig. 3. Universal curve of
σ_p(300 K) vs ΔE. Same f and
λ as Fig. 2.

of σ_o = 200 Ω^{-1}cm^{-1}, consistent with calculations by Mott,[6] and invert
the Arrhenius equation, obtaining an effective activation energy,

$$\Delta E(T) \equiv E_c - E_F(T) = kT \, \ell n[\sigma_o/\sigma_d(T)] \quad .$$

Figure 1 shows plots of $\Delta E(T)$ vs 1000/T for six samples with different
dopant concentrations. Values of ΔE(300 K) provide an energy scale
which will be used for comparison of samples in the next section.
This scale is only weakly dependent on the arbitrary choice of σ_o.
The broken curves show that if ΔE(300 K) > 0.4 eV, E_F moves toward the
conduction band edge E_v with increasing T. This would cause the tra-
ditional Arrhenius plot to yield a value $E_\sigma > E_c - E_F$ and unphysically
high values of σ_o, sometimes as high as 10^8 Ω^{-1}cm^{-1}. The solid lines
show that if ΔE(300 K) < 0.4 eV, E_F moves away from E_c with increasing
T. This behavior indicates[7] that there must be a minimum in n(E) in
the upper half of the gap. Our measurements estimate this minimum to
be at 0.4 eV below E_c.

PHOTOCONDUCTIVITY σ_p(T)

Figure 2 shows plots of log σ_p vs 1000/T for four samples with
different Fermi levels. Values of E_σ and ΔE(300 K) obtained from
σ_d(T) are shown for these samples. The complicated shapes of these
curves have been discussed in some detail[1,2] using a model containing
three sets of gap states with different electron-capture cross sec-
tions, σ_n. Curve "a" is typical of a lightly doped n-type film in
which E_F lies high in the gap. The recombination centers are mostly
filled, and electron lifetimes are long. Curves "b" and "c" show that
when E_F is lower in the gap the room temperature recombination rate
increases, as centers we call "states 2" become vacant. However, at
low temperatures, holes are transferred from states 2 to a set of
states la with very low σ_n. This reversible transfer gives rise to
the phenomena of thermal quenching, infrared quenching, and supra-
linear dependence on light intensity.[1-3] Curve "d" indicates that

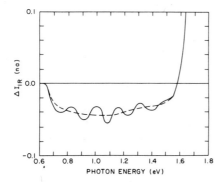

Fig. 4. Infrared quenching spectrum at 140 K for a sample similar to "c" in Fig. 2.

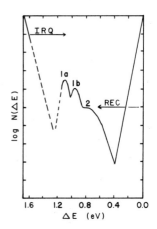

Fig. 5. Schematic of gap states.

when E_F moves still lower in the gap another valley appears, indicating the existence of another set of states 1b.

The dependence of $\sigma_p(300\ K)$ on $\Delta E(300\ K)$ is demonstrated in Fig. 3 for a large number of specimens. The highest values of σ_p are measured for films with $\Delta E \approx 0.4$ eV. This is a second indication that the minimum in n(E) is 0.4 eV below E_c. For $\Delta E > 0.4$ eV, σ_p falls by a factor of $1/e$ every 0.03 eV, suggesting that states 2 have an exponential tail with this characteristic slope. Similarly for $\Delta E < 0.4$ eV, σ_p decreases by a factor of $1/e$ every 0.02 eV, providing an estimate of the slope of the conduction band tail. Heavy doping may also introduce additional states in the gap that reduce σ_p. The solid points indicate samples with $\Delta E > 0.73$ eV that show two valleys like curve "d", Fig. 2.

Time resolved measurements of $\sigma_p(t,T)$ show that samples similar to film "a", Fig. 2, with high values of $\sigma_p(300\ K)$ have long response times ($t_r > 10^{-3}$ s). Films like "b" and "c" have short response times ($t_r < 10^{-5}$ s) at T = 300 K and long response times at low temperature. These measurements confirm that the differences between samples can be explained by electron lifetime effects, rather than mobility effects.

INFRARED QUENCHING

Films similar to sample "c" (Fig. 2) exhibit the phenomenon of IR quenching at low temperatures.[3] When a steady state has been achieved with a beam of visible light, the photocurrent is reduced by the application of a second beam of photons in the near IR. These photons excite electrons from the valence band into vacant states in level 1a, thereby freeing holes that diffuse to states 2 where they recombine rapidly. The spectrum of such excitations at 140 K, shown in Fig. 4, is very similar to the spectrum of light-induced absorption reported by O'Connor and Tauc.[8] In both cases, the threshold of such transitions around 0.65 eV is interpreted as the energy difference between the valence band edge E_v and the quasi-Fermi level for holes trapped in states la. This measurement gives an approximate location of states la.

DENSITY OF STATES PICTURE

Figure 5 is a pictorial summary of the above findings about the states in the gap of a-Si:H. Starting at the dominant conduction pathway at the righthand side, an exponential tail is shown with a slope of 0.02 eV. At 0.4 eV below E_c there is a deep minimum in n(E). Rising from this minimum is the exponential tail of states 2, which have a high σ_n. Between mid-gap and E_v are two more sets of hole traps, la and lb with low σ_n. The region between states la and E_v is now being investigated using statistical shifts of p-type films, and little data are as yet available.

SPECTRAL RESPONSE AND DEFECTS

Modifications in n(E) induced by either low levels of PH$_3$ or N$_2$ and O$_2$ impurities in the plasma have been inferred from analysis of the spectral response of Pd MIS photovoltaic devices. In attempting to model the experimental results we found it necessary to account for the fall-off in collection efficiency Y(λ) for λ<550 nm observed by our group and others.[9] At short wavelengths, electron-hole pairs are created in close proximity to the Pd/a-Si:H interface; diffusion against the field of "majority" carriers (electrons) to the interface is then a significant process that subtracts from the "minority" carrier (hole) drift current entering the metal. By solving the continuity equation for photogenerated electrons, under the simplifying assumption of a constant field F, we have shown[4] that $\Delta Y(\lambda) =$
$= -\{s_n/(s_n + v_{d,n})\}\{\alpha_\lambda \Lambda_F/(2 + \alpha_\lambda \Lambda_F)\}$ due to this majority carrier effect, where s_n is the effective surface recombination (or collection) velocity for majority carriers, $v_{d,n} = \mu_n F$ and $2/\Lambda_F = eF/kT$. We therefore write Y(λ) as the sum of three terms:

$$Y(\lambda) = \{\alpha_\lambda L_{F,p}/(1 + \alpha_\lambda L_{F,p})\}\{1 - \exp(-W(\alpha_\lambda + L_{F,p}^{-1}))\}$$
$$+ \{\alpha_\lambda L_p/(1 + \alpha_\lambda L_p)\} \exp(-W(\alpha_\lambda + L_{F,p}^{-1}))$$
$$- \{s_n/(s_n + v_{d,n})\}\{\alpha_\lambda \Lambda_F/(2 + \alpha_\lambda \Lambda_F)\} \quad . \tag{1}$$

The first two terms represent the collection of holes generated in the space charge region (width W), and field-free region respectively, where the hole drift length $L_{F,p} = \mu_p \tau_p F$ and the hole diffusion length $L_p = (\mu_p \tau_p kT/e)^{1/2}$.

In each of Figs. 6a, 6b, and 6c we show the following curves for three MIS cells fabricated without an AR coating: (i) the measured external quantum efficiency QE(λ)$_{ext}$; (ii) the internal quantum efficiency (collected carriers per absorbed photon) calculated from QE(λ)$_{int}$ = QE(λ)$_{ext}$/T(λ), where T(λ), the optical transmission into the a-Si:H, was determined in a separate experiment;[4] (iii) the theoretical collection efficiency (collected carriers per free, or separated, carrier) Y(λ), computed from Eq. (1) above and fitted to curve (ii); and (iv) the theoretical Y(λ) obtained if the majority carrier effect de-

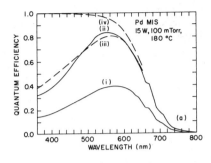

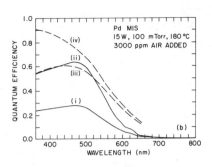

a

b

Figs. 6a, b, and c. Fitting of
theoretical curves of collection
efficiency to experimental data
to extract W and $\mu_p\tau_p$.

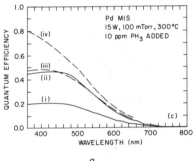

c

scribed above is ignored. Assuming that geminate recombination is
negligible, $QE(\lambda)_{int} = Y(\lambda)$. The following impurities were introduced
into the plasma during the deposition of the bulk a-Si:H layer of the
three cells: a) nothing added, b) 3000 ppm air, and c) 10 ppm PH_3
(140 ppm P incorporated according to SIMS). Comparing $QE(\lambda)_{int}$ in
Fig. 6b to that in Fig. 6a we note: 1) the response for $\lambda > 500$ nm has
fallen dramatically with the addition of air, 2) the response for
$\lambda < 450$ nm has risen and the fall-off almost disappeared, and 3) the
peak response is smaller in magnitude and shifted to a shorter wavelength.

Table I lists the values of W, F, and $\mu_p\tau_p$ obtained by fitting Eq.
(1) to the experimental curves (ii). The fits show that the presence
of air: 1) collapses the depletion width W, thereby accounting for
the drop in red response, and 2) severely degrades $\mu_p\tau_p$ and hence L_p.
The higher blue response in Fig. 6b is due to a suppression of major-
ity-carrier diffusion as a result of the stronger drift field (smaller
$\Lambda_F \sim 1/F \sim W$ in Eq. (1)). (As a result, the conversion efficiency of
SiO/Pd/p-i-n solar cells was reduced from 3.1% to 1.5% under AM1 illumination.) These results receive a natural explanation if we assume
that the air impurity in the plasma led to an increase of the positive
space charge density ρ in the depletion region of the a-Si:H alloy.
Quite similar results can be seen in Fig. 6c for the cell containing
140 ppm P. In this cell, the increase in ρ results from ionized
donors (i.e. substitutional P), while the reduction of $\mu_p\tau_p$ presumably
results from hole traps introduced by doping-associated defects.

Table I Space Charge Region and Hole Transport Parameters

Impurity in Plasma	W(cm)	F(V cm^{-1})	$\mu_p\tau_p$(cm^{2}V^{-1})	L_p(cm)	Λ_F(cm)
nothing added	5×10^{-5}	1.2×10^4	3.0×10^{-8}	2.8×10^{-5}	4.3×10^{-6}
3000 ppm air	1.2×10^{-5}	2.8×10^4	5.5×10^{-10}	3.8×10^{-6}	1.8×10^{-6}
10 ppm PH$_3$	1.0×10^{-5}	3.8×10^4	1.5×10^{-10}	1.9×10^{-6}	1.4×10^{-6}

We now discuss the effects of air on $n(E)$. At high substrate temperatures T_s we have conclusively demonstrated[2] that 3000 ppm air added to the plasma results in n-type doping ($\Delta E = 0.35$ eV, $S = -1.1$ mV/°K). The donor species appears to be either substitutional N, or an N-O complex. However, the collapse of W in the air leak devices does not noticeably depend on T_s, whereas the alloy doping does. Hence the shallow donors just mentioned cannot be principally responsible for ρ. We postulate that, for all T_s, and independently of the other effects, air introduces deep states roughly 0.8 eV below E_c i.e. below E_F in the bulk. These states do not affect σ_p since they are filled. In the space charge region these centers change their charge state as they cross E_F, thereby increasing ρ. For these air leak alloys we have established that the photoluminescence at 78°K is not quenched. The dark ESR signal at $g = 2.0055$ ($N_s \approx 10^{15}$ spins cm^{-3}) is likewise unaffected.[10] So dangling bonds do not seem to have been created. However, O_1^- or O_2^- defects have been detected in x-irradiated air leak alloys.[10] (These states are presumably associated with some other defects X^+.) As in the chalcogenides such deep-lying states are expected to act as hole traps. Their density ($\approx 10^{16}$ cm^{-3}) is sufficient to account for the observed collapse in W but further work is in progress to determine the exact nature of the states responsible.

REFERENCES

1. R.W. Griffith, F.J. Kampas, P.E. Vanier, and M.D. Hirsch, J. Non-Cryst. Solids 35/36, 391 (1980).
2. P.E. Vanier, A.E. Delahoy, and R.W. Griffith, to appear.
3. P.E. Vanier and R.W. Griffith, Bull. Amer. Phys. Soc. 25, 330 (1980), and to appear.
4. A.E. Delahoy and R.W. Griffith, to appear.
5. W. Beyer, R. Fischer, and H. Overhof, Phil. Mag. B39, 205 (1979).
6. N.F. Mott and E.A. Davis, Electronic Processes in Noncrystalline Materials, (Oxford: Clarendon Press), p. 31 (1971).
7. W. Beyer, H. Mell, and H. Overhof, Proc. 7th Int. Conf. Amorphous and Liquid Semiconductors, (Edinburgh), p. 328 (1977).
8. P. O'Connor and J. Tauc, Solid State Comm. (to be published).
9. C.R. Wronski, B. Abeles, G.D. Cody, D.L. Morel and T. Tiedje, Proc. 14th IEEE Photovoltaic Specialists Conf., San Diego, 1057 (1980).
10. P.C. Taylor, private communication.

SPIN POLARIZATION EFFECTS IN THE PHOTOCONDUCTIVITY OF a-Si:H#

E.A. SCHIFF

The University of Chicago, Chicago, Illinois 60637

ABSTRACT

The influence of electron spin resonance and of magnetic field on the photoconductivity of plasma-deposited a-Si:H has been studied. New dynamics measurements are interpreted as evidence for a spin-dependent trapping process, and the relationship between the ESR and magnetic field effects is established. It is also proposed that geminate recombination is required to account for the optical flux dependence of these effects.

INTRODUCTION

Electron spin resonance is an important approach to characterizing defects in semiconductors. However, in the best grade a-Si:H spin densities are too low ($N_s < 10^{16} cm^{-3}$) to be useful for characterizing typical thin film samples ($d \sim 1 \mu m$). The discovery by Solomon, et al[1] that electron spin resonance can be readily detected in the photoconductivity of a-Si:H even though the spin density is unobservable with direct measurements suggests that this spin-dependent photoconductivity (SDPC) may be a useful alternate approach to characterizing the defects involved in recombination.

A second, related effect with a simpler experimental configuration is the magnetic field dependent photoconductivity (HDPC) first reported in a-Si:H by Mell, et al[2]; this effect also promises to provide important information about recombination processes. The exact relationship between these two effects has not been established for the photoconductivity of a-Si:H, although there has been considerable progress with the analogous effects in low-temperature luminescence[3]

In this paper I report the first measurements of dynamics and optical flux dependence of the HDPC and SDPC effects. These measurements show that there are two components to the SDPC resonance lineshape, and that the dynamics of SDPC are not compatible with the dynamics expected solely from generation or recombination effects. To account for the anomolous dynamics a spin-dependent trapping mechanism is proposed. The measurements also address two questions. First, which of the theories for spin-dependent recombination[4-6] accounts best for the observed relationship of the HDPC and SDPC effects? Second, are these effects due to geminate recombinations?

EXPERIMENTAL DETAILS

The specimens used in the present work were prepared by RF plasma decomposition from a 10:1 argon/silane mixture without doping gases. Specimens were deposited on Corning 7059 glass substrates held at 260°C; the growth rate was approximately 1.5 Å/s and the specimens were 1.5 μm thick. The largest spin-dependent photoconductivity effects were observed in cathode specimens. Measurements were performed with 3000 V/cm bias in a commercial microwave cavity and ESR bridge system operating at ~9.5 GHz. The full microwave power

ISSN:0094-243X/81/730233-05$1.50 Copyright 1981 American Institute of Physics

of this system (300mW) was normally employed; the cavity Q was 1500 with the specimen in place. Specimens were illuminated using a 75W tungsten halogen bulb and appropriate filters and were at 300 K.

Both the magnetic-field dependence of the photoconductivity and the spin resonance effects were detected using magnetic field modulation; the spectra measured as a function of the magnetic field are thus proportional to the derivative of the photoconductivity with respect to the field. Both the in-phase and quadrature spectra were recorded. A light emitting diode was used to measure the specimen's photoconductive response as a function of modulation frequency while the specimen was simultaneously illuminated by the main light source.

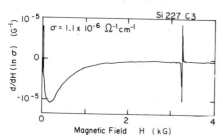

Fig. 1: Magnetic field derivative spectra of photoconductivity in the presence of 9.5 GHz microwaves.

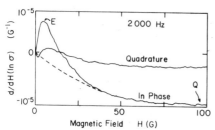

Fig. 2: Low magnetic field derivative spectra at 2000 Hz modulation frequency E-enhancing, Q-quenching.

MEASUREMENTS

The magnetic-field derivative spectrum in the presence of microwave radiation is illustrated in Fig. 1. The sharp feature at 3.25 kG is due to electron spin resonance; the low field features are not influenced by the microwaves. The ESR effect decreases the photoconductivity, as does the broad magnetic field effect. Close to the magnetic-field origin an enhancement of the photoconductivity is observed. These effects have been reported earlier.[1-2]

A closer examination of the low-field region of the spectrum in Fig. 1 is presented in Fig. 2. Fig. 2 was taken at a magnetic-field modulation frequency which is somewhat lower than the frequency at which the specimen's response to light modulation has fallen by 3 db. It is evident in Fig. 2 that the quadrature and the in-phase spectra of HDPC are not identical. We account for this behavior with the following picture. The extrema E (enhancement) and Q (quenching)are associated with two distinct frequency independent spectra with different relaxation behavior. For the conditions of Fig. 2 the enhancing effect shows little relaxation relative to the quenching effect, accounting for the relative absence of the enhancing feature in the quadrature spectrum. The dashed line in Fig. 2 is an extrapolation of the quenching spectrum and was used to establish a baseline for the enhancing spectrum.

A similar approach has been used to interpret the SDPC spectrum near 3.25 kG shown in Fig. 3. The quadrature spectrum is associated with a g-value of 2.0093. The best estimate for the g-value of spec-

trum remaining after removal of the g=2.0093 line is g=2.0057. I spe-
culatively assign the g=2.0093 line to trapped holes near the valence
band edge, in accord with ESR on B-doped specimens.

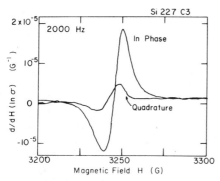

Fig. 3: ESR derivative spectra
of the photoconductivity at
2000 Hz.

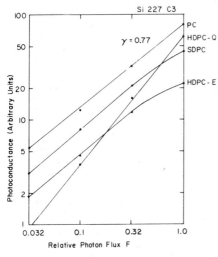

Fig. 4: Photoconductance
response vs. photon flux(100Hz).
PC: photoconductance
HDPC-Q: low-field quenching
feature.
HDPC-E: low-field enhancing
feature.
SDPC:ESR-effect.

A clear correlation was found between the sharp enhancing HDPC feature at small fields and the SDPC
amplitude. In Fig. 4 the magnitudes
of these two effects, as well as of
the broad HDPC quenching effect and
the photoconductivity are plotted
logarithmically as a function of the
photon flux. The modulation frequency for these data was 100Hz, well below the -3db frequencies for this
specimen at these flux levels. The
contributions of the two SDPC lines
were not separated. The correlation
seen in Fig. 4 between the SDPC and
the enhancing HDPC feature was also
found in the dependence of the two
effects on modulation frequency.
The broad HDPC quenching effect is
quite superlinear with photon flux.
It is uncertain at this time whether
this quenching HDPC effect can be
related to part of the SDPC effects.
It is also noteworthy that the SDPC
effect and the photoconductivity are
nearly proportional.

Perhaps the most surprising observation in the present work is
that the dynamics of the SDPC effect
is quite different from that observed with light modulation. The dynamics data obtained for two different illumination levels are illustrated in Fig. 5. For both levels
the light modulation data (LED)show
the monotonic decrease with increasing frequency expected for generation rate modulation. The observed
relaxation times are much longer
than typical recombination times
(<1 μ sec) and are due to trapping
effects. The SDPC data obviously
have very different dynamics; a model for the dynamics will be presented in the next section. Preliminary
excitation spectrum experiments show
that, for a given specimen photoconductivity, the SDPC modulation is
twice as large for 3 eV excitation than for broadband excitation.

236

This effect may be due to the effects of the surface or of geminate pair formation and is under investigation. Surface sensitivity for SDPC has been noted by Solomon.[4]

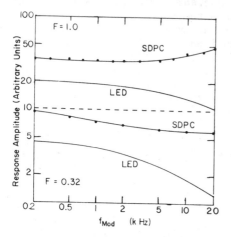

Fig. 5: Photoconductance response to light modulation (LED) and ESR (SDPC) as a function of modulation frequency. F: relative photon flux.

DISCUSSION

All extant models for spin-dependent recombination are closely related to the "radical pair" approach long known to scientists studying chemically induced magnetic polarization. Recombination of an electron-hole pair is assumed to occur principally when the spin wavefunction of the pair has some spin singlet character. In the version of this theory described recently by Haberkorn and Dietz[6] all thermalization times are assumed longer than the pair life-time and exchange is neglected. At H=0 all spin states are degenerate; only singlet pairs S recombine, with the triplet states T_{+1}, T_0, and T_{-1} being dissociated thermally. A magnetic field lifts this degeneracy and couples the S and T_0 eigenstates; the recombination rate thus increases, but the T_{+1} and T_{-1} states still don't recombine. Electron spin resonance on either the electron or hole spins then couples the T_{+1} and T_{-1} eigenstates to the remaining eigenstates, increasing the recombination rate again.

This theory predicts that the SDPC effect and the HDPC quenching effect should be related; in fact, we have shown that the HDPC enhancing effect is correlated with SDPC. This observation has been accounted for by Mell, et al,[2] who invoke magnetic field dependent thermalization times to destroy the coherence of the H=0 eigenstates, but leave the high magnetic field eigenstates unchanged.

This model describes recombination; however, any photoconductive response due to modulation of either the recombination or generation rates must decrease monotonically as the f_{mod} exceeds the reciprocal response time of the photoconductor.[7] In contrast, the SDPC magnitude actually increases at this response frequency at high photon flux (Fig. 5). I propose here that these anomolous dynamics are due to spin-dependent trapping. Thus, the spin resonance effect acts to increase the cross-section for capture of a photocarrier at a center from which it is ultimately detached thermally. The modification of the trapping parameters does not modify the steady state photoconductivity of a material in the absence of extensive optical charge transfer in the gap states.[7] However, if the modulation of the trapping parameter is faster than the material's photoconductive response time an effect will be observed and can account for the anomolous dynamics.

The process which I propose to account for spin-dependent trapping is an extension of the recombination process described above. A photocarrier interacts weakly with a singly occupied center in the gap with spin. Capture of the carrier results in a doubly occupied spin singlet center; the cross-section for the capture process is clearly spin-dependent and can in principle lead either to recombination or trapping.

Returning to the low f_{mod} processes, the near proportionality of the SDPC effect and the photoconductivity is prima facie evidence for geminate recombination. The recombination lifetime in the specimen examined here depends strongly on the optical flux, as evidenced by the fact that the slope of the linear logarithmic relationship between the photoconductivity and the photon flux is .77 (Fig. 4). The importance of a normal spin-dependent recombination process can thus in principle also vary with photon flux, as evidenced in the present work by the HDPC quenching effect and the strong flux dependence of the SDPC dynamics. Any modulation of the recombination probability for a geminate pair, however, should be independent of the optical flux and thus give rise to a response which is proportional to the photoconductivity. The hypothesis of geminate recombination is also required to account for preliminary SDPC temperature-dependence measurements; this model postulates that geminate recombination plays a fairly minor role in the room-temperature photoconductivity, for which the temperature dependence is dominated by recombination lifetime effects. Finally, if geminate recombination does account for the SDPC effect, it is evident that the thermalized pair cannot be in its singlet state; I suggest that intersystem crossing involved in the triplet mechanism developed for chemically induced magnetic polarization[8] might provide the required spin polarization of the geminate pair.

The author gratefully acknowledges conversations with H. Fritzsche and P. D. Persans.

Supported by the NSF (DMR 80-09225) and by the NSF-MRL at The University of Chicago. Additional support from USDOE 03-79-ET-23034.

REFERENCES

1. I. Solomon, D. Biegelson and J. C. Knights, Solid State Comm. 22, 505 (1977).
2. H. Mell, B. Movaghar, and L. Schweitzer, Phys. Stat. Sol. (b) 88, 531 (1978).
3. D. K. Biegelson, J. C. Knights, R. A. Street, C. Tsang, and R. M. White, Phil. Mag. B, 37, 477 (1978).
4. I. Solomon, J. Non-Cryst. Sol. 35/36, 625 (1980).
5. B. Movaghar, B. Ries, and L. Schweitzer, Phil. Mag. B 41, 159 (1980).
6. R. Haberkorn and W. Wietz, Solid State Comm. 35, 505 (1980).
7. A. Rose, Concepts in Photoconductivity and Allied Problems (Krieger, N.Y. 1978).
8. P. W. Atkins, in Chemically Induced Magnetic Polarization, edited by L.T. Muus, et al (D. Reidel, Dordrecht, 1977), p. 191.

INFRARED QUENCHING OF PHOTOCONDUCTIVITY: RECOMBINATION IN a-Si:H*

P.D.Persans and H.Fritzsche

University of Chicago, Chicago, IL 60637

ABSTRACT

We report dual beam photoconductivity measurements on undoped and lightly doped glow discharge a-Si:H. Infrared quenching of photoconductivity is observed for T<200K. A temperature and sample independent optical quenching threshold of 0.5-0.6eV is found which indicates a low energy cutoff in the distribution of gap states which give rise to quenching. The electron capture coefficient of these states is estimated to be $4 \times 10^{-13} cm^3 sec^{-1}$ at 133K.

INTRODUCTION

The distribution of gap states in a-Si:H allows a variety of recombination paths for photogenerated carriers. In the present study we wish to identify different groups of recombination centers by means of dual beam photoconductivity modulation. This technique involves the use of a steady pump light beam with $h\nu>1.5$ eV and a modulation beam with 0.6 eV$<h\nu<1.5$ eV. The pump beam establishes a steady state photoconductivity and, besides producing free carriers, causes a change in the occupancy of gap states which act as recombination centers. The occupancy of recombination centers in selected energy ranges is altered by the second chopped monochromatic light beam. These changes are detected as a modulation of the photocurrent. The modulation spectrum of the photoconductivity changes with sample temperature, pump beam intensity, and the wavelength and chopping frequency of the infrared modulation beam, indicating the presence of different groups of recombination centers. We shall discuss here only a few aspects of the dual beam spectroscopy. A more complete description of the results and their analysis will appear elsewhere.[1,2] In the following we describe measurements of infrared quenching of photoconductivity in the temperature range from 100K to 200K on undoped and lightly doped films.

The existence of infrared quenching implies that there are at least two distinct groups of recombination centers, one having a smaller majority photocarrier recombination coefficient than the other.[3] We assume that the majority photocarriers are electrons. At low pump light levels recombination takes place primarily through states close to the dark Fermi level E_F which we designate as r-type centers with recombination coefficients b_{rn} and b_{rp} for electrons and holes, respectively. At high pump light levels s-type centers below the dark Fermi level also act as recombination centers. If $b_{sn} < b_{rn}$ $b_{sp} \backsim b_{rp}$ then the electron lifetime will increase as the trap quasi-Fermi level E_{tp}^s for holes passes downwards through the s-type centers and their occupation becomes recombination controlled.[4] An electron can then be excited by the infrared modulation beam from the valence band to an unoccupied s-type center. Some of the holes generated in the valence band by the infrared beam will be captured by r-type states. Since unoccupied r-type states are more efficient electron recombination centers than s-states, a decrease in electron photocurrent results. The distribution of r-type and s-type states can be explored by varying the temperature and the pump light intensity which determine the occupancy of the states and the positions of the electron and hole trap quasi-Fermi levels.

EXPERIMENTAL DETAILS

Amorphous Si films were deposited from an RF plasma discharge of SiH_4 mixed in the ratio 1:3 in Ar buffer gas. Details of preparation will be discussed elsewhere.[2] The samples in this study were deposited under the following conditions onto Corning 7059 glass substrates clamped to the plates of a capacitively coupled system: T = 530K; gas pressure = 150 mTorr; gas flow rate = 30 sccm; RF peak to peak voltage = 250 V; dc bias voltage = 100 V. Films were doped by premixing PH_3 or B_2H_6 into the SiH_4. Samples were 2 μm thick. Cr contacts with a length of 1 cm and a gap of 0.05 cm were evaporated on top of the films. All films exhibited ohmic photocurrent up to 10^4 V cm^{-1}. Measurements were usually made in a two probe configuration.

The dc pump light source was a tungsten-halide lamp focused onto the sample through a Corning #69 heat filter. The modulation beam consisted of chopped light passed through a glass prism monochromator. Current through the sample was measured using a Keithley 616 electrometer which was also used as a current preamplifier for an HR8 lock-in amplifier used to detect the photocurrent modulation signal.

RESULTS AND DISCUSSION

The temperature dependence of the dc photoconductance of undoped and lightly doped films is shown in Fig. 1 for a pump beam flux of 2×10^{16} photons cm^{-2} sec^{-1}. The doping levels and the activation energies E_σ and E_{ph} of the dark and photoconductivities, respectively, are listed for these films in Table 1. Temperature activated photoconductivity is attributed to a decrease in the free carrier lifetime as T is decreased.[5,6] This is due either to i) an increase in the number of recombination centers as T is decreased and the free carrier

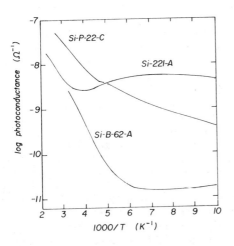

Table 1. Sample Parameters

Sample	Dopant [Gas Ratio]	E_σ (eV)	E_{ph} (eV)
Si-221-A	------	0.9	0.20
Si-P-22-C	PH_3 [3ppm]	0.67	0.12
Si-B-62-A	B_2H_6 [3ppm]	0.9	0.22

Fig. 1. Temperature dependence of the dc photoconductance excited by 2×10^{16} photons cm^{-2} sec^{-1} for the samples listed in Table 1.

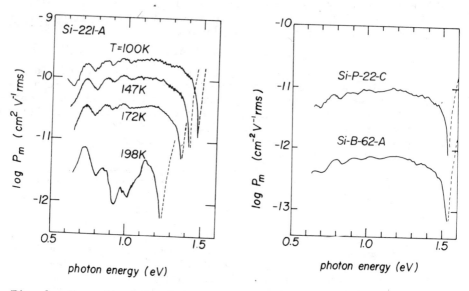

Fig. 2. Normalized in phase modulation photoconductance $P_m(h\nu_m)$ for 5Hz chopping speed with the same pump conditions as in Fig. 1: (a) Undoped sample Si-221-A at several temperatures; (b) Lightly doped samples Si-P-22-C and Si-B-62-A at T = 100K. Solid lines indicate negative and dashed lines indicate positive modulation sign.

Fermi levels E_{fn} and E_{fp} spread apart and enclose more states or to ii) temperature dependent recombination coefficients. The increase in photoconductance observed in sample Si-221-A below 250K is surprising because it implies that either new recombination centers with smaller recombination coefficients are being enclosed within the trap quasi-Fermi levels as T is decreased or that the recombination coefficient for a single type of center reaches a maximum at 250K and then decreases. Anomalous photoconductance temperature dependence has previously been observed by other groups.[7] One can distinguish between these possibilities using dual beam photoconductivity; the observation of infrared quenching verifies the existence of two types of recombination center.

In Fig. 2a we show the in-phase modulation spectrum $P_m(h\nu_m)$ of Si-221-A for several temperatures. P_m is the modulation photoconductance normalized linearly by the incident modulation beam photon flux. The pump beam had a photon flux of about 2×10^{16} photons cm^{-2} sec^{-1}. The absolute magnitude of the decrease in photoconductance shown in Fig. 2 is much smaller than the total photoconductance of the sample, thus the spectra shown represent only a small perturbation on the pump photoconductance. As the modulation beam photon energy is increased above 1.4 eV the sign of the modulation photoconductance changes to positive as expected since additional band gap light causes an increase in the total photoconductance. The change in sign of P_m appears as a sharp downward spike because of the logarithmic scale of Fig. 2a. The infrared quenching signal decreases with increasing temperature until it is unobservable above 210K.

Infrared quenching of photoconductivity is also observed in samples SiP-22-C and Si-B-62-A at low temperature, as shown in Fig. 2b. The temperature dependence of the photoconductivity is radically different in these films from that of the undoped film. The presence of s-states alone is not sufficient to observe thermal quenching; we conclude that they exist in sufficient relative number below E_f in Si-221-A to cause an increase of the photoconductance by at least a factor of two at 250K.

The optical quenching threshold E_q can be used to determine whether the s-states are distributed or localized in energy below mid-gap. The dependence of P_m on photon energy is given by:[2,8]

$$P_m \cdot h\nu_m \propto \int_0^\infty \eta_q |M|^2 N_v(E) N_s(E+h\nu_m) [1-f_s(E+h\nu_m)] dE \qquad (1)$$

where η_q is the quantum efficiency; $N_v(E)$ and $N_s(E)$ are the valence and s-state densities of states; M is the optical matrix element; and f_s is the occupation function for s-states. The threshold energy for optical quenching thus depends upon the distribution and occupation of s-states. The quenching threshold should shift with E_{tp}^s if the trap quasi-Fermi level is moving within the s-state distribution. If E_{tp}^s is below the s-state distribution in energy then the threshold for quenching should not shift with light level and temperature.

In order to determine the infrared quenching threshold we assume that η_q and M are independent of $h\nu_m$ and that $N_v(E) \propto (E_v-E)^{1/2}$. Assuming a sharp distribution of s-states at E_s, Eq. (1) reduces to $(P_m \cdot h\nu_m)^2 \propto (h\nu_m-(Es-Ev))$. A uniform distribution of s-states gives $(P_m \cdot h\nu_m)^{3/2} \propto (h\nu_m-(E_{tp}^s-E_v))$. We have plotted $(P_m \cdot h\nu_m)^{3/2}$ versus $h\nu$ for sample Si-221-A in Fig. 3 at T = 100K, 148K, and 172K. A temperature independent threshold energy of $E_q = 0.58\pm0.05$ eV is found. A shift in E_q of 0.2 eV is expected if E_{tp}^s is moving through a distribution of s-states as T increases from 100K to 172K. We also note that E_q for both samples Si-P-22-C and Si-B-62-A is 0.55 eV$\pm$0.05 eV. The steady state photoconductivity of the three samples varies by over three orders of magnitude at 100K; it is expected in a distributed states model that the threshold should differ in the three films by about 0.1 eV. On the basis of the absence of T dependence and sample dependence of E_q we propose that the small capture coefficient states which give rise to infrared quenching have a lower cutoff energy of 0.5 eV to 0.6 eV above Ev. So far we have neglected the possibility of a Franck-Condon shift. This might lower the relative threshold for thermal excitations by 0.1 to 0.2 eV.

An estimate of the electron capture coefficient for unoccupied s-type centers can be made by analyzing the rate equation for the occupation of the s-states in the presence of quenching radiation Fq:

$$dn_s/dt = nb_{sn}(N_s-n_s) - pb_{sp}n_s + F_q S_q \eta_q (N_s-n_s) \qquad (2)$$

where S_q is the optical cross section for the excitation of a hole to the valence band from an s-center, and N_s and n_s are the densities of s-states and occupied s-states, respectively. When the optical release rate for holes (third term on right) becomes comparable to either of the other terms, the magnitude of the quenching signal will become nonlinear in Fq. Setting the first and third terms equal at

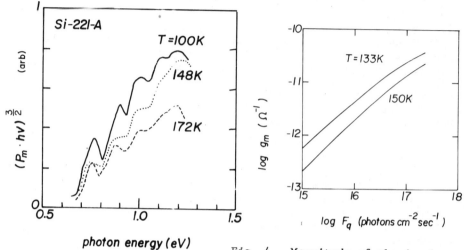

Fig. 3. $(P_m \cdot h\nu_m)$ vs $h\nu_m$ for Si-221-A at T=100, 148, and 172K.

Fig. 4. Magnitude of the in-phase modulation photoconductance at 3Hz plotted vs F_q at 1.0 eV. Pump photoconductance was $4 \times 10^{-10} \Omega^{-1}$.

the onset of nonlinearity F_q' we find $b_{sn} = F_q' S_q \eta_q / n$. The F_q dependence of the negative modulation photoconductance g_m for T=133K and 150K is shown in Fig. 4. If we use $F_q' \sim 10^{17} cm^{-2} sec^{-1}$ and calculate $n = 1.5 \times 10^{12} cm^{-3}$ for a mobility of 1 $cm^2 V^{-1} sec^{-1}$ and we assume $S_q = 10^{17} cm^2$ based on photoinduced absorption data,[8] we estimate $b_{sn} = 4 \times 10^{-13} cm^3 sec^{-1}$. Recombination coefficients for sensitizing centers in crystals[9] range from 10^{-12} to $10^{-15} cm^3 sec^{-1}$. Typical coefficients for neutral centers are $10^{-8} cm^3 sec^{-1}$.

We have demonstrated that dual beam photoconductivity modulation techniques can be used to extract new information about recombination in a-Si. The existence of a small capture coefficient center has been established. Further measurements and analysis using this important tool will soon be published.

REFERENCES

*Supported in part by the NSF-MRL program at The University of Chicago and by NSF Grant DMR-8009225.
1. P. D. Persans, Solid State Commun. <u>36</u>, 851 (1981).
2. P. D. Persans, to be published.
3. A. Rose, <u>Concepts in Photoconductivity and Allied Problems</u> (Interscience, New York, 1980).
4. G. W. Taylor and J. G. Simmons, J. Phys. Chem. <u>9</u>, 1013 (1976).
5. C. R. Wronski and R. E. Daniel, Phys. Rev. <u>B23</u>, 794 (1981).
6. W. Fuhs, M. Milleville, and J. Stuke, Phys. Status Solidi <u>B89</u>, 495 (1978).
7. R. W. Griffith, F. J. Kampas, P. E. Vanier, and M. D. Hirsh, J. Non-Cryst. Solids <u>35/36</u>, 391 (1980).
8. P. O'Connor and J. Tauc, Solid State Commun. <u>36</u>, 947 (1981).
9. R. H. Bube and F. Cardon, J. Appl. Phys. <u>35</u>, 2712 (1964).

OPTICAL PICOSECOND STUDIES OF CARRIER

THERMALIZATION IN AMORPHOUS SILICON

Z. Vardeny and J. Tauc*
Division of Engineering and Department of Physics
Brown University, Providence, RI   02912

C. J. Fang**
Max-Planck-Institut, Stuttgart, FRG

ABSTRACT

Thermalization of photogenerated hot carriers in a-Si, a-Si:H and a-Si:H:F was studied using the pump and probe method with sub-picosecond resolution. The process is optically observable because the absorption cross-section of the hot carriers depends on their excess energy. It was found that the energy dissipation rate to phonons is the maximum possible in a-Si while in a-Si:H it is slower and can be described by Fröhlich interaction with polar phonons.

EXPERIMENTAL RESULTS

We used the pump and probe technique (Fig. 1a) with a passively mode locked dye laser for studying the ultrafast dynamics of photo-generated carriers in a-Si, a-Si:H (C_H = 4 to 24 at %), a-Si:F (C_F = 12 at %) and a-Si:H:F (C_F = 10 to 18 at %). The dye laser and experimental set up have been described elsewhere[1,2]. The laser produces linearly polarized light pulses of t_p = 0.6 to 0.8 ps duration at $\hbar\omega_p$ = 2eV, with about 2 nJ per pulse, and repetition rate of $10^6 s^{-1}$. The probe beam was passed through a polarization rotator and its polarization was either parallel ($\parallel$) or perpendicular ($\perp$) to that of the pump beam. The photoinduced carrier densities were estimated to be about $10^{19} cm^{-3}$ and 1 to 4 x $10^{18} cm^{-3}$ per pulse in a-Si and a-Si:H respectively.

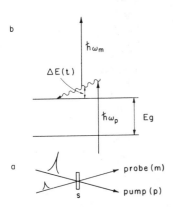

Fig. 1 - a) Pump and probe technique.
b) Proposed mechanism for photo-induced absorption.

The observed changes ΔT in the transmission T_r correspond to induced absorption $\Delta\alpha$ =$\Delta T/T_r d$ where d is the sample thickness (in the range of 0.3 to 2.5μm). Typical results for $\parallel$ polarizations are shown in Fig. 2. Most a-Si:H and a-Si:H:F samples show an initial nonsymmetric response around t = 0 that decays fast to a lower value $\Delta\alpha_s$ persisting over 50ps independently

244

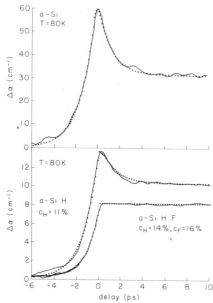

Fig. 2 – Time dependence of
the photoinduced absorption in
a-Si, a-Si:H (C_H = 11% and
a-Si:H:F (C_H = 14%, C_F = 16%),
for parallel polarization.
Solid curves – experimental,
dotted curves – calculated.

of temperature; this behavior is
observed in a-Si only at low T.
When $\perp$ polarization is used the
peak in $\Delta\alpha$ is reduced; this is
ascribed to the reduction of the
coherent artifact component[3].
The depolarization ratio at long
times (up to 30 ps at least)
$\Delta\alpha_s(\perp)/\Delta\alpha_s(\parallel)$ is equal to 1 in
non-hydrogenated samples at 300K
but is between 0.6 and 0.8 in
hydrogenated samples at
all T[3].

The proposed mechanism for explaining the data shown in Fig. 2 is
described in Fig. 1b. Hot carriers
(with excess energy ΔE) are excited
across the band gap E_g by the pump
pulse of energy $\hbar\omega_p$. These carriers thermalize to the bottom of
the band by loosing their energy
due to the electron-phonon interactions. During this process they
can absorb light ($\hbar\omega_m$). The optical cross-section σ for the absorption of hot carriers depends on the
instantaneous excess energy of the
carriers[4]. This makes the thermalization process observable by optical
methods. The response $\Delta\alpha_s$ corres-
ponds to carriers at the bottom of the band. These carriers can subsequently be removed either by trapping or recombination. This
effect has been observed at room temperature in a-Si[2] and recently
we observed it also in a-Si:F. However, in the hydrogenated samples
$\Delta\alpha_s$ persists over 50ps at all T; this behavior is observed in a-Si
at low T. In this paper, we concentrate on the fastest component
of the decay which we associate with thermalization.

We can exclude some possible origins of the fastest component
of the observed decay. It is easy to see that it cannot be due to
coherent artifact alone. Using the $\parallel$ and $\perp$ polarizations we determined the contribution of the coherent artifact and reconstructed[3]
the true impulse response function A(t). It is a step function at
t = 0 followed by a fast decay down to $\Delta\alpha_s$ which can be approximated
by a linear function of time. The fast decay cannot be due to two
photon absorption which would give a symmetric peak, should not
depend on C_H and at our light intensity of 0.3 GW/cm^2 is estimated[5]
to give $\Delta\alpha$ two orders smaller than observed.

The relative height of the measured peak at t = 0 is closely
related to the average initial excess energy $\overline{\Delta E}(0) = (\hbar\omega_p - E_g)/2$.

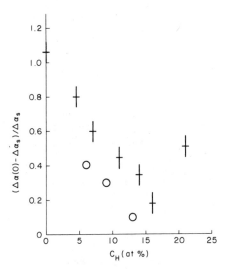

Fig. 3 - Variation of the relative height of the induced absorption peak at t = 0 with hydrogen concentration. Crosses for a-Si:H, circles for a-Si:H:F.

This is seen in Fig. 3 where $\Delta = (\Delta\alpha(0) - \Delta\alpha_s)/\Delta\alpha_s$ is plotted against C_H. Δ decreases with C_H until C_H = 16%; this can be related to the increase of E_g produced by increasing the hydrogen content. In a-Si:H:F Δ is smaller than in a-Si:H with the same C_H, in agreement with the higher E_g of a-Si:H:F[6].

We can explain the fast component as well as the residual one by phonon assisted free carrier absorption (FCA). The generation of free carriers in these materials was demonstrated by the picosecond photoconductivity studies of Johnson et al[7]. In addition, $\Delta\alpha_s$ scales with the density of photogenerated carriers (Fig. 2). The optical absorption cross-section σ calculated from $\Delta\alpha_s$ is $3 \times 10^{-18} cm^2$ which is close to σ of free carriers in a-Si[5] ($2 \times 10^{-18} cm^2$ at 2eV and 80K).

The data indicate that the excess energy dissipation rate by interaction of electrons with phonons $d\Delta E/dt$ is the fastest possible[8] $h\nu^2$ in a-Si while it is slower in hydrogenated samples. The calculated average of $h\nu^2$ over the phonon spectrum was found to be 0.5eV/ps and this gives in a-Si a thermalization time t_0 = 0.6 ps but only 0.2 ps in a-Si:H with C_H = 11%, which is much shorter than the decay time seen for this sample in Fig. 2. A possible slower dissipation mechanism is by coupling to polar phonons only (Fröhlich coupling)[9]. This coupling is possible because of the presence of ir active vibrations in these materials[10]. We calculated the maximum $d\Delta E/dt$ for this interaction and found 0.1 eV/ps. This rate is smaller than the carrier-carrier energy dissipation rate[9] (0.3 eV/ps) and, therefore, a hot carrier temperature T_e can be defined in this case but not in a-Si.

For a-Si:H, we calculated the average $(d\Delta E/dt)_{pol}$ using a Boltzmann distribution $\exp(-\Delta E/kT_e)$ integrated over the ir active phonon spectrum[10]; the dependence of $(d\Delta E/dt)_{pol}$ on T_e is shown in Fig. 4. The rate increases sharply with T_e up to $T_e \simeq 1500K$, suggesting that in this region the thermalization time t_0 and the thermalization radius r_0 depend only weakly on the excitation photon energy. The time dependence of T_e was obtained by numerically solving the equation $(3/2)kdT_e/dt = -[d\Delta E(T_e)/dt]_{pol}$ with $T_e(0) = 2/3\overline{\Delta E}(0)/k = 800K$ in a-Si:H with C_H = 11%, T = 80K.

246

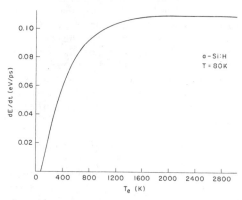

Fig. 4 – Calculated hot carrier excess energy dissipation rate $(d\Delta E/dt)_{pol}$ due to Fröhlich interaction with polar phonons in a-Si:H (T = 80K) as a function of carrier temperature T_e.

$T_e(t)$ could be approximated as $T_e(t) - T = 800(1-t/t_o)$ with $t_o = 1.2$ ps. The experimental curve could be fit by taking $A(t) \sim \sigma(t) = \sigma_o[1+aT_e(0)(1-t/1.2)]$ for $t < 1.2$ ps, and $\sigma = \sigma_o$ for $t > 1.2$ ps, with one adjustable parameter a (enhancement). a was found to be approximately independent of C_H; its value $1.7 \times 10^{-3}K^{-1}$ is close to the theoretical value of $1.3 \times 10^{-3}K^{-1}$ for FCA at 2eV assisted by optical deformation potential scattering in crystals[4].

A different approach was used for a-Si where T_e is not defined. We replace the Boltzmann distribution by an initial non-equilibrium distribution $f_i(\Delta E) \sim \sqrt{\Delta E} \sqrt{\hbar\omega_p - E_g - \Delta E}$ which was assumed to be proportional to the product of the densities of states of the initial and final states during generation. We assumed that the enhancement in the absorption cross-section of hot carriers depends linearly on the excess energy $\Delta\sigma = b\Delta E$ and calculated $\Delta\sigma(t)$ using the distribution $f_i(\Delta E)$ in which ΔE decreases with time according to $d\Delta E/dt = 0.5$ eV/ps. We could approximate $\Delta\sigma(t)$ by a linearly decreasing function of 0.7 ps duration. The fit shown in Fig. 2 was obtained with $b = 1.2 \times 10^{-3}K^{-1}$ (to be compared with $a = 1.7 \times 10^{-3}K^{-1}$ for the hydrogenated samples).

The general agreement with the data, self-consistency and reasonable values for the adjustable parameters point out the plausibility of the proposed explanation of the ultrafast decay of the photoinduced absorption as due to hot carrier phonon-assisted mechanism.

We thank J. Strait for his help with computer calculations.

*The work at Brown was supported in part by NSF grant DMR79-09819 and the NSF-MRL program at Brown University.

**On leave from Chinese University of Science and Technology, Beijing, People's Republic of China.

REFERENCES

1. E. P. Ippen and C. V. Shank, in Ultrafast Light Pulses (ed. by S. L. Shapiro) Springer, NY, 1977, p. 83.
2. D. E. Ackley, T. Tauc and W. Paul, Phys. Rev. Lett. 43, 715 (1979).
3. An explanation of polarization effects will be given in a forthcoming paper.
4. K. Seeger, Semiconductor Physics, Springer, New York, 1973, p. 374.
5. T. F. Reintges and T. C. McGroddy, Phys. Rev. Lett. 30, 901 (1973).
6. A. Madan and S. R. Ovshinsky, J. Non-Cryst. Sol., 35, 171 (1980).
7. A. M. Johnson, P. H. Auston, P. R. Smith, J. C. Bean, J. P. Harbison and D. Kaplan, in Picosecond Phenomena II (ed. by R. M. Hochstrasser et al.) Springer, NY, 1980, p. 71 and 285.
8. D. M. Pai and R. C. Enck, Phys. Rev. B11, 5163 (1975).
9. E. M. Conwell, Solid State Physics, Supp. 9 (ed. by F. Seitz et al.) Acad. Press, NY, 1967.
10. M. H. Brodsky and A. Lurio, Phys. Rev. B9, 1646 (1974).

PICOSECOND TIME-RESOLVED PHOTOCONDUCTIVITY

IN AMORPHOUS SILICON

A. M. Johnson,[*] D. H. Auston, P. R. Smith
J. C. Bean, J. P. Harbison, and A. C. Adams.

Bell Laboratories, Murray Hill,
New Jersey, 07974, USA

ABSTRACT ·

An initial mobility of approximately 1 cm^2/Vs has been measured in three types of amorphous silicon by picosecond photoconductivity. The photocurrents are observed to decay at rates from 4 ps to 200 ps depending on the method of sample preparation. The initial mobility of a-Si:H was found to be thermally activated with an activation energy of approximately 60 meV and a pre-factor of 8 cm^2/Vs.

- - -

The relaxation of non-equilibrium carriers in amorphous semiconductors spans a time scale which extends from picoseconds to seconds and involves many different processes including thermalization, capture and emission by localized states, and recombination. The early time history is especially interesting since it relates more closely to the transport properties of the extended and localized states associated with the intrinsic disorder of the random atomic network, whereas the slower event tend to be influenced by the deeper states associated with structural defects and depend on the method of preparation. It is especially important to have more detailed information about the magnitude and temperature dependence of the mobility of carriers in extended states and to determine the magnitude and energy distribution of the shallow localized states.

To investigate these effects, we have developed a measurement technique[1] which enables us to directly observe transient photocurrents with a time resolution of approximately 10 ps. As illustrated in figure 1, the basic feature of this technique is to correlate the response of two photoconductors, each of which is

* Physics Dept., City College, CUNY, New York, NY 10031.

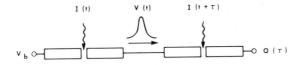

Figure 1.

mounted in a high speed circuit and illuminated by an
optical pulse of a few picoseconds duration($\hbar\omega$ = 2.2 eV).
One of the photoconductors has a dc bias applied to it
and the output signal from it is used to bias the second
photoconductor. The total charge, $Q(\tau)$, produced at the
output of the second photoconductor is measured as a
function of the time delay, τ , between the two optical
pulses. It is proportional to the convolution of the
two photoconductances, $g_1(t)$, and $g_2(t)$:

$$Q(\tau) \propto V_b Z_0 \int_{-\infty}^{+\infty} g_1(t)\, g_2(t+\tau)\, dt$$

When the two photoconductors are identical, the measurement gives an autocorrelation of the photoresponse. If,
however, one of the photoconductors is much faster than
the other, the measurement, which we call a cross-
correlation, acts similar to a sampling technique. This
approach has the additional advantage that problems due
to non-ohmic contacts can be avoided if the bias pulse
applied is very short relative to the dielectric relaxation time.

An example of this technique is illustrated in
figure 2 which is a plot of the autocorrelation of the
photoresponse of an amorphous silicon sample prepared by
low pressure chemical vapor deposition (CVD). The decay
of the photocurrent is non-exponential with an initial
slope of 16 ps/Neper (the wiggle on the right is an
electrical reflection from the edge of the circuit). A
calibration of the measurement permits us to estimate
the initial mobility to be 1 cm^2/Vs. A similar measurement of an evaporated (EV) a-Si sample had an initial
decay of approximately 4 ps and the same initial mobility
of 1 cm^2/Vs. The more rapid decay rate in the EV sample
is expected from the higher defect density(approximately
10^{20}/cm^3 vs 10^{19}/cm^3 for the CVD sample).

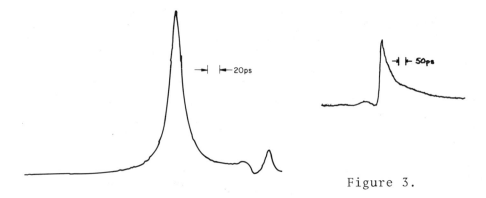

Figure 3.

Figure 2.

In figure 3 , the transient photocurrent of an
a-Si:H sample prepared by RF glow discharge is shown
as obtained by a cross-correlation measurement with a
very fast radiation-damaged silicon-on-sapphire
photoconductor[2]. The decay is highly non-exponential and
much slower than the CVD and EV samples, as would be
expected for this lower defect density material. The ini-
al mobility, however, is 0.8 cm^2/Vs, comparable to the
other two samples, which suggests that the transport
mechanism responsible for the initial photocurrent is
due to the intrinsic disorder of the a-Si network and
is not strongly affected by the density of structural
defects arising from the different methods of preparation.
A possible interpretation of this result is that the
initial photocurrent arises from carriers in extended

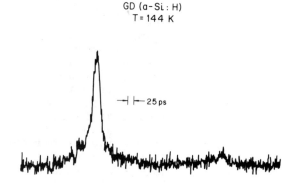

GD (a-Si:H)
T = 144 K

states prior to
capture by localiz-
ed states. To det-
ermine if this is
the case, we have
repeated this exp-
eriment at lower
temperatures and
found that the
decay rate became
more rapid as
illustrated in
figure 4.The
initial mobility
was observed to
have an activated

Figure 4.

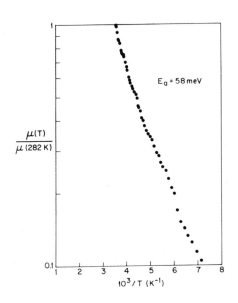

$$\frac{\mu(T)}{\mu(282\,K)}$$

$E_a = 58\,meV$

$10^3/T\ (K^{-1})$

Figure 5.

behavior with a charactistic energy of 0.058 eV as illustrated in figure 5. Although it is difficult to see in figure 4, there is a slow component to the signal corresponding to a mobility of 6 x 10^{-3}. If we extrapolate the temperature dependance of the initial mobility to infinite temperature, we obtain a prefactor of 8 cm^2/Vs, which is comparable to the theoretical mobility expected for extended states. this suggests that within our time resolution of 25 ps, a considerable fraction of the free carriers have already been captured by shallow localized states. The activation energy of 0.058 eV is an approximate measure of the average depth of these states from the mobility edge. Thermal emission from these states could account for the non-exponential decay observed at room temperature similar to the multiple trapping recently observed by Hvam and Brodsky[5] in phosphorous doped a-Si:H on much longer time scales. It is not clear, however, why the initial transient is so much faster at lower temperatures. It is possible that that this fast component(which is not completely resolved in this case) arises from the initial capture process. A capture time of approximately 1 ps would give a $\mu\tau$ product having the same area as the fast component in figure 4.

In summary, it is clear that improved time resolution can provide a unique insight into the transport properties of amorphous semiconductors. We are currently improving our measurement technique to provide more detail about the specific shape of the photocurrent decay so that comparisons can be made with multiple trapping and other theoretical models.

252

REFERENCES:

1. D. H. Auston, A. M. Johnson, P. R. Smith, and J. C. Bean, Appl. Phys. Lett. $\underline{37}$,371 (1980).
2. P. R. Smith, D. H. Auston, A. M. Johnson, and W. M. Augustyniak, Appl. Phys. Lett. $\underline{38}$,47(1981).
3. J. M. Hvam and M. H. Brodsky, Phys. Rev. Lett. $\underline{46}$, 371(1981).

RELAXATION OF PHOTOINDUCED SUB-BANDGAP ABSORPTION IN a-Si:H

S. Ray, Z. Vardeny and J. Tauc
Department of Physics and Division of Engineering
Brown University, Providence, RI   02912

T. Moustakas and B. Abeles
Exxon Research and Engineering Company, P.O. Box 45
Linden, NJ   07036

ABSTRACT

The decay of photoinduced sub-bandgap absorption (PA) following pulsed excitation was studied in the temperature range 80 - 305K, in a-Si:H samples prepared by glow discharge and sputtering. The decay was interpreted in terms of bimolecular diffusion limited recombination involving dispersive transport of electrons and was used for the determination of the dispersion parameter α. It was found to be a linear function of T in the glow-discharge sample while it was weakly T-dependent in the sputtered sample. In addition, a first measurement of the time evolution of the PA spectrum is reported.

INTRODUCTION

Photoinduced sub-bandgap absorption (PA) under steady illumination has been observed in tetrahedrally bonded amorphous semiconductors.[1] A first study of the relaxation of PA in doped and undoped a-Si:H following pulsed excitation has also been recently reported.[2] In this work the recombination of excess carriers was found to follow a diffusion limited bimolecular kinetics with a time dependent rate coefficient $b = B/t^{1-\alpha} (0 < \alpha < 1)$. This is a consequence of the dispersive nature of the transport characteristic of amorphous materials.[3] In this paper we extend the previous work to PA decay studies in a-Si:H as a function of sample preparation. We found different temperature dependences of the dispersion parameter α in the samples prepared by glow discharge (GD) and sputtering (SP); this indicates different modes of carrier transport in the two kinds of materials. We also measured time evolution of the PA spectrum in the sputtered a-Si:H sample at 305K. The shift of the band with increasing time towards higher energy is consistent with the idea of thermalisation of trapped carriers.

EXPERIMENT

The photoinduced absorption was excited by a dye laser pumped with a N_2 laser with the following parameters: photon energy $\simeq$ 2.1eV, repetion rate 20Hz, pulse energy 15μJ, pulse duration 10ns. The estimated carrier density produced by each exciting pulse is $\simeq 10^{18} cm^{-3}$. The transient absorption was probed with radiation from a tungsten lamp in the energy range from 0.7 to 1.4eV. The detection system consisted of a Ge photodiode (Judson J-16 LD), a broad

ISSN:0094-243X/81/730253-05$1.50 Copyright 1981 American Institute of Physics

band preamplifier followed by a boxcar integrator (PARC 162) and an x-y recorder. The time resolution of the experiment was 500ns. For measuring the time evolution of the PA spectrum, a monochromator was placed between the sample and the detector. The average energy resolution in the spectral range of interest was ≈ 0.03eV.

We report the results obtained on a GD sample with 16 at % H_2 and a SP sample with 19 at % H_2.

RESULTS AND DISCUSSION

Figure 1 shows a log-log plot of the fractional transmission change, $-\Delta T/T$, as a function of the delay time after the laser pulse for several temperatures between 80 and 306K. We note that for both the GD and SP samples the curves approximate a straight line, indicating a power law response, for almost three decades in time. The decay is faster at higher temperatures and is weaker than t^{-1} at all temperatures in both samples.

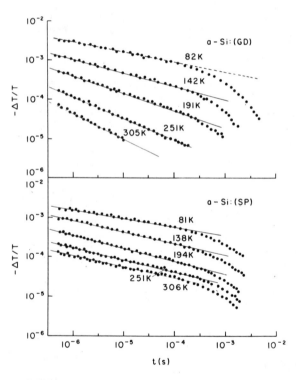

The straight line portions of the curves in Fig. 1 are followed by a faster decay at longer times. This decay is exponential and its time constant does not depend on temperature. We will not consider these last decays in this paper and in the following will discuss the origin of the decay represented by the straight lines in Fig. 1.

It was proposed that the PA band is due to photo-induced transitions of holes trapped in states close to the valence band into the valence band.[4] In this model, the decay of the PA band is due to the disappearance of the holes by recombination with electrons. Since the mobility of electrons is much higher than that of holes the decay characteristics give us information about the transport of electrons.

Fig. 1 - PA decay in (a) glow discharge and (b) sputtered a-Si:H as a function of temperature. The dashed line in (a) is a theoretical fit to equation (5) in Ref. 2 with $N_0 = 5 \times 10^{18} cm^{-3}$, $B = 2.0 \times 10^{-17}$ and $\alpha = 0.24$.

Both steady state[1] and transient[2] PA measurements in a-Si:H have indicated that the recombination is diffusion limited bimolecular at the carrier densities produced in the present experiment and obeys the equation

$$dN/dt = -bN^2 \qquad (1)$$

If the coefficient b is constant (time-independent) then N(t) decays as t^{-1} at long times, in contradiction with experimental results. As shown in Ref. (2) we obtain good agreement with experiment if we assume that b is time dependent. The time dependence of b is due to the same dispersive mechanism as that of the mobility μ (b$\sim\mu$)[5]. Taking b$\sim$ t $^{-(1-\alpha)}$ gives at long-times -ΔT/T $\sim$ t$^{-\alpha}$. Therefore, the values of α could be determined from the slope of the lines in Fig. 1; they are plotted in Fig. 2 as a function of temperature and sample preparation. In a-Si:H sample prepared by glow discharge α was found to be a linear function of temperature α = 0.075 + 1.9 x 10^{-3}T in the range 82 $\leq$ T $\leq$ 306K. At 6K the measured α was 0.14; this suggests a saturation of α at low temperatures (T < 80K) indicated in Fig. 2 by the dashed line. In the sputtered sample, α was only weakly temperature dependent.

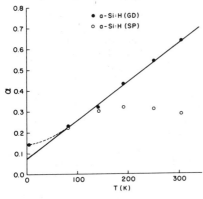

Fig. 2 — Temperature dependence of the dispersion parameter for glow discharge and sputtered a-Si:H.

In the dispersive regime, electron transport occurs either through multiple trapping or hopping. In the GD sample the fairly strong temperature dependence of α shows that trap controlled transport dominates.[6,7] However, the saturation of α at low temperatures and the fact that α (T) curve does not pass through the origin indicate that hopping transport persists as a parallel mode even at the highest temperatues. The dominating linear temperature dependence in the GD sample is consistent with an exponential distribution of trapping states under the conduction band edge, in accordance with the recent observation by Hvam and Brodsky in a-Si:H:P prepared by glow discharge.[8]

The weak temperature dependence of α in SP samples can be attributed to a predominantly hopping mode of transport. The dominance of the hopping transport may be associated with a higher overall density of traps in SP films, perhaps with non-exponential distributions.

The PA spectrum was measured for the sputtered a-Si:H sample at delay times 2μs, 20μs, 0.2ms and 2ms (Fig. 3) The structures which appear in the curves are due to thin film interference fringes which could not be completely averaged out. The spectrum shifts to

256

higher energy with increasing delay time t and the shifts are
approximately equal when t changes by a decade.

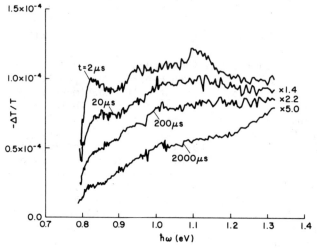

$-\Delta T/T$

$t=2\mu s$

$20\mu s$

$\times 1.4$
$\times 2.2$
$\times 5.0$

$200\mu s$

$2000\mu s$

$\hbar\omega$ (eV)

Fig. 3 - Time evolution of the PA-spectrum
in sputtered a-Si:H at 305K. Curves at
20 s. 0.2ms and 2ms have been multiplied
by factors shown in the figure.

This is in agreement
with the model that
we proposed for the
PA band and the
suggestion by Tiedje
and Rose, and
Orenstein and Kastner
(to be published)
that the highest
occupied trap state
of energy (measured
from the band edge)
moves with time
according to the
relation

$$E_d = kT \ln (\nu t) \qquad (2)$$

where ν is a vibra-
tional frequency.
The energy $E_d(t)$ is
the absorption edge
for the photoinduced
transitions of

carriers from traps into the band (in our case of holes into the
valence band); the observed logarithmic dependence of E_d with t is
consistent with Eq. (2). Let us note that our model in which the
time dependence of the PA band spectrum is explained by the thermalization of holes in traps, is not in contradiction with the observation of temperature independent α in SP samples (suggesting a hopping
transport mechanism) because α is associated with the transport of
electrons.

    In conclusion, we have measured the decay of the photoinduced
absorption in a-Si:H and interpreted the result with bimolecular
diffusion limited kinetics with dispersive transport. The temperature dependence of the dispersion parameter α shows that the transport is predominantly trap-controlled in glow-discharge samples
while in sputtered samples hopping transport dominates. The main
advantage of this method for determining α over the usual transient
photocurrent or drift mobility measurements is that the temperature
dependence of α could be measured to very low temperatures. A
measurement of the time evolution of the PA spectrum was performed
on the SP sample and could be qualitatively explained by thermalization of trapped holes.

    The work at Brown was supported in part by NSF grant DMR79-09819
and the NSF-MRL program at Brown University.

REFERENCES

1. P. O'Connor and J. Tauc, Phys. Rev. Lett. 43, 311 (1979).
2. Z. Vardeny, P. O'Connor, S. Ray and J. Tauc, Phys. Rev. Lett. 44, 1267 (1980).
3. H. Scher and E. W. Montroll, Phys. Rev. B 12, 2445 (1975).
4. P. O'Connor and J. Tauc, Sol. St. Commun. 36, 947 (1980).
5. K. L. Ngai and Fu-sui Liu, Phys. Rev. B (in print).
6. G. Pfister and H. Scher, Phys. Rev. B 15, 2062 (1977).
7. Recently, Tiedje and Rose, and Orenstein and Kastner proposed a model in which the dispersive transport is explained by multiple trapping in exponential trap distributions. M. Kastner (private communication) pointed out that in this model recombination occurring simultaneously with the trapping that determines should change the dispersive transport with respect to the case where no recombination takes place.
8. J. M. Hvam and M. H. Brodsky, Phys. Rev. Lett. 46, 371 (1981).

PHOTOACOUSTIC SPECTRA OF P-DOPED AND UNDOPED GD a-Si:H FILMS

S.Yamasaki, K.Nakagawa, H.Yamamoto, A.Matsuda, H.Okushi
and K.Tanaka
Electrotechnical Laboratory, 1-1-4 Umezono, Sakuramura,
Niiharigun, Ibaragi 305, Japan

ABSTRACT

Photoacoustic spectroscopy (PAS) was employed on a-Si:H films for the first time, and optical absorption spectra extending to $\alpha = 1$ cm^{-1} were determined absolutely. Undoped a-Si:H shows a long Urbach tail in its spectrum while P-doped a-Si:H has an additional absorption over a wide photon-energy range below 1.7 eV. It is demonstrated through the comparison between PAS and photoconductivity methods that the PAS is an extremely useful tool for determining α of a-Si:H below the optical gap.

INTRODUCTION

Optical absorption coefficient (α) in the range below the optical gap (E_o) involves an important information on band tailing and defect states near the mobility edge. Crandall measured the primary photocurrent in a-Si:H solar-cell structure and determined the absorption coefficient down to 10^{-1} cm^{-1}, while Cody et al. inferred the optical absorption from the measurement of the secondary photocurrent.[1,2] Both measurements have indicated that the optical absorption coefficient α below the optical gap E_o has an exponential dependence on photon energy E of the form $\alpha \propto \exp(E/E_c)$, although there exists a considerable difference in the obtained values of E_c between two groups. Their photoelectric measurements are, however, inherently accompanied by the ambiguities originated in surface states and/or photon-energy dependence of $\mu\tau$ product. In order to eliminate such uncertainty we have employed the photoacoustic spectroscopy (PAS) for determining the absorption spectra below E_o.[3]

In this report we present the first data on the PAS of the a-Si:H films, both of undoped and P-doped specimens, and discuss their below-gap absorption spectra obtained by analyzing the PAS data in comparison with those inferred from the secondary photocurrent measurements. We also touch upon the dependence of $\eta\mu\tau$ product on photon energy.

EXPERIMENTAL

Used samples in the present work, undoped and P-doped a-Si:H films, were deposited on glass substrates (Tempax) in a 13.56-MHz induction plasma chamber at a low power density from pure SiH$_4$ and 1 % PH$_3$/SiH$_4$, respectively.[4] A flow rate of 5 SCCM, a gas pressure of 100 mTorr and a substrate temperature of 300°C were maintained during the deposition of both samples. These samples contain around 14 at.% of bonded H, mainly in the monohydride bonding configuration, which were determined by ir stretching absorption of Si-H bond.[4]

ISSN:0094-243X/81/730258-05$1.50 Copyright 1981 American Institute of Physics

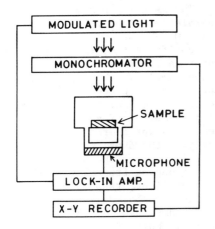

MODULATED LIGHT

↓↓↓

MONOCHROMATOR

↓↓↓

SAMPLE

MICROPHONE

LOCK-IN AMP.

X-Y RECORDER

Fig.1. Block diagram of the
measurement system of the PAS.

EPMA analysis has shown that the
P-doped specimen involves around
0.7 at.% of P.[4] The optical gap
E_0 is 1.7 eV, the same value for
both samples, being determined
graphically using the empirical
relation $\sqrt{\alpha h\nu} \propto h\nu - E_0$ in high α
range.

Figure 1 shows a block diagram of the measurement system of
the photoacoustic spectrum (PAS).
The thin film sample to be studied
is placed inside a closed cell
containing air and a sensitive
microphone, and then illuminated
with a modulated monochromatic
light. The periodic heating
caused by the nonradiative processes associated with optical
absorption gives a periodic heat
flow to the air gas and the
resultant acoustic signal is
detected by the microphone as a function of the photon energy of the
incident light. Actual PAS signals of a-Si:H films were traced
using the PAR model 6001 photoacoustic spectrometer. A 1-kW xenon
arc was provided as a light source at a chopping frequency of 40 Hz,
and all the signals were normalized to the carbon black standard.

The secondary photocurrent measurements were also carried out
against a 40-Hz chopped light at room temperature on the same samples
using coplanar electrode configurations of evaporated Al.

RESULTS AND DISCUSSION

Figure 2 shows the PAS signals (Q) obtained both for undoped
and P-doped a-Si:H films, 9 μm in thickness, as a function of wavelength. The spectrum of the undoped specimen drops abruptly down to
the background level in the wavelength range longer than 800 nm,
while that of the P-doped specimen has a long tail extending to
longer wavelengths. Q takes a maximum value around at 660 nm for
both specimens. The decrease in Q in shorter wavelengths which correspond to photon energies below E_0 has been considered to originate
from a change in the reflectivity.[5]

In order to get the optical absorption spectra from the above
PAS data we need a theoretical interpretation of the PAS as a function of α. Rosencwaig and Gersho (RG) have first presented a quantitative derivation for the PAS of solid samples in terms of the
optical, thermal and geometric parameters of the system.[3] The RG
theory, however, is essentially for a bulk sample and does not take
into account the multiple-reflection of a light within a thin film
sample. We have extended the RG theory to the case of a thin film
and derived a more general expression for the PAS accounting
multiple-reflection effect.

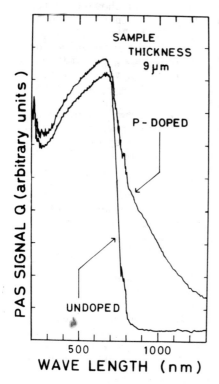

Fig.2. PAS of a-Si:H films

The main factors affecting the relationship between the PAS signal Q and the optical absorption coefficient α, to a first approximation, are the thickness of the sample ℓ, the penetration depth of the incident light α^{-1} and the thermal diffusion length of the sample μ_s ($= \sqrt{2\kappa/\omega\rho c}$), where κ is the thermal conductivity, ρ the density, c the specific heat of the sample and ω the chopping frequency of the incident light, respectively. In high α range, Q(α) is saturated independent of whether the sample is bulk ($\ell \gg \mu_s$) or thin film ($\ell \ll \mu_s$) since both ℓ and μ_s are much larger than α^{-1}, i.e.,

$$Q(\alpha) = Q_s = \text{const.}; \qquad (1)$$
$$\text{for } \ell, \mu_s \gg \alpha^{-1}.$$

As an actual value of Q_s we can use the maximum value of Q around at 660 nm in Fig.2. In low α range ($\ell \ll \alpha^{-1}$) for a thin film sample ($\ell \ll \mu_s$), the PAS signal is nearly proportional to α and is reasonably approximated by the following equation if normalized to Q_s,

$$q = Q(\alpha)/Q_s = (1 + r_2^2)\, \alpha\ell/(1 - r_1^2 r_2^2) \; ; \text{ for } \ell \ll \mu_s , \alpha-1, (2)$$

where r_1^2 and r_2^2 are the reflectivities for the normal incidence of a light from the sample to the gas and the sample to the backing material, respectively. It should be noted that eq.(2) does not involve μ_s which is directly associated with the thermal parameters of the specimen. Namely, the normalized PAS signal q of a thin film sample is independent of its thermal constants, which is one of the big advantages for the PAS of a thin film structure when compared with a bulk form. Details of these calculations will be published elsewhere.

Figure 3 shows the optical absorption spectra below E_o of the a-Si:H films, undoped and P-doped, which we obtained from the PAS data of Fig. 2 using eq.(2). The spectrum of the undoped a-Si:H reveals a steep exponential drop in α over nearly three orders of magnitude in 0.38 eV, which has a minimum less than 10 cm^{-1} around at 1.4 eV. A quantity E_c giving a measure of the steepness of the exponential tail $\alpha \propto \exp(E/E_c)$ is (0.06 ± 0.01)eV, being coincident with the data of Cody et al. determined on the GD a-Si:H$_{0.16}$ using

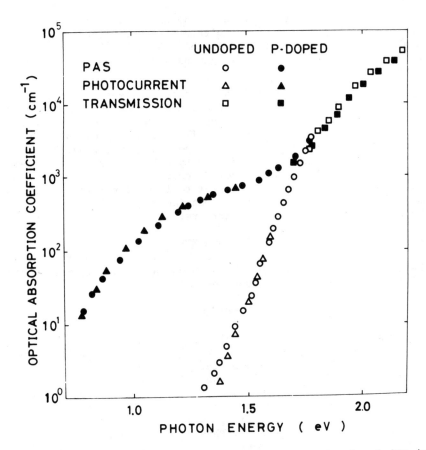

Fig.3. Optical absorption spectra for undoped and P-doped (PH$_3$/SiH$_4$: 1 %) a-Si:H films derived from photoacoustic spectroscopy (PAS), secondary photocurrent and transmission measurenents.

the secondary photocurrent method.[2] Zanzucchi et al., Tsai and Fritzsche independently observed the broad absorption tails amounting to $\alpha = 10^2$–10^3 cm^{-1} in the range from 1.4 eV to 1.6 eV, which are likely due to scattering losses.[6,7] On the other hand, the P-doped a-Si:H film has an additional optical absorption over a wide energy range below 1.7 eV, indicating that the introduction of P atoms produces the states deep in the gap as well as possible donor states near the conduction band. Essential feature of the absorption spectra of our P-doped GD a-Si:H is close to that of P-doped rf-sputtered a-Si:H reported by Freeman and Paul.[8]

The data of α determined from the transmission and the secondary photocurrent measurements are also plotted in the figure. As shown in the figure, values of α in low α range are in good agreement with each other between PAS and photoconductivity methods. It means that the $\eta\mu\tau$ product involved in the expression for the secondary photocurrent is kept constant within a factor difference over a wide photon–energy range studied in the present work. This result throws doubt upon the presence of a geminate recombination at the room temperature in this system.

In summary, we have employed a photoacoustic spectroscopy (PAS) on a-Si:H films and obtained the optical absorption spectra below optical gap down to 1 cm^{-1}. The undoped a-Si:H film shows a steep and long Urbach tail in its spectrum while P-doped specimen has an additional broad absorption over a wide photon–energy range below 1.7 eV. The PAS and the photoconductivity data have suggested that $\eta\mu\tau$ has no strong dependence on photon energy below E_0. It has been demonstrated that the PAS is a powerful tool for determining α below E_0 and is free from any problems accompanied by the transport phenomena of the photo–generated carriers.

ACKNOWLEDGMENTS

We gratefully acknowledge N.Hata, H.Oheda, K.Nozaki, H.Tokumoto and T.Ishiguro for helpful discussions.

REFERENCES

1. R. S. Crandall, J. Non–Cryst. Solids 35&36, 381 (1980).
2. G. D. Cody, B. Abeles, C. R. Wronski, B. Brooks and W. A. Lanford, J. Non–Cryst. Solids 35&36, 463 (1980).
3. A. Rosencwaig and A. Gersho, J. Appl. Phys. 47, 64 (1976).
4. K. Tanaka, K. Nakagawa, A. Matsuda, M. Matsumura, H. Yamamoto, S. Yamasaki, H. Okushi and S. Iizima, Proc. 12th Conf. on Solid State Devices (Tokyo, 1980) (in press).
5. H. Tokumoto and T. Ishiguro, J. Phys. Soc. Jpn 50, (1981) (in press).
6. P. J. Zanzucchi, C. R. Wronski and D. E. Carlson, J. Appl. Phys. 48, 5227 (1980).
7. C. C. Tsai and H. Fritzsche, Solar Energy Materials 1, 29 (1979).
8. E. C. Freeman and W. Paul, Phys. Rev. B20, 716 (1979).

DIRECT MEASUREMENT OF THE ABSORPTION
TAIL OF a-Si:H IN THE RANGE OF
2.1 eV > hν > 0.6 eV

Warren B. Jackson and Nabil M. Amer
Applied Physics and Laser Spectroscopy Group
Lawrence Berkeley Laboratory
University of California
Berkeley, CA 94720

ABSTRACT

The absorption edge of a-Si:H has been measured in the 0.6 - 2.1 eV (or $\alpha\ell = 5 \times 10^{-4}$) range using a sensitive technique of photothermal deflection spectroscopy which measures the optical absorption directly and is insensitive to scattering. Absorption edges were measured for films formed under a variety of deposition conditions. An absorption shoulder was found in materials with high defect densities and is strongly correlated with spin densities.

INTRODUCTION

The complete characterization of the shape of the optical absorption edge and tail of a-Si:H at and below the absorption edge yields information on the nature of the joint density of states. Furthermore, since the absorption tail in, for example, the chalcogenides has been attributed to transitions associated with defect centers, it would be of interest to investigate the applicability of this conclusion to a-Si:H films. However, published optical transmission measurements have been restricted to absorption coefficient values of $\alpha > 10$ cm^{-1}. This limitation is set by the inability of conventional techniques to measure small values of $\alpha\ell$.

We have recently developed a new technique, photothermal deflection spectroscopy (PDS)[1], which enables us to extend the sensitivity of determining α by two orders of magnitude over published values. PDS is highly insensitive to scattering and does not involve the use of experimentally unverified assumptions.

EXPERIMENTAL CONSIDERATIONS

When an intensity-modulated light beam (pump beam) is absorbed by a medium, heating will ensue. This heating causes a periodic index of refraction gradient in a thin layer adjacent to the sample surface. A second beam (probe beam), propagating through this thin layer, will then experience a periodic deflection which can be quantitatively related to the optical absorption. We have shown that the magnitude of the deflection ϕ is related to optical absorption in the following manner

$$\phi \propto (1-e^{-\alpha\ell}) \tag{1}$$

where ℓ is the film thickness. The experimental arrangement is

ISSN:0094-243X/81/730263-05$1.50 Copyright 1981 American Institute of Physics

shown in Fig. (1). Our pump beam was the monochromatized output of Hg-Xe arc lamp (0.01 eV bandwidth), and the deflection of the He-Ne laser probe beam was monitored with a conventional position sensor whose output was detected with a lock-in amplifier and normalized for the intensity variations of the pump beam as the wavelength was changed. The absolute absorption coefficient was obtained by using measured values of reflection and transmission at 1.96 eV in the formulae for reflectance and transmittance for thin films. These equations were then solved for the absorption coefficient and the index of refraction using a numerical routine.

To verify that PDS spectra are identical to those obtained by conventional techniques, we measured the absorption spectra of crystalline silicon, Nd^{3+} doped glasses, and graphite and found that our PDS results accurately reproduced those reported in the literature.

One important advantage of PDS over conventional transmission measurements is its insensitivity to elastic scattering of light by imperfections in the sample. Using the one-dimensional equation for radiation transport in an isotropically scattering slab and the heat diffusion equation, we find that[2]

$$\phi \propto (1-R-T) \qquad (2)$$

where R (T) is the reflection (transmission) coefficients for diffuse and specular beams. Fig. (2) shows that PDS signal is independent of scattering up to $\lambda\alpha\ell = 1$, where λ is the fraction of light scattered, α is the total extinction coefficient (scattering plus absorption), and ℓ is the film thickness. Hence, if the transmitted flux is reasonably collimated, PDS will be independent of scattering.

The a-Si:H samples used were obtained from the Xerox and RCA research groups. The RCA samples were produced by the d.c. discharge decomposition of silane and were deposited on SiO_2 substrate. Xerox samples were deposited by r.f. decomposition of silane on quartz and 7059 glass substrates. A summary of the characteristics and deposition parameters is given in Table I.

RESULTS AND DISCUSSION

Figs. 3-5 summarize our results for the absorption coefficient as a function of photon energy for films deposited at various substrate temperatures, r.f. powers, and for samples doped with phosphorous. Note in Fig. 3 that for low substrate temperature ($\sim100°C$), a pronounced shoulder appears at 1.3 - 1.4 eV which is not exhibited by samples deposited at higher temperatures. As one would expect, samples prepared at 230°C show the lowest tail absorption. The dependence of the absorption tail on deposition power is given in Fig. 4. Again, for deposition conditions known to produce large defect densities and columnar morphology, a discernable shoulder is observed. Similarly, the effect of doping (P) is to give rise to a clear shoulder at ~1.3 eV. In Fig. (5), we plot the absorption at 1.4 eV as a function of spin density.

From these results, the following tentative conclusions can be drawn:

1. Deposition parameters play a dominant role in the nature and number of states in the pseudo-gap. Furthermore, the tail absorption appears to be strongly correlated with unpaired spins.

2. By comparing luminescence data[3] with our absorption results, it appears that strong luminescence is inversely related to the observation of a shoulder on the absorption tail. In fact, one can argue that such a structure on the absorption tail appears to compete with radiative transitions. Thus models of radiative recombination of carriers need not be based on the presence of such a shoulder.

3. Since the size of the shoulder shows significant variations with deposition parameters, this suggests that it is caused by defects rather than being an intrinsic property of the film.

We are currently measuring the photoconductivity as a function of photon energy and comparing these results with the absorption measurements to deduce the dependence of $\eta\mu\tau$ on photon energy.

Table I. Sample Parameters

Sample	Deposition Conditions	Substrate	Thickness (μm)
	Xerox		
1	1 W rf 5% SiH$_4$ in Ar	100°C-7059 glass	2.27
2	1 W rf 100% SiH$_4$	230°C-Quartz	0.7
3	2 W rf 10^{-3} P	230°C	1.1
4	2 W rf 5% SiH$_4$ in Ar	230°C-Quartz	1.15
5	5 W rf 10% SiH$_4$ in Ar	230°C-Quartz	1.01
6	15 W rf 5% SiH$_4$ in Ar	230°C-Quartz	1.825
7	30 W rf 10% SiH$_4$ in Ar	230°C-Quartz	2.29
8	40 W rf 5% SiH$_4$ in Ar	230°C-Quartz	1.55
	RCA		
9	DC Proximity discharge	250°C-SiO$_2$	2.8
10	DC Proximity discharge	330°C-SiO$_2$	.95

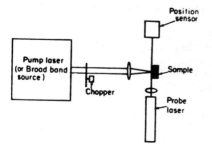

Fig. 1. Experimental configuration. The broad band output is passed through a monochromator before the chopper.

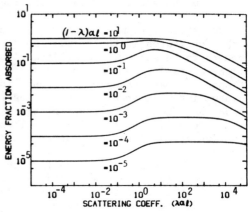

Fig. 2. Theoretical PDS signal vs. scattering ($\lambda\alpha\ell$) for different absorptions. λ is the fraction of light scattered and α is the total attenuation coefficient.

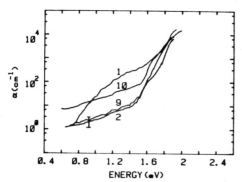

Fig. 3. Absorption vs. photon energy for various substrate temperatures.

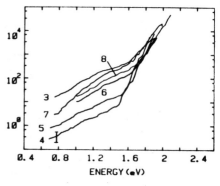

Fig. 4. Absorption vs. photon energy for various rf powers. 3 is phosphorous doped.

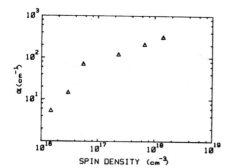

Fig. 5. Absorption vs. spin density (provided by the Xerox group).

ACKNOWLEDGEMENTS

We wish to thank Drs. Robert Street, David Carlson, and John Knights for generously providing us with samples; and Drs. Claude Boccara and Danielle Fournier for their contribution to the development of PDS.

This work was supported by the Assistant Secretary for Conservation and Solar Energy, Photovoltaic Energy Systems Division, of the U. S. Department of Energy under Contract W-4705-ENG-48, and by contract DS-0-8107-1 from the Solar Energy Research Institute (which is funded by DOE contract EG-77-C-01-4042).

REFERENCES

1. W. B. Jackson, N. M. Amer, A. C. Boccara and D. Fournier, Appl. Optics (April).
2. Z. Yasa, W. B. Jackson and N. M. Amer (to be published).
3. R. A. Street, J. C. Knights and D. K. Biegelsen, Phys. Rev. B, 18, 1880 (1978).

INFLUENCE OF COMPRESSION ON RADIATIVE RECOMBINATION IN a-Si:H

Bernard A. Weinstein

Xerox Webster Research Center, Webster, New York 14580

ABSTRACT

Photoluminescence (PL) in hydrogenated amorphous silicon (a-Si:H) was measured in the range 0-75kbar, 10-110K. Whereas the PL intensity is strongly quenched by pressure, the peak position is only weakly shifted to lower energy. This interesting dichotomy indicates that compression affects radiative and non-radiative processes differently. The quenching is interpreted as evidence for pressure induced structural changes. This discourages a direct connection between pressure shifts in a-Si:H, and c-Si.. Simple tunneling cannot explain the pressure dependence of the radiative decay rate.

INTRODUCTION

High pressure optical properties of amorphous silicon were investigated by Connell and Paul[1], and Welber and Brodsky[2]. Despite extensive 1 atm. PL work on a-Si:H, the effect of compression on PL was not studied by previous researchers.[3-7] Considering the productive history of high pressure research on crystals, and in view of the internal stress exhibited by as-deposited films (sometimes sufficient to shatter their substrates[8]), a more complete understanding of pressure effects in amorphous silicon seems desirable. The work discussed here includes measurements of the PL spectrum, quantum efficiency, temperature dependence, and time-decay in the regime 0-75kbar, 10-110K.[9]

PL was excited by 0.1mJ pulsed (10ns width) unfocused radiation at 6080A.[10] Samples of a-Si:H, supplied by J.C. Knights, were prepared by glow-discharge decomposition of silane gas. They were estimated to contain an excess spin density of $\sim 10^{16} cm^{-3}$.[11] The diamond-cell pressure environment around the sample was quasi-hydrostatic, with estimated stress gradients not exceeding 15kbar.[9]

RESULTS AND DISCUSSION

Figure 1 shows typical measured PL spectra. The peak at 1.72eV is part of the background and exhibits no pressure dependence. An intriguing dichotomy is evident. Compression strongly quenches the PL intensity, but only weakly shifts the peak to lower energy. The line width did not change within an uncertainty of 0.01eV.

Pressure-induced quenching of the PL (Figs. 1 and 2) is a strong effect. It was repeatedly observed using different samples in measurements to 75kbar, at which pressure the PL could no longer be detected above background. Upon pressure release, the PL only partially returned. This sharp decrease in PL efficiency cannot be due to the red-shift of the excitation spectrum,[10] which could account for only a 20% drop at 50kbar.[9] Likewise, the decrease is not solely due to changes in the radiative recombination rate, as this is not monotonic with pressure (Fig. 5), is not large enough, and probably would not be irreversible. Rather, the quenching is attributed to an increase in the concentration of non-radiative centers. One can estimate this increase after the measurement series in Fig. 2 using the non-radiative tunneling picture of Street et al.,[11] in which the quantum efficiency is given by, $Y_L \sim \exp(-V_c N)$,

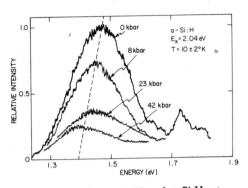

Fig. 1 Measured PL of a-Si:H at various pressures (10K) using a $2\mu s$ gate and $8\mu s$ delay. Spectra were subsequently corrected for background and throughput, and fit to a Gaussian profile. Dashed line indicates red-shift.

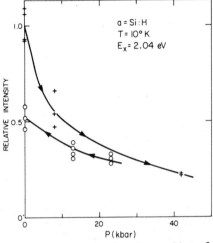

Fig. 2 Pressure induced quenching of peak PL intensity for a single measurement sequence on the same sample at 10K, with 2 μs gate and 8 μs delay. The direction of pressure change is distinguished by crosses (up) and circles (down).

where $V_c \sim 5 \times 10^{-18} cm^3$. Assuming that V_c is pressure in-dependent, one finds an increase in defect density of $\Delta N \sim 10^{17} cm^{-3}$.

In contrast to the PL efficiency, the pressure-induced energy-shift of the PL peak (Fig. 3) is a weak and reversible effect. The measured rate of shift is -2.0 ± 0.5 meV/kbar, essentially the same as for the absorption edges in crystalline (-1.5meV/kbar[12]) and amorphous (-1.0 ± 0.5meV/kbar[2]) silicon.[1] The simplest interpretation of this result is that radiative recombination occurs between levels ultimately derived from intrinsic c-Si band-edge states. However, this interpretation must be regarded with caution.

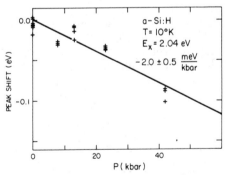

Fig. 3. Energy-shift of PL peak with pressure. Data includes measurements for both increasing and decreasing pressure. No irreversibility was detected to 42 kbars.

The temperature dependence of the PL quantum efficiency in the regime 10-110K, 0-42kbar exhibited no strong pressure effects (Fig. 4). The rate of thermal quenching for T > 55K was similar to that previously observed at 1atm.[5,7,13] At low temperature, the initial intensity increase was weaker than observed in Ref. 6. However, we note that varied behavior, including intensity saturation, has been observed in this temperature range.[5-7,13]

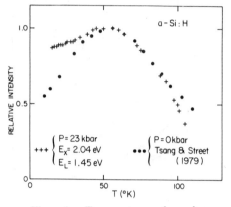

Fig. 4. Temperature dependence between 10-110K of peak PL intensity at 23kbar (crosses) compared to previous 1atm. results (dots) of Ref. 6.

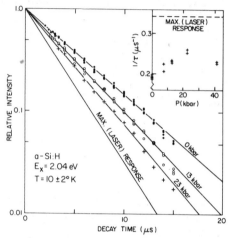

Fig. 5. Semilog plot showing pressure dependence of PL time-decay in μs regime. The insert plots decay rate vs. pressure; preamplifier limited maximum response to $\sim 3\mu$s.

Figure 5 shows the influence of pressure on the PL time-decay measured at the spectral peak (for each pressure) with a 1μs window scanned from 2 to 20μs. The 1atm. result is in agreement with previous reports.[5,6] The decay rate first increased and then decreased, with a maximum observed change of $\sim$25% at 23kbar (Fig. 5 insert). There was no irreversibility, as the same 1atm. decay returned after pressure release. This behavior can be attributed to radiative recombination alone, since non-radiative decay, should be largely completed before the microsecond observation period.[5,6]

The pressure data demonstrate an important result. A dichotomy exists between the catastrophic loss of PL efficiency, and the small change in PL (and absorption) energies. Thus, pressure effects radiative and non-radiative recombination processes in quite different ways. This suggests that radiative and non-radiative centers could be surrounded by very different structural environments.

The strong compression-induced quenching (Figs. 1 and 2) has been interpreted as an increase of $\sim 10^{17}$cm^{-3} in the defect density. This order of magnitude increase is consistent with observed defect concentrations in low-substrate-temperature samples exhibiting reduced PL intensity.[11] The increase is not due solely to a volume reduction, because this would require (on the basis of the Street et al[11] picture) a compressibility two orders of magnitude softer than the crystalline value.[14] Instead we conclude that new defects have been created through structural changes. This interpretation supports a structural model in which the amorphous network is pocked by various species of vacancies,[15] and larger voids.[8,16] Under compression these relatively soft regions should become focal points for locally inhomogeneous strains that could cleave bonds reconstructed across internal void surfaces, thereby producing strongly non-radiative centers.

A small negative pressure coefficient is quite rare for bandgaps in crystalline tetrahedral semiconductors. Generally, it is associated only with indirect $E_{\Gamma\Delta}$ transitions from the top of the valence band to the conduction band minima along $\langle 100 \rangle$. The difference between the pressure dependence of $E_{\Gamma\Delta}$ and that of most other bonding-antibonding gaps has been related to the different pseudocharge distributions for the corresponding conduction band states.[17] For the amorphous case disorder should strongly mix different crystalline states,[1] and the levels (band-tail or defect) below the mobility edge are expected to posses varying degrees of localization. Therefore, although some contribution of crystalline band-edge states is likely, it is difficult to presume a direct relation between the pressure dependence of $E_{\Gamma\Delta}$ in c-Si, and that of emission and absorption energies in a-Si:H.

Another explanation of the pressure-shift results is that they also reflect structural changes, and thus are not to be compared with behavior in c-Si.[2] Again we consider the implications of numerous voids in the amorphous network. If enough energy of compression is absorbed, through pressure induced bond-distortion and/or bond-breaking at internal void surfaces, a reduced effect on the bulk network may be expected. This is a possible explanation for the small pressure coefficients, regardless of sign, of the PL peak and absorption edge. A more extreme situation, corresponding to disconnected macromolecular units, has recently been discussed for a-As$_2$S$_3$, in which nearest neighbor (intramolecular) bonds are insulated from compression.[18] Although the 3d-network of a-Si:H cannot be considered topologically disconnected, Phillips[16] has pointed out that it may be near the open porosity threshold.

For a-Si:H strong electron-phonon coupling has been proposed to explain the ~0.5 eV Stokes shift between the PL, and PL-excitation peaks.[6,10] In a simple strong coupling model, the effect of pressure on the Stokes shift Δ can be estimated by scaling the network distortion amplitude x_0 according to the proper microscopic compressibility κ_0, which may differ from the bulk value κ_B.[9] According to Zallen's Gruneisen scaling law,[19] the ratio $\kappa_0/\kappa_B \approx \gamma_0$, where γ_0 is the relevant phonon Gruneisen parameter. This leads to,[9] $\gamma_\Delta \approx 4/3\, \gamma_0$. The present measurements (and those of Ref. 2) indicate $\gamma_\Delta \approx 2.0 \pm 1.4$, so that we estimate $\gamma_0 \approx 1.5 \pm 1.0$. This value of γ_0 marginally overlaps the known Gruneisen parameter range in c-Si, $-1.5 \lesssim \gamma_0 \lesssim 1.5$.[20] Thus the Stokes shift model and the pressure results are only marginally compatible. However, given the Stokes shift hypothesis, negative γ_0 are excluded. This rules out coupling to zone boundary TA (bond-bending) modes,[20] which have been proposed as the dominant distortions for self-trapping and vacancies in crystalline III-V materials.[21]

The simple donor-acceptor type radiative tunneling picture of Ref. 6 may be used to estimate the influence of pressure on the PL time-decay. This model predicts that an electron and hole separated by R will recombine with rate,[22] $W = W_o \exp(-2R/R_o)$, where R_o is the larger wavefunction radius and $W_o \approx 10^8 \text{ sec}^{-1}$.[6] Using the c-Si compressibility[14] one finds that the decrease in R corresponding to 23kbar can account for only a 5% increase in W. This is much less than the observed 25% increase at this pressure (Fig. 5). Furthermore, to obtain other than monotonic behavior, W_o or R_o would have to exhibit highly nonlinear pressure variation. Thus, a more detailed picture of the radiative tunneling process seems necessary. Recently a chemical rate treatment of small polaron hopping between inequivalent sites has been applied to the pair recombination problem.[23] It was found that this model could account for the observed non-monotonic behavior, but the final result would depend on the details of the initial pair distribution.

1. G.A.N. Connell and W. Paul, J. of Non-Crystalline Solids 8-10, 215 (1972).
2. B. Welber and M.H. Brodsky, Phys. Rev. B16, 3660 (1977); these authors measure absorption edge pressure coefficients of -1.0 ± 0.5 meV/kbar for a-Si, and -0.7 to -2.0meV/kbar (growing more negative as pressure is increased to 70kbar) in a-Si:H. This differs from the value +0.25 meV/kbar of Ref. 1 for a-Si. Therefore, the compromise value -1.0 ± 0.5meV/kbar was adopted for our a-Si:H. (See text.)
3. D. Engemann and R. Fischer, Phys. Stat. Sol. (b)79, 195 (1977).
4. J.I. Pankove and D.E. Carlson, Appl. Phys. Lett. 29, 620 (1976).
5. I.G. Austin, T.S. Nashashibi, T.M. Searle, P.G. Le Comber and W.E. Spear, J. of Non-Crystalline Solids 32, 373 (1979).
6. C. Tsang and R.A. Street, Phys. Rev. B19, 3027 (1979).
7. M.A. Paesler and W. Paul, Phil. Mag. B41, 393 (1980).
8. J.C. Knights, J. of Non-Crystalline Solids 35-36, 159 (1980); J.C. Knights, G. Lucovsky and R.J. Nemanich, J. of Non-Crystalline Solids 32, 393 (1979).
9. B.A. Weinstein, Phys. Rev. B23, 787 (1981); B.A. Weinstein, to be published.
10. R.A. Street, Phil. Mag. B37, 35 (1978).
11. R.A. Street, J.C. Knights and D.K. Biegelsen, Phys. Rev. B18, 1880 (1978).
12. R. Zallen and W. Paul, Phys. Rev. 155, 703 (1967).
13. R.W. Collins, M.A. Paesler, G. Moddel and W. Paul, J. of Non-Crystalline Solids 35-36, 681 (1980).
14. H.J. McSkimin and P. Andreatch, Jr., J. Appl. Phys. 35, 2161 (1964); the crystalline compressibility is used; no data exists for a-Si:H films.
15. A. Madan, P.G. Le Comber and W.E. Spear, J. of Non-Crystalline Solids 20, 239 (1976).
16. J.C. Phillips, J. of Non-Crystalline Solids 35-36, 1157 (1980).
17. J.C. Phillips in Bonds and Bands in Semiconductors (Academic Press, N.Y., 1973) pp. 147-50.
18. B.A. Weinstein, R. Zallen and M.L. Slade, J. of Non-Crystalline Solids 35-36, 1255 (1980).
19. R. Zallen, Phys. Rev. B9, 4485 (1974).
20. B.A. Weinstein and G.J. Piermarini, Phys. Rev. B12, 1172 (1975).
21. D.V. Lang, J. Phys. Soc. Japan 49, Suppl. A, 215 (1980).
22. D.G. Thomas, J.J. Hopfield and W.M. Augustiniak, Phys. Rev. 140A, 202 (1965).
23. H. Scher and T. Holstein, Philos. Mag., to be published.

SUPER-BANDGAP RADIATION IN a-Si

B. A. Wilson

Bell Laboratories, Murray Hill, N.J. 07974

ABSTRACT

The nature of the super-bandgap radiation observed in a-Si and a-Si:H is investigated. This broad spectrum postulated to arise from localized states above the mobility gap exhibits many remarkable features.[1] These same features occur in radiation from porous quartz, but in that case the effect is known to be surface related.[2] Using the Raman spectrum for calibration, the strength of the signal from a-Si has been studied as a function of surface preparation. The results suggest the possibility that the radiation is a surface contaminant effect unrelated to the bulk states of the material.

A broad emission band has been reported recently in a number of amorphous semiconductors,[1] including amorphous silicon, which remarkably extends 1 eV or more above the optical absorption gap of the material. The peak position depends on the exciting laser frequency, ν_{ex}, shifting to higher frequency as ν_{ex} is increased, but with a shift that is somewhat smaller than the change in ν_{ex}. The decay after pulsed excitation is fast, < 10 ns, and the intensity is linear in laser power. The spectrum is essentially independent of temperature, except for an anti-Stokes tail that grows with temperature, and the intensity exhibits only a weak dependence. Thus the emission behaves neither like a scattering process nor a simple fluorescence, and these remarkable features have been thought to indicate unique properties of the electronic states in amorphous solids, such as localized states above the mobility gap. Unfortunately, the results reported here indicate the plausibility of an alternate explanation: the emission may simply be fluorescence from surface contaminants present in the laboratory environment.

The widespread speculation on the nature of the electronic states responsible for this emission has been due, at least in part, to the apparent novelty of its characteristics. In fact, however, rather similar behavior has been reported in Vycor[2] (porous quartz) and other high surface area materials used in catalysis,[3] when pumped with Ar laser lines. The spectra are similar to those observed in a-Si and the chalcogenides, and they also broaden, intensify and shift with laser frequency. In the case of quartz, however, the intensity can be reduced by orders of magnitude by appropriate surface preparation. As a result, organic surface contamination has been postulated to be responsible. Although the reported signal from a-Si or the chalcogenides is orders of magnitude weaker, the effective surface area is comparatively smaller. Consequently, in order to investigate the possibility that the amorphous semiconductor emission is also due to surface contamination, I have

ISSN:0094-243X/81/730273-05$1.50 Copyright 1981 American Institute of Physics

studied the intensity of the emission from a-Si as a function of surface preparation.

The a-Si films used in this investigation include 6 samples grown by RF glow discharge on crystalline Si and quartz substrates, and 2 UHV evaporated films. The samples were excited with a 10 Hz Nd:YAG pumped dye laser with a 10 ns pulse length and ∿ 2 mW average power, lightly focused to a 1 mm × 2 mm spot. The beam was passed through a monochromator to remove broadband dye fluorescence. The radiation from the samples was dispersed with a double monochromator and detected with an S-20 photomultiplier with a 20 ns response time, followed by a gated boxcar integrator whose 15 ns gate was set coincident with the laser pulse. The strength of the radiation was calibrated by comparison with the Raman phonon peak at ∿ 480 cm⁻¹,[4] using 70 cm⁻¹ resolution. As it became apparent that similar broadband emissions are ubiquitous in the laboratory, and many sources are much stronger than the sample itself, extreme care was taken to shield the collection optics from any other surfaces illuminated by scattered laser light.

All off-the-shelf samples, both UHV evaporated and glow discharge, exhibited a broad emission as shown in Fig. 1. The emission behaved as described in the literature. The peak intensity was

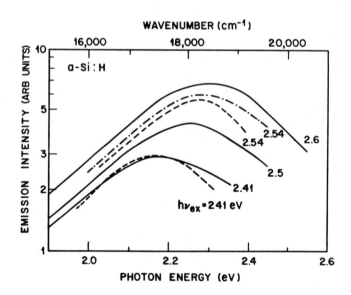

Fig. 1. Above bandgap emission spectra in a-Si:H. Solid curves from reference 1, dashed curves this study. Dash-dot curve is a bulk sample of pump oil. The relative strengths of the dashed and dash-dot curves are arbitrary.

comparable to or greater than the Raman phonon mode (at 70 cm⁻¹ resolution), also in agreement with earlier work.[1] As found for porous quartz, however, the emission intensity could be greatly reduced by appropriate surface preparation, in this case by cleaning.

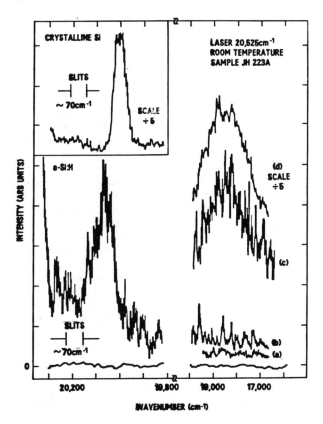

Fig. 2. Strength of above bandgap emission in a-Si:H relative to the Raman phonon spectrum as a function of cleaning procedures. a) After vapor degreasing, b) after methanol cleaning, c) off-the-shelf and d) beam hitting dust speck. At upper left a crystalline Si Raman spectrum is shown for comparison.

As shown in Fig. 2, careful cleaning with methanol in which the solvent is pulled off the sample with a lens tissue, reduced the broadband signal considerably in a-Si:H. Vapor degreasing with trichloroethylene reduced the signal level below background noise levels – factors of at least 15 and 25 below the Raman phonon peak at pump frequencies of 20,500 cm⁻¹ (∿ 4880 Å) and 19,450 cm⁻¹ (∿ 5145 Å) respectively. The reference Raman phonon spectrum shown in Fig. 2 was unchanged by cleaning, or by the laser excitation during the measurement of the broadband spectrum. If the sample was subsequently allowed to sit for a few days in the laboratory environment, or if any methanol was allowed to dry on the sample during cleaning, the signal returned. Care also had to be taken to avoid any dust on the sample which can result in a tenfold increase in the signal strength, as indicated in Fig. 2.

This sensitivity to cleaning procedures strongly suggests that the anomalous emission in a-Si is due to surface contamination, and unrelated to bulk states in the amorphous film. Any remanent broadband emission originating from the bulk of the film must apparently be exceedingly weak — < 1/25th of the Raman phonon intensity at 19,450 cm^{-1}, and would itself be suspect — bulk contamination of the film is also possible during sample growth. The similarity of the emission reported in chalcogenide glasses suggests that it too may be due to surface contaminants.

Surface contaminants could easily reproduce the essential features of the anomalous emission. The composite spectrum of a mixture of many fluorescing organics would be a broad featureless band whose peak would shift with ν_{ex} due to selective excitation of different subsets of the mixture. The observed intensity and width increase when pumping in the blue is consistent with the less extensive variety of organic species which absorb in the red. Some well known samples of organic mixtures that behave in precisely this fashion are fore pump oil, finger oil and wood or cloth fibers — all common contaminants in the laboratory environment. The spectrum of a bulk pump oil sample is shown for comparison in Fig. 1. The fluorescence from bulk samples is quite strong — only miniscule amounts on the sample surfaces could account for the observed weak signal levels.

Although it seems clear that the source of the above bandgap emission is some form of surface contamination, this particular model leaves a few unanswered questions. First, the decay time is rather fast for many fluorescing organics such as naphthalene derivatives whose lifetimes are more commonly in the tens of ns. Secondly, although the generally weak temperature dependence is consistent with high quantum efficiency fluorescing species, the reported <u>rise</u> in intensity of the emission[1] from a-Si:H between 2 K and 50 K is difficult to reconcile with this model. Since the sub-band luminescence in a-Si:H follows this same pattern,[5] some involvement of the underlying substrate would seem to be implied. There are also slight, but reproducible differences in the spectra from different materials, although this may merely indicate a sample dependence of the affinity to adsorb certain species.

In summary, I have examined the nature of the super-bandgap radiation in a-Si. The unusual characteristics of this emission have led to much speculation on the nature of the electronic states in amorphous semiconductors, but the data presented here indicate the plausibility of an entirely different explanation. The signal intensity in a-Si was shown to be extremely sensitive to the cleanliness of the surface. This is a strong indication that the emission originates from surface contaminants, rather than bulk states in the amorphous film, and a simple model of a mixture of fluorescing organic species was shown to reproduce the essential features.

ACKNOWLEDGMENTS

Samples of a-Si were grown by J. P. Harbison (RF glow discharge) and J. C. Bean (UHV evaporated). I thank D. H. Auston and A. M. Johnson for communication of results prior to publication. The technical assistance of T. P. Kerwin is gratefully acknowledged.

REFERENCES

1. J. Shah and M. A. Bosch, Phys. Rev. Lett. 42, 1420 (1979); J. Shah and M. A. Bosch, Solid State Commun. 31, 769 (1979); J. Shah and P. M. Bridenbaugh, Solid State Commun. 34, 101 (1980); J. Shah, F. B. Alexander, Jr. and B. G. Bagley, Solid State Commun. 36, 195 (1980); and J. Shah, private communication.
2. Cherry Ann Murray and Thomas J. Greytak, Phys. Rev. B 20, 3368 (1979).
3. T. A. Egerton and A. H. Hardin, Catal. Rev. - Sci. Eng. 11, 71 (1975).
4. J. E. Smith, Jr., M. H. Brodsky, B. L. Crowder and M. I. Nathan, Phys. Rev. Lett. 26, 642 (1971).
5. J. Shah, B. G. Bagley, F. B. Alexander, Jr., Solid State Commun. 36, 199 (1980); C. Tsang, R. A. Street, Phys. Rev. B 19, 3027 (1979).

PHOTOLUMINESCENCE EXCITATION SPECTROSCOPY OF HYDROGENATED AMORPHOUS SILICON[*]

S. G. Bishop, U. Strom and P. C. Taylor
Naval Research Laboratory, Washington, D.C. 20375

William Paul
Harvard University, Gordon McKay Laboratory, Cambridge, MA 02138

ABSTRACT

Photoluminescence excitation (PLE) spectra have been obtained at 77K for compacted samples of both glow discharge deposited and reactively sputtered a-Si:H. In all cases the low energy PLE spectra parallel the slope of the higher energy band edge absorption curves obtained from thin films without change in slope down to ~1.3 eV. The absence of a slope change or shoulder in the PLE spectra at energies $\leq$ 1.5 eV indicates that the low energy below gap absorption processes which give rise to the ~1.3 eV shoulder observed in photoconductivity spectra of a-Si:H <u>do not</u> contribute to the excitation of the ~1.3-1.4 eV luminescence band.

INTRODUCTION

Studies of the optical absorption edge in amorphous semiconductors can provide a measure of the energy distribution of the joint valence band-conduction band density of states and an indication of the extent of band tailing into the pseudo-gap. However, in amorphous semiconductors such as hydrogenated silicon (a-Si:H), which are usually prepared as thin films $\lesssim$10 μm thick, the determination of the absorption coefficient α from transmission measurements at low energy (and low αd) is limited to $\alpha \sim 10$ cm^{-1} or, in most cases, to photon energies $\gtrsim$ 1.6 eV for a-Si:H.

Several workers[1-4] have taken advantage of the high sensitivity of photoconductivity for the detection of weak absorption processes (e.g. impurity absorption in crystalline semiconductors) to study the weak below-band gap optical absorption in a-Si:H, that is, for α as low as 0.1-1 cm^{-1}, which corresponds to energies as low as 0.8 eV. These measurements have revealed that while the exponential part of the optical absorption edge extends down to about 1.5 eV, there is a distinct shoulder in the absorption spectrum at an energy of about 1.2-1.3 eV in both glow discharge deposited and reactively sputtered films of a-Si:H. This shoulder has been interpreted in terms of transitions from localized states in the gap between the Fermi energy and the top of the valence band to the conduction band.

Photoluminescence excitation (PLE) spectroscopy can also provide a measure of the shape of the optical absorption spectrum for those absorption processes which lead to the excitation of luminescence. In the PLE technique the intensity of a selected luminescence band

[*]Supported in part by SERI under DOE Contract No. DE-AI02-80CS83116.

ISSN:0094-243X/81/730278-05$1.50

is measured as a function of the wavelength of monochromatic exciting light from a tunable source. Previous studies[5,6] of PLE in a-Si:H obtained broadly peaked spectra in the vicinity of the absorption edge similar to those obtained in chalcogenide glasses.[7] These spectra exhibited the expected fall off in excitation efficiency at low energy due to the decreasing absorption coefficient, and at energies well above the ~ 1.8-2.0 eV peak in PLE, an approximate α^{-1} dependence[5] which appears to be a general property of low mobility materials (e.g. chalcogenide glasses[7]) in which photoabsorption must occur within a diffusion length of a radiative center in order for radiative recombination to occur. The ~0.5-0.6 eV shift between the peak in the PLE spectrum and the usual 1.3-1.4 eV peak in the photo-luminescence spectrum has been interpreted[6] as a Stokes shift which occurs when the electron phonon interaction causes photo-excited excitons bound to band tail states to lower their energy and to become self-trapped before recombining radiatively.

The present work is primarily concerned with the PLE spectrum in the low energy spectral range where the shoulder is observed in photoconductivity spectra. We find that the absence of a slope change or shoulder in the PLE spectra in this spectral range indicates that the low energy absorption processes responsible for the shoulder in the PC spectra do not contribute to the excitation of PL.

EXPERIMENTAL PROCEDURE

PL and PLE spectra have been obtained at 77K for samples of glow discharge deposited and reactively sputtered a-Si:H obtained from three independent sources. In all cases, the a-Si:H was undoped and the single, relatively efficient 1.3-1.4 eV PL band characteristic of such material was observed.[5,6,8] Hence the PLE spectra reported here are representative of this "intrinsic" PL band and not the weaker ~ 0.9 eV band reported in doped[9-12] a-Si:H. In order to extend the practicable range of PLE to somewhat lower values of α than can normally be reached with thin film samples, we used com-pacted samples (with effective thickness ~1 mm) of a-Si:H which had been removed from the Aℓ foil substrate. Comparison of PL and PLE spectra from the compacted samples with those obtained from their thin film counterparts indicates that the compacted sample spectra are representative of the as-deposited films aside from obvious thickness dependent effects discussed below.

The PLE spectra were excited by light from a tungsten-halogen lamp which was passed through a 3/4 meter single grating monochroma-tor, a water filter, and appropriate Corning glass filters. The exciting light was focussed onto the sample which was immersed in liquid nitrogen. PL was detected by a cooled S-1 photomultipler and the detected PL wavelengths were those which lie between the short wavelength limit of the transparency of a Si filter (~1.0 μm) and the long wavelength limit of the photomultiplier response (~1.15 μm). PL spectra were excited by 6471Å light from a Krypton laser and detected by a 77K PbS photoconductive cell.

The two sputtered samples employed in this study were made under similar conditions (argon partial pressure $P_{Ar}=5\times10^{-3}$ Torr; substrate temperature $T_s=325°C$) at hydrogen partial pressure P_H which differed by an order of magnitude. The values of P_H are 4×10^{-4} Torr and 4×10^{-3} Torr for samples SiS-159 and SiS-186, respectively. The NRL and RCA samples were made by the glow discharge technique under the following growth parameters: for NRL, $T_s=250°C$, silane pressure of 0.1 Torr, and growth rate of ~350Å/min, for RCA, $T_s=330°C$, silane pressure of 0.5 Torr, and growth rate of ~300Å/min. The hydrogen content of all three films is approximately 10-15 at.%.

RESULTS AND DISCUSSION

Figure 1 compares PLE spectra obtained from a thin film sample and a compacted sample of reactively sputtered a-Si:H (Harvard, SiS-186). The relative intensities of the two spectra have been normalized at their peak intensities. The shape of the thin film spectrum is consistent with previously reported PLE spectra (as described in the INTRODUCTION), and its fall off due to decreasing absorption coefficient occurs at significantly higher energy than that of the compacted sample. Comparison of these two PLE spectra in the 1.5-1.8 eV energy range clearly illustrates the additional signal strength provided at longer wavelengths by the compacted sample because of its greater effective thickness.

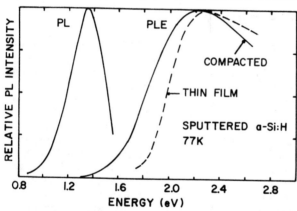

Fig. 1. PL and PLE spectra for thin film (~3μm) and compacted samples of reactively sputtered a-Si:H (Harvard, SiS-186)

In Fig. 2 the PLE spectra for two samples of glow discharge deposited a-Si:H and another reactively sputtered sample (Harvard SiS-159) are plotted on a logarithmic scale. These three spectra have been displaced arbitrarily on the logarithmic scale for the sake of clarity. Clearly, the experimentally observed relative intensities are expected to be a strong function of the film deposition parameters (especially thickness) as well as the reproducibility of the experimental conditions. However, we are only concerned with the spectral line shape, particularly the low energy exponential portion. Also plotted for purposes of comparison are the photoconductivity data of Moddel et al.[1] The photoconductivity data display a distinct deviation in slope at ~1.4 eV which corresponds to the

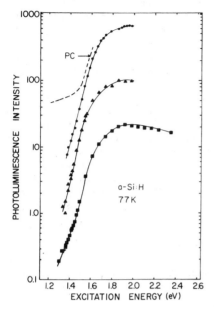

Fig. 2. PLE spectra for compacted samples of reactively sputtered a-Si:H (-Δ-, Harvard, SiS-159) and glow discharge deposited a-Si:H from RCA (-O-) and NRL (-□-). Photoconductivity data for 200K are from ref. 1.

beginning of the low energy shoulder reported in the photoconductivity spectrum.[1-4] In contrast, the PLE spectra exhibit no such inflection or kink in the vicinity of 1.4 eV. The approximately exponential fall off (with 0.05 eV activation energy) in PLE efficiency extends, without significant deviation, from about 1.6 eV to the lowest energy attainable, 1.30 eV. This behavior parallels that exhibited by the band edge absorption curves[1-4] obtained at higher energies from thin films of a-Si:H.

It is significant that the reactively sputtered samples employed in the PLE spectroscopy were deposited under conditions identical to those for films which exhibited the 1.3 eV shoulder in their photo-conductivity spectra. The absence of a slope change or shoulder in the PLE spectra of these films indicates that the low energy, below-gap absorption processes which are responsible for the 1.3 eV photo-conductive shoulder do not contribute to the excitation of the 1.4 eV luminescence band. The fact that we have found this to be true for both glow discharge and sputtered films from several laboratories indicates that the exponential shape of the PLE spectrum for the 1.4 eV PL band is an intrinsic or general feature of a-Si:H.

The 1.3-1.4 eV PL band has been attributed[6] to a Stokes shifted transition between band tails, and the continued exponential decrease in the PLE efficiency for this band at low excitation energy (with slope corresponding to the intrinsic absorption edge, Fig. 2), is certainly consistent with this finding. The apparently extrinsic absorption shoulder observed in the photoconductivity spectra does not contribute to the excitation of the 1.3-1.4 EV PL band. A positive correlation has been observed[13] between the low energy photoconductivity shoulder and the density of ESR centers ("defect states"), but the 1.3-1.4 eV band is quenched[8] by the presence of singly occupied (paramagnetic) defects. In contrast, the 0.9 eV PL band is observed[9-12] in doped samples or undoped samples with high spin density ($\sim 10^{18} cm^{-3}$) and has been attributed[9,14] to recombination at native defects. Comparison of the low energy photoconductivity and PLE data of Fig. 2 indicates that at ~ 1.3 eV, the component of absorption which leads to the 1.4 eV PL and which exhibits the exponential dependence on photon energy, is nearly an order of magnitude weaker than the absorption which excites the photoconductivity shoulder. Significantly, the 0.9 eV PL band can be excited[14] by photon energies corresponding to the 1.3 eV photoconductivity shoulder which do not efficiently excite the 1.4 eV PL band. (The low quantum efficiency of the 0.9 eV PL band precludes PLE spectroscopy.) An obvious suggestion is that the 1.3 eV absorption shoulder may be associated with the defects which give rise to the 0.9 eV PL band.

ACKNOWLEDGEMENTS

The authors gratefully acknowledge D.E. Carlson and J. Dresner (RCA), and P. Reid (Naval Research Laboratory) for supplying well-characterized films of a-Si:H.

REFERENCES

1. G. Moddel, D.A. Anderson, and W. Paul, Phys. Rev. B 22, 1918 (1980); R.W. Collins, M.A. Paesler, G. Moddel and W. Paul, J. Non-Cryst. Solids 35-36, 681 (1980).
2. T.D. Moustakas, Solid State Commun. 35, 745 (1980).
3. B. von Roedern and G. Moddel, Solid State Commun. 35, 467 (1980).
4. B. Abeles, C.R. Wronski, T. Tiedje, and G.D. Cody, Solid State Commun. 36, 537 (1980).
5. T.S. Nashashibi, I.G. Austin, and T.M. Searle, Philos. Mag. 35, 831 (1977).
6. R.A. Street, Philos. Mag. B 37, 35 (1978).
7. R.A. Street, Advances in Physics 25, 397 (1976).
8. R.A. Street, J.C. Knights, and D.K. Biegelsen, Phys. Rev. B 18, 1880 (1978), and references therein.
9. R.A. Street and D.K. Biegelsen, Solid State Commun. 33, 1159 (1980).
10. W. Rehm, D. Engemann, R. Fischer, and J. Stuke, Proc. 13th Int. Conf. on the Physics of Semicond., ed. F.G. Fumi (Tipografia Marves) 1976, p. 525.
11. I.G. Austin, T.S. Nashashibi, T.M. Searle, P.G. LeComber, and W.E. Spear, J. Non-Cryst. Solids 32, 373 (1979).
12. D.A. Anderson, G. Moddel, R.W. Collins, and W. Paul, Solid State Commun. 31, 677 (1979).
13. J. Stuke, Proc. 6th Int. Conf. on Amorphous and Liquid Semiconductors, ed. B.T. Kolomiets (Leningrad, 1976), p. 193.
14. R.A. Street, Phys. Rev. B 21, 5775 (1980).

GEMINATE AND NON-GEMINATE RECOMBINATION IN a-Si:H

J. Mort, I. Chen, S. Grammatica and M. Morgan
Xerox Corporation, Webster Research Center, Webster, N.Y. 14580

and

J.C. Knights and R. Lujan
Xerox Palo Alto Research Center, Palo Alto, California 94304

ABSTRACT

A number of recent measurements including xerographic discharge and a delayed-collection field technique have indicated that the photogeneration process in a-Si:H is controlled by a geminate recombination process. This results in the primary quantum efficiency being field dependent which could limit performance of solar cells using a-Si:H. An extension of the delayed-collection experiment has also allowed a direct study of the non-geminate recombination process (i.e., the recombination of free electron-hole pairs that avoid geminate recombination). The analysis of the experimental data shows that the non-geminate recombination is diffusion-controlled and that both bulk and surface losses are extremely slow. The effective recombination lifetimes, under the conditions of these experiments, can be as long as 10 milliseconds.

Recent work has suggested that the photogeneration process in a-Si:H may be controlled by geminate recombination.[1,2] The luminescence decay measurements[1] were carried out at low temperatures and so only apply to this temperature regime. The initial observations, which were somewhat indirect, by Crandall[3] indicated zero-field quantum efficiencies between 0.3-0.4, but no values of quantum efficiency at intermediate fields, nor correlation to Onsager's theory were reported. Xerographic discharge studies[2] also were consistent with a geminate process but the possibility of surface recombination and/or bulk trapping effects prevented a direct measurement of the zero field quantum efficiency and therefore could not be considered conclusive evidence. Despite the critical role that carrier recombination play in any photoconductive material, questions remain about the microscopic nature of this phenomenon in amorphous materials in general. Although some measurements have been reported for a-Se,[4] the most detailed studies have been by Spear, et al[5] which dealt directly with steady-state secondary photoconductivity in a-Si:H surface cells. In this paper we report experimental studies of both geminate and non-geminate recombination processes in a-Si:H.

The experiments to study geminate processes involve the combined use of xerographic discharge and delayed-collection field techniques[6] to make absolute quantum efficiency measurements as a function of field, wavelength and temperature and study the recombination of photogenerated carriers. The samples used in these studies were prepared using an rf diode deposition onto substrates held at 230°C with (a) rf power 18w, silane concentration 5% in He or (b) rf power 2W 100% silane.[7] The samples were deposited on 2 in. x 2 in. aluminum substrates. The xerographic discharge techniques for determining photogeneration efficiency are described elsewhere[2] and require no top electrode. For the pulsed-field photogeneration technique a top electrode of 200A of Bi was evaporated with the simultaneous deposition on quartz substrates for precise calibration of its transmission characteristics. All experiments were performed with positive bias on the illuminated surface so that the photogeneration of holes is involved.

The delayed-collection field technique was performed in the following way. The sample was exposed to a 10 nanosecond light pulse of variable wavelength from a N_2 pumped dye laser while a field adjustable from zero upwards was applied. Within 50 nanoseconds of the light flash the field increases from its initial value to a field sufficiently high to sweep out all the photogenerated holes. This was confirmed by the direct time resolution of the transit of the holes. In order to evaluate the quantum efficiency the transit signal was integrated using a Biomation 8100 transient recorder in conjunction with Nicolet 1170 Signal Processor. Since hole transport in a-Si:H is dispersive[2] particular care was taken in the integration procedure to ensure that the integration was carried to completion. This was done by comparing the values of integrals for integration times of 1, 10 and 100 transit times (transit time here refers to fiduciary observed in log current - log time transit pulses). In order to take account of variability in the laser pulse each intensity data point involved the average of four pulses and the careful substraction of the background signal produced by the pulsed field sequences without the light pulse. This can be done with great accuracy with the electronic capability of the signal processer. In order to ensure that no carriers were lost during the minimum delay of 50nsecs the integrated charge displacement was studied as a function of larger delays. This confirmed that no carrier loss occurred during the unavoidable 50nsec delay. This study of the number of surviving carriers as a function of delay time also allows a direct measure of non-geminate recombination processes as discussed below. The overall accuracy of the quantum efficiency measurement was checked by measuring the absolute responsivity of a photodiode by integration of the photocurrent produced by the laser pulse and comparing with calibrated values made by the National Bureau of Standards. An absolute accuracy of $\pm 6\%$ was achievable.

Figure 1 shows a composite plot of the quantum efficiency measured by the xerographic discharge technique (open symbols) and the delayed-field pulse experiments (solid symbols) for samples prepared with rf power of 18W and a silane concentration of 5% in He. Results were obtained for two samples prepared in nominally the same way and essentially the same results were obtained. As can be seen the xerographic discharge measurements indicate a sharp drop in quantum efficiency for fields less than $\sim 5 \times 10^4$V/cm. By contrast, although the quantum efficiency measured by the delayed-collection field technique agrees very well with the xerographic data at the highest fields, for fields less than $\sim 5 \times 10^4$V/cm the quantum efficiency becomes independent of field and equal to the zero field value for these samples of ~ 0.4. The delayed-collection field technique data at low fields allows us to measure the quantum efficiency of photogeneration at low field while avoiding any trapping or recombination processes that occur at time $>$50nsecs. Together with high field data from both measurements this gives an absolute measurement of the photogeneration efficiency from zero to 2×10^5V/cm in these a-Si:H samples.

The data shown in Fig. 1 have the general features of a photogeneration process controlled by geminate recombination. The solids lines are plots of the well-known Onsager formula[8] evaluated to all terms with $\Phi_0 = 1$ and the dielectric constant for a-Si of 11.5. The lines correspond to the indicated values of the thermalization length r_0. The best fit appears to be for $r_0 \sim 45A$. The experimental deviation of about 15% from the low and zero field values for this value of r_0 may be indicative of some build-in field $\sim 10^4 V/cm$ at the metal-a:Si contact. An important feature of the Onsager formalism is that once the values of Φ_0, r_c and r_0 are fixed the quantum efficiency and field dependence are uniquely determined on an absolute scale. In addition this further determines what the temperature dependence of the quantum efficiency at a fixed field must be. The experimental points are found to conform very closely to the

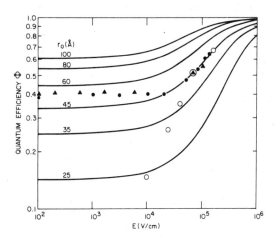

Figure 1 - Plot of quantum efficiency for photogeneration Φ versus electric field with log-log axes. The solid lines are theoretical plots of the Onsager theory with $\Phi_0 = 1$, $\varepsilon = 11.5$ and the indicated values of the thermalization distance r_0. The open symbols refer to xerographic discharge measurements. The closed symbols refer to the delayed-collection field pulse experiments. In the latter case two samples $\sim 15\mu m$ thick were studied. The measurements were made at an excitation wavelength of 4950A.

predicted temperature dependence for a value of $r_0 = 40A$. This important independent check gives further support for the identification of a geminate recombination process in a-Si:H. Data on a sample made with 100% silane gives a zero-field efficiency of 0.55 and an estimated thermalization length of $\sim 80A$. These values of r_0 are in reasonable agreement with estimates from luminescent decay experiments.[1] Previous measurements of the photosensitivity by xerographic[2] and other techniques[5] have established that the quantum efficiency edge in a-Si:H coincides with the absorption edge. This implies that the thermalization distance r_0 in a-Si:H has at most every weak dependence of wavelength. This is fundamentally different from the well-documented case of a-Se where r_0 is strongly wavelength dependent.[9] The implication of this process for a-Si:H photovoltaic cell performance, discussed in detail elsewhere,[10,11] are that a geminate recombination-controlled photogeneration process with r_0 values varying from 40-80A can account for observed photovoltaic conversion efficiencies.

Subsequent recombination of photogenerated electrons and holes after their creation (i.e. the electron-hole pairs that evaded geminate recombination) is obviously an equally important recombination process that occurs in this technologically important material. As indicated earlier a variation of the delayed collection field technique can be used to explore recombination processes. In this case photogeneration is chosen to occur in zero field since the geminate process is now known to result in ~50% of the absorbed photons creating free carriers. After a time delay of variable and controlled duration, a high positive bias is applied with a rise time of <50 nanoseconds that results in all the remaining holes free in the excitation region transiting the sample. By integrating this transit signal one can monitor directly the dependence of the number of surviving holes as a function of the time they co-exist with free electrons in zero field in the excitation region.

The experimental results of the collected charge Q as a function of the delay time t, for a number of temperatures are shown in Fig. 2.

An analysis based on carriers diffusing in a semi-infinite slab with a diffusion constant D, a surface recombination velocity v and a bulk free carrier lifetime of τ allows a fit of the shape of Q versus delay time as indicated by the solid lines in Figure 2.[6] This gives estimates of the surface recombination velocity and the bulk lifetime. At room temperature value of surface recombination velocities of ~5cm/sec and recombination lifetimes ~10 mseconds are observed. In addition, both these parameters have activation energies similar to those of the hole drift mobility suggesting that the recombination process at these intensities are monomolecular diffusion controlled. The possible implication and relation of these long lifetimes to solar cell performance and to the much shorter ones reported are discussed elsewhere.[11]

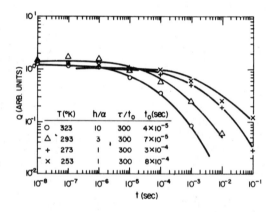

Figure 2 - Experimental results of collected charge Q vs delay time t. The solid curves are calculated values obtained with the parameter values shown in the insert.

References

1. D. Engemann and R. Fischer, *Phys. Status Solidi* B79, 195 (1977); J. Noolandi, K.M. Hong and R.A. Street *J. Non-Cryst. Solids* 35 - 36, 669 (1980).

2. J. Mort, S. Grammatica, J.C. Knights ands R. Lujan, *Solar Cells.*

3. R. Crandall, *Appl. Phys. Letters* 36(7), 607 (1980).

4. G. Pfister and R.C. Enck, Photoconducting and Related Phenomena (edited by J. Mort and D. Pai), Elsevier Scientific Publishng Co, Amsterdam 1975).

5. R.J. Loveland, W.E. Spear and A. Al-Sharbaty, *J. Non-Cryst. Solids* 13, 55 (1973/74).

6. J. Mort, I. Chen. A. Troup, M. Morgan, J.C. Knights and R. Lujan, *Phys. Rev. Letters* 45 1348 (1980).

7. J.C. Knights AIP Conference Proc. 31, 296 (1976).

8. L. Onsager, *Phys. Rev.* 54, 554 (1938).

9. D.M. Pai and R.C. Enck, *Phys. Rev.* B11, 5163 (1975).

10. I. Chen and J. Mort, *Appl. Phys. Letter* 37(10), 952 (1980).

11. I. Chen and J. Mort (in this publication).

STUDIES ON PRIMARY PHOTOCURRENT OF a-Si:H USING
XEROGRAPHIC AND VIDICON TECHNIQUES

I. Shimizu, S. Oda, K. Saito, H. Tomita and E. Inoue
Tokyo Institute of Technology, Yokohama, Japan

ABSTRACT

The primary photocurrent of a-Si:H prepared by glow discharge of SiH_4 was investigated with VIDICON and ELECTROPHOTOGRAPHIC techniques. The photoresponse current depends greatly upon the device structures used and an excellent photoconductivity gain of unity is attainable if the leakage current in the dark is excluded. All results in this study can be interpreted in terms of field-independent efficiency for carrier-generation in a-Si:H.

INTRODUCTION

Amorphous Si (a-Si) prepared by glow discharge of SiH_4 has received much attention from the technical point of view. Solar-cells[1] and photoreceptors[2] for imaging techniques using its excellent photoconductivity are the most promising. A lot of difficulties in designing such photoelectric devices with a-Si arise from either the small mobility or the dispersive relaxation of its photo-induced carriers.

Crandall et al [3] suggested the existence of geminate recombination in the carrier-generation step of a-Si in consequence of primary photocurrent study with a Schottky-type solar-cell. Recently, Mort et. al. presented some experimental support for the interpretation.[4] On the other hand, Tiedje et. al. predicted the carrier-generation efficiency to be independent of the electric field down to 10^3 V/cm in their transient photocurrent study.[5]

In this study, we present measurements of the primary photocurrent of a-Si using the imaging techniques (Xerographic and Vidicon technique) and conclude that "great care must be paid in the experimental work to avoid the complexities caused by space-charge when we study the primary photocurrent of a-Si."

EXPERIMENTAL

The film of a-Si used in this study was prepared by RF glow discharge of SiH_4 with an apparatus described elsewhere.[6] We will refer to the doping levels as the vol % in vppm of the dopant gas added to SiH_4 and express them with a symbol (B-10). An insulative silicon nitride (a-SiN) was prepared by RF glow discharge of a gaseous mixture of N_2 and SiH_4 in a ratio (100:1 in volume).

The structures of a-Si vidicon target are schematically illustrated in Fig. 1. In TYPE 1, n-type a-Si thin layer was inserted between a transparent electrode (In_2O_3:Sn, ITO) and a-Si photoconductive layer to prevent injection of carriers from the electrode. A thin film of a-SiN in TYPE 2 could play the same role as the

ISSN:0094-243X/81/730288-05$1.50 Copyright 1981 American Institute of Physics

doped a-Si in TYPE 1.

In Xerographic receptors, these blocking contacts are essentially required to give a sufficient charge acceptance when the receptors are sensitized with corona.

The photocurrent behaviors of the a-Si targets were measured with a demountable vidicon tester and

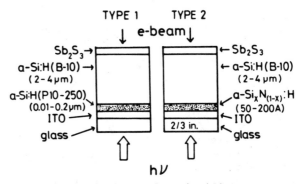

Fig. 1.   Structures of a-Si Vidicon Targets

more accurate measurements were carried out with an image pick-up tube in which the a-Si target was sealed off. Xerographic measurements were made by the conventional method described previously.

RESULTS

VIDICON STUDIES

Some typical current curves of a-Si in the dark and under light illumination plotted as a function of the target voltages (V_T) are shown in log-log plot in Fig. 2. In a target without the blocking-layer, the dark current is proportional to V_T. In TYPE 1, there is no corresponding increase in the dark current despite the increase in the V_T until a certain voltages (broken lines) and abrupt increase in current is observed immediately after exceeding the threshold voltages (V_T^S). The V_T^S value depends greatly upon either the thickness or the doping-level of the blocking layer. The level of the dark current showed in this figure (left) involved some errors arising from light emitted from the filament of the e-gun of the demountable vidicon tester. A low current level

(1--2 nA) was attainable in these targets sealed in an image pick-up tube. In Type 2 target (right), the current was measured with an imaging tube. It is noteworthy that the dark current behavior as a function of the V_T is almost independent of the thickness of the a-SiN in

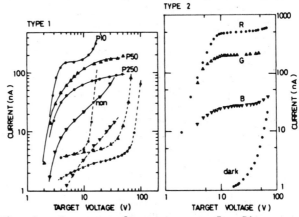

Fig. 2.   Current-voltage curves of a-Si Vidicon targets

TYPE 2. Except for the non-blocking target, the photoresponse current rises rapidly with an increase in the V_T and is saturated at the high level by applying a field of 2×10^4 -- 10^5 V/cm. A constant intensity of light (2 lux cm^{-2}) from W-lamp (3000°K) impinged upon the target in case of

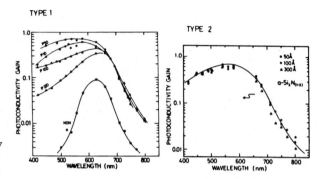

Fig. 3. Photoresponse spectra of a-Si Vidicon

TYPE 1. A TYPE 2 target was illuminated with blue (B), green (G), and red (R) light with W-lamp (3200°K, 10 lux cm^{-2}) fitted with the color filters. The photoresponse behaves in a fashion similar to that of TYPE 1. Only the non-blocking target showed a different behavior. The photoconductive gain derived simply from photocurrent flux divided by incident photon flux is plotted as a function of wavelength (see Fig. 3). With regard to spectral response, a great difference can be seen between TYPE 1 and 2. Here we did not make any corrections for errors anticipated from the optical reflection and absorption. The photoresponse in TYPE 1 decreases dramatically for light of the short wavelengths, which is a consequence of the optical interference due to the optical absorption of the blocking layer. In TYPE 2, no significant changes are seen in the spectra despite the change in the thickness of a-SiN for the blocking, implying that incident light can pass through the layer.

XEROGRAPHIC STUDY

The blocking structure must be required to give a sufficient charge acceptance for the Xerographic receptor. The blocking layers described above are applicable. The type of the doped a-Si depends upon the polarity of the corona, i.e., n-type a-Si is for the positive corona and p-type for the negative corona. The insulative thin film (50--300 Å thick) of a-SiN is applicable to both polarities. The surface of a-Si can retain the positive charges but not the negative ones. Therefore, the top of the receptor must be covered with thin films for negative corona.

By providing these blocking structures, the charge acceptance about 40 V/μm is achievable in the a-Si receptor and consequently about 400 volt is attained as a saturated surface voltage in a receptor with 10μm thick. A half decay time of about 10 sec. was attained in the receptor comprised of undoped a-Si. Illumination with light causes the discharge and the photo-discharge current is deduced from the time derivative of the surface voltage (V_S). Typical photo-discharging current starting at different initial voltages are plotted as a function of V_S in log-log plot and shown in Fig. 4. The photoconductivity gain derived from the initial photo-discharge current is close to unity and independent of the

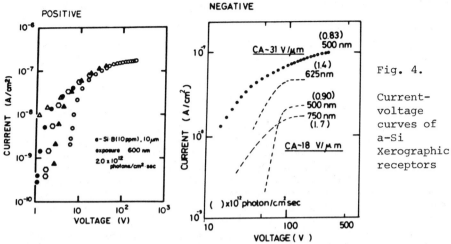

POSITIVE

NEGATIVE

Fig. 4.

Current-voltage curves of a-Si Xerographic receptors

photon energy (hν) when the receptor is illuminated with light of strong absorption. For the negative (right) corona, lower charge acceptance (--18 V/μm) is attained in a receptor with the blocking-layer only at the contact with the electrode, which is affected greatly by the atmospheric condition. This behavior is antici-pated from the leak of charge at the surface of a-Si. The photo-discharge current depends greatly upon the voltages and the wave-lengths of the incident light (broken line). The current-voltage relation for the receptor with an insulative a-SiN layer on the top becomes similar to that for the positive corona (left). By provid-ing such a dielectric layer for the top, the charge acceptance rises to more than 30 V/μm and the photo-discharge behavior is improved dramatically.

DISCUSSION

THE ROLE OF THE BLOCKING

The blocking effect by the n-type a-Si in TYPE 1 Vidicon is interpreted in terms of a short Schubweg (μτE) of holes in the layer deducing from the fact that the threshold voltage correlated with the onset of rising the dark current depends greatly upon the thickness and the doping level of the n-type a-Si. In case of TYPE 2 Vidicon, on the other hand, the amount of carriers emitted from the electrode is decreased by providing the a-SiN thin layer, resulting from a potential barrier at the contact with the elec-trode. It is another important function of the blocking layer that the photo-carriers generated in the a-Si must be passed through the layer to avoid collecting the space-charge. The doped a-Si satisfies this requirement and the thickness of the a-SiN layer would be an important factor from this point of view. Unfavorable phenomena such as "blooming or charge-up" appeared in the devices with a-SiN of more than 0.1 μm thick. No significant increase in the dark current is observed in the a-Si vidicon when the chalcogenide layer on the top is excluded. The top layer is required to avoid lateral conduction and smearing of the picture.

PHOTOCURRENT RESPONSE

Referring to Fig. 2 for TYPE 2 Vidicon, the current-voltage relation may be divided into three regions[7]: one carrier-SCLC in the region of low voltages (i), the saturated current region at high voltages where the photoconductivity gain approaches towards unity (ii), and the intermediate voltage region (iii). The Xerographic receptor for the positive corona showed analogous behavior to the TYPE 2 Vidicon. In case of the Xerographic receptor with a thick a-Si, the photo-discharge current corresponding to the intermediate voltages can be categorized into two; the space-charge free current (a) and the space-charge perturbed current due to traps (b). According to the results shown in Fig. 4 (left), the current curve corresponding to the envelope of the plots is interpreted in terms of range-limited-current and the $\mu\tau$ product of 2×10^{-8} cm^2/V was obtained for the photoholes since the initial photo-discharge current is the case (a). These interpretations are based upon an assumption of the field-independent carrier-generation efficiency.

The current-voltage relation of the TYPE 1 Vidicon and the receptor for the negative corona are more complicated. In case of TYPE 1 Vidicon, the P-doped a-Si used as the blocking-layer may partly interfere the incident light flux due to its strong optical absorption and the degree of the optical interference depends on the field, wavelengths of light, the doping level and the thickness. In Xerographic study, considerable care must be taken to avoid the leakage of the carriers from the contacts since the photoresponse current and its field-dependence are affected greatly as shown in Fig. 4. The charge acceptance of the receptors is a powerful tool to evaluate the leakage of charge.

Within the framework of our experimental work, we conclude that a decrease in photoresponse current in low fields is mainly attributed to the effect of the space-charge and the field-dependence of the carrier generation efficiency is not significant factor of a-Si when it is applied to imaging devices.

This work was supported in part by a Grant-in-Aid for Scientific Research from the Ministry of Education, Science and Culture and by the HOSO-BUNKA Foundation.

REFERENCES

1. D. L. Staebler and C. R. Wronski, Appl. Phys. Lett. 31, 292 (1977).

2. I. Shimizu, T. Komatsu, K. Saito and E. Inoue, J. Non-crystalline Solids 35 & 36, 773 (1980).

3. R. S. Crandall, R. Williams and B. E. Tompkins, J. April. Phys. 50, 5506 (1979).

4 J. Mort, A. Troup, M. Morgan, S. Grammatica, J. Knights and R. Lujan, to be published in App. Phys. Lett.

5. T. Tiedje, C. R. Wronski, B. Abeles and J. M. Cebulka, to be published in Solar Cells.

6. J. C. Knights, G. Lucovsky and R. J. Nemanich, Phil. Mag. B37, 467 (1977).

7. F. J. du Chatenier, Philips Res. Repts. 23, 142 (1968).

Dispersive Diffusion-Controlled Bimolecular
Recombinations in a-Si:H*

K. L. Ngai
Naval Research Laboratory, Washn, D.C. 20375

Abstract

The time evolutions of dispersive diffusion-controlled bimolecular reactions and recombinations are considered in the light of a universal time correlation function $\psi_n(t)$ which comes from a recently proposed fundamental process. The predictions are in excellent agreement with available experimental data for electron-hole recombinations in a-Si:H while those of another currently accepted event-time distribution function fails to agree.

Recently, evidence for dispersive diffusion of electrons in sputtered a-Si:H has been found in diffusion-controlled electron-hole (bimolecular) recombination studies by Vardeny et al.[1] They found that the observed time evolution of the photoinduced midgap absorption can be explained by bimolecular recombination with time-dependent rate $K(t)$ of the form Bt^{-n} and that n has the same value as that determined by transient transport measurements. The latter strongly suggests that both dispersive diffusion and transient transport are due to the same cause. Thus one expects that any model which can describe transient transport must also be able to derive the dispersive diffusion controlled bimolecular recombination rate $K(t) = Bt^{-n}$.

In this work we present the study of non-Markovian diffusion controlled recombinations caused by the jump time distribution $\psi_n(t)$ derived from a recent microscopic model[2-3] that has been applied to a number of areas. The predictions of the model based on $\psi_n(t)$ are in excellent agreement with the experimental data of Vardeny et al.,[1] while those of another widely accepted event-time distribution function[4] fails to agree.

Of central importance in the present work is the jump-time distribution function $\psi_n(t)$ given[2] by

$$\psi_n(t) = (1-n)\, a_n t^{-n} \exp(-a_n t^{1-n}); \quad a_n = e^{-n\gamma}/(1-n)\tau_o E_c^n \quad (1)$$

where $\gamma = 0.577$, E_c is an upper cut-off energy defined earlier and n, referred to as the infrared divergence exponent, is a constant whose value can range from zero to unity. Good agreement of the predictions of our model based on $\psi_n(t)$ with experimental data is achieved for diverse low frequency responses and for materials of different physical and chemical structures. Besides dispersion,

---

*Work supported in part by ONR.

the unified theory offers predictions on quantities including activation energics.[2,3]

Unimolecular and bimolecular reactions involve the calculations[5] of the reaction rate $K(t)$, a conditional probability distribution, which is related to an unconditional one $F(t)$. Both $K(t)$ and $F(t)$ are first-encounter distributions appropriate for irreversible reaction, but $F(t)$ is immediately amenable to calculation by the continous time random walk (CTRW) formalism of Montroll and Weiss[6] once the jump-time distribution is specified. This has been carried out for unimolecular (UM) and pseudo-unimolecular (PUM) reaction.[5] We have rederived the result, which in the notation of Montroll is[6]

(Laplace Transform:) $F(t) = (1/(V-1)) \{ [(1-\psi_n^*(u)) G(\underset{\sim}{0}, z = \psi_n^*(u))]^{-1} - 1 \}$ (2)

where $G(\underset{\sim}{0}, z)$ for $\ell = \underset{\sim}{0}$ that has already been evaluated earlier for various lattices, and extend it to consider bimolecular (BM) reaction which has not been done before. Here we follow Shlesinger[5] and divide the system into $N_A(t=0)$ identical unit cells each containing V sites, one A reactant at its origin and one B reactant which at t=0 has equal probability of occupying all sites in the unit cell except the origin. We consider here a bimolecular reaction A+B→C where $N_A(t=0) = N_B(t=0)$ and the A's diffusing so slowly compared with the B's that the A's can be considered stationary at the origins of their unit cells. This is appropriate for electron-hole recombination in a-Si:H where although both electrons and holes diffuse, yet they have very different mobilities. The stochastic master equation approach leads to the equation for bimolecular decay.

$$d\langle N_A(t) \rangle / dt = -K(t) \langle N_A(t) \rangle^2$$ (3)

From the mathematics of CTRW it is more direct to calculate $F(t)$. $K(t)$ can be obtained once $F(t)$ is known through the relation $K(t) = F(t)/\int_t^\infty F(\tau) d\tau$.

Note that the random walk generating function $G(\underset{\sim}{0}, z)$ as appeared in Eq. (2) has already been evaluated by Montroll[6] for various lattices in different dimensions. Hence we can obtain $F(t)$ by substitution of the Laplace transform $\psi^*(u)$ of our model $\psi_n(t)$ into Eq. (2). For a simple cubic lattice it has been shown that

$$G(0, z = \psi^*(u)) = \{V(1-\psi^*(u))\}^{-1} + (1/V) \sum_{k_1=0}^{N-1} \sum_{k_3=0}^{N-1} {}'$$

$$\{(1-\psi^*(u) [\cos(2\pi k_1 N) + \cos(2\pi k_2 N) + \cos(2\pi k_3 N)]\}^{-1}$$ (4)

where the prime at the summation signs means that the origin $k_1 = k_2 = k_3 = 0$ is to be omitted.

At very long times $t \to \infty$ ($u \to 0$) we can readily obtain $\psi_n^*(u)$ by the expansion $\psi_n^*(u) = 1 - u\langle t \rangle + \dfrac{u^2}{2} \langle t^2 \rangle + \ldots$ where $\langle t^p \rangle \equiv \int t^p \psi_n(t)dt$. Substitution into $G(\underset{\sim}{0},z)$ for a simple cubic lattice, Eq. (4), yields

$$F(t) = [1/(VW)^{1-n}](1-n)a_n t^{-n} \exp\{-[1/(VW)^{1-n}]a_n t^{1-n}\} \tag{5}$$

Here W is the Watson integral which for a simple cubic lattice has the value of 1.516. It then follows,

$$K(t) = [1/(VW)^{1-n}](1-n) \, a_n t^{-n} \tag{6}$$

This is exactly the same as the time-dependent bimolecular recombination rate $K(t) = Bt^{-n}$ as assumed by Vardeny et al.[1] which gives, as they have already shown, a good account of the time dependence of the electron-hole recombination decay in a-Si:H. It would be interesting to compare this (Eq. (6)) with the corresponding predicted $K(t)$ that follows from the Scher-Montroll[4] form of the jump-time distribution function

$$\psi_{SM}(t) \propto A[\Gamma(1-\alpha)]^{-1} t^{-1-\alpha}$$

on the bimolecular recombination rate. The jump-time distribution $\psi_{SM}(t)$ was proposed originally to explain the dispersive transient transport in amorphous systems. At large times where $\psi_{SM}(t)$ has been proposed to apply for dispersive transient transport,[4] the Laplace transform of $\psi_{SM}(t)$ is given by $\psi^*(u) \sim 1 - Au^\alpha$ for $u \to 0$. Substituting this into $G(\underset{\sim}{0},z)$ for a simple cubic lattice we obtain

$$F(t) = \{\alpha AWV/\Gamma(1-\alpha)\}t^{-1-\alpha} \quad .$$

Then, Eq. (3) yields

$$K_{SM}(t) = \alpha t^{-1} \quad .$$

The decay $N_A(t)$ and the decay rate $dN_A(t)/dt$ are very different for the two models. For BM reaction, as $t \to \infty$ our $\psi_n(t)$ model predicts that $\langle N_A(t) \rangle \propto t^{-1+n}$, while the $\psi_{SM}(t)$ model gives $\langle N_A(t) \rangle \propto (\ln t)^{-1}$. In actual experiments[1] the $N_A(0)$ depends on the distance x from the sample surface due to the attenuation $e^{-\alpha_L x}$ of the exciting laser light in a sample of thickness d such that $N_A(0,x) = N_A(0) \exp(-\alpha_L x)$. Then the BM reaction Eq. (3) must be integrated over x as well. This being taken into account and in terms of a reduced time $\tau = t a_n^{1/(1-n)}/VW$, the $\psi_n(t)$ model predicts that $\langle N_A(t) \rangle = (N_A(0)/(1-n)\tau^{1-n})\ln\{(1+\tau^{1-n})/(1+\tau^{1-n}\exp(-\alpha_L d))\}$, in agreement with the results of Vardeny et al.[1] and their experimental data of excess carrier recombination in aSi:H. On the other hand the ψ_{SN} model with $\psi_{SM} = t^{-1-\alpha}$ gives $N_A(t) = (\alpha_L \alpha \ln(t/t_o)) \ln\{[1+\alpha N_o \ln(t/t_o)]/[1+\alpha N_o \ln(t/t_o) \exp(-\alpha_L d)]\}$, where $N_o = N_A(t=t_o)$ and t_o is a reference time. This prediction of the ψ_{SM} model is in contradiction with experimental data.

For pseudounimolecular reaction, the $\psi_n(t)$ model leads to the decay $N_A(t)$ of the form $\exp(-B_n'Mt^{1-n})$ for both the earlier and the long time regimes where M and B' are constants. This is consistent with pulse radiolysis experimental results of Miller[7] and of Baxendale and Sharpe[7] on the decay of trapped electrons in aqueous glasses by reaction with impurity molecules whose concentration is much larger than that of the electrons (M >> 1).

In summary in this work we have extended our unified theory of low frequency (long time) fluctuation-dissipation properties of condensed matter to the consideration of diffusion-controlled bimolecular recombination. The entire consideration is based on the same universal correlation function $\psi_n(t)$ that has been derived microscopically and applied successfully in several areas of low frequency responses. The important results we have derived here include diffusion-controlled bimolecular reaction rate and its time dependence that is in accord with experimental data. In contrast the Scher and Montroll's $\psi_{SM}(t)$ fails to reproduce the observed behavior of the bimolecular electron-hole recombination decay in a-Si:H which shows also dispersive transient transport.

It is important to emphasize that we address our discussion here to sputtered a-Si:H, the material studied by Vardeny et al.[1] They have found that n which appears in $K(t) = Ct^{-n}$ is independent of temperature. Glow discharged a-Si:H may behave differently. The recombination observed by Vardeny et al.[1] is definitely bimolecular as supported by measurements and one should not be confused with the different situation of diffusion and unimolecular recombination studies by Mort et al.[8] Note also that Vardeny et al. have assumed, and correctly so, that the rate K(t) has the time dependence of t^{-n}. Their assumption is based on the dispersive transient transport data with mobility $\mu \sim t^{-n}$ and a generalized Nernst-Einstein relation between mobility and diffusion constant. Although the Scher-Montroll function is sufficient to explain $\mu \sim t^{-n}$, yet it may not be necessary. Vardeny et al. are guided by the data and the Nernst-Einstein relation to arrive at the assumption of $K(t) \sim t^{-n}$. They certainly have not justified that the Scher-Montroll function is necessary for the t^{-n} mobility or for the $K(t) \sim t^{-n}$ relation. In our work, we show that when K(t) is calculated by CTRW, it turns out that Scher-Montroll function does not give $K(t) \sim t^{-n}$. Not only Scher-Montroll's hopping time distribution function model but also alternate models such as (1) multiple trapping from an exponential distribution of traps[9] and (2) progressive thermalization of carriers in an exponential distribution of traps[10] will not be consistent with Vardeny et al.'s data in sputtered a-Si:H. The latter model gives the distribution of release times $\psi(t) \sim t^{-1-\alpha}$ of the same form as that of Scher and Montroll and hence the same difficulty of its prediction on long time bimolecular recombination decay will arise at least for sputtered a-Si:H.

REFERENCES

1. Z. Vardeny, P. O'Connor, S. Ray and J. Tauc, Phys. Rev. Lett. 44, 1267 (1980).
2. K.L. Ngai, Comments Solid State Phys. 9, 127 (1979) Part I; 9, 141 (1980) Part II.
3. K.L. Ngai, Xiyi Huang and Fu-sui Liu, to appear in Proceedings of the Conference on the Physics of MOS Insulators, Raleigh, North Carolina (1980), ed. G. Lucovsky and S. Pantelides, Plenum, N.Y.
4. H. Scher and E.W. Montroll, Phys. Rev. B12, 2455 (1975).
5. M.F. Shlesinger, J. Chem. Phys. 70, 4813 (1979).
6. E.W. Montroll, Proc. Symp. Math. Am. Math. Soc. 16, 193 (1964); J. Math. Phys. 10, 753 (1969); E.W. Montroll and G.H. Weiss, J. Math. Phys. 6, 167 (1965).
7. J.R. Miller, J. Phys. Chem. 79, 1070 (1975); J.H. Baxendale and P.H.G. Sharpe, Chem. Phys. Lett. 39, 401 (1976).
8. J. Mort, I. Chen, A. Troup, M. Morgan, J. Knights and R. Lujan, Phys. Rev. Lett. 45, 1348 (1980).
9. F.W. Schmidlin, Phys. Rev. B 16, 2362 (1977).
10. T. Tiedje and A. Rose, to be published.

COLLECTION EFFICIENCY OF PHOTOGENERATED CARRIERS IN SILICON HYDRIDE a-SiH$_x$ MIS SOLAR CELL STRUCTURES

B. Abeles, C. R. Wronski, Y. Goldstein*, H. E. Stasiewski,
D. Gutkowicz-Krusin, T. Tiedje and G. D. Cody
Exxon Research and Engineering Company
P. O. Box 45, Linden, NJ 07036

ABSTRACT

The collection efficiency in a-SiH$_x$ Schottky barrier solar cell structures is enhanced at short wavelengths by a thin oxide layer at the metal semiconductor interface due to reduction in diffusion of electrons from the semiconductor into the metal. Interpretation of the experimental results yields a diffusion length for holes of 0.2μm and a depletion width of 0.26μm.

Metal-insulator-semiconductor (MIS) solar cells afford convenient and versatile structures to investigate electrical transport properties of the semiconductor and of the semiconductor insulator interface. In a previous paper[1] it was shown that in a-SiH$_x$ Schottky barrier solar cells, diffusion of electrons from the semiconductor into the metal contact can significantly reduce the collection efficiency, especially at short wavelengths, for which the optical absorption coefficient is large. The experimental results and the theoretical model in the previous paper were for the case of thin semiconductor films (thickness less than the diffusion length of the minority carriers (holes)), for which the bulk recombination time of photogenerated carriers could be neglected. In a subsequent paper, Gutkowicz-Krusin[2] extended the model to include the effects of bulk recombination so as to make it applicable to films of arbitrary thicknesses. In this paper we report experimental results for the effect of surface oxide on the collection efficiency in a-SiH$_x$ MIS structures and compare the results to the theoretical model.

The a-SiH$_x$ films were prepared by RF glow discharge decomposition of SiH$_4$ under conditions described previously.[3] The substrates were 7059 glass with a 1000Å thick evaporated Cr film. A 500Å thick phosphorous doped SiH$_x$ film formed ohmic contact to the undoped SiH$_x$ film which was typically 1μm thick. When we wished to achieve an intimate metal insulator contact, we either transferred the films within several minutes after preparation to the vacuum system in which metal contacts were evaporated, or the films were etched in buffered HF and rinsed in deionized water just prior to metalization. No significant differences in the collection efficiencies were found in solar cell structures produced by the two methods. Oxidations were performed in air or in pure oxygen from room temperature up to 300°C prior to metalization. The metal contacts were Pd or Pt dots 100Å thick, 2mm^2 in area.

*Permanent Address: Racah Institute of Physics,
The Hebrew University, Jerusalem 91000, ISRAEL

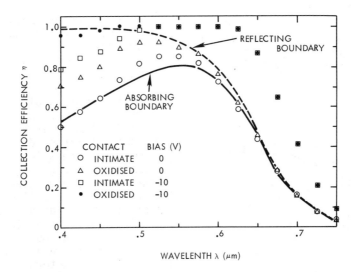

Fig. 1. Collection efficiencies $\eta(\lambda)$ for Pd-SiH$_x$ MIS
structures with "intimate" metal-semiconductor contact
(circles and squares) and with oxidized metal-semiconductor contact (triangles and dots). Measurements
are given for zero bias and for a 10V reverse bias
voltage. The film thickness L = 1.5μm. The two calculated curves are for reflecting and absorbing electron boundaries using L_p = 0.20μm, x_0 = 0.26μm,
V_0 = 0.45 V and $\alpha(\lambda)$ from ref. 3.

Collection efficiency measurements were made with monochromatic
light flux of 10^{13} photons/cm^{2}sec. Details of the technique have been
published[4]. The collection efficiency $\eta(\lambda)$ (defined as the ratio of
charge carriers collected to photons transmitted through the top metal
contact) is shown as a function of λ in Fig. 1 for two solar cell
structures. The circles and triangles in the figure were obtained
under short circuit current conditions, the circles on a cell with
intimate metal-semiconductor contact and the triangles on one in
which the SiH$_x$ film was exposed to oxygen at 240°C for 30 minutes.
The corresponding results for a reverse bias of 10V are shown by
the squares and dots. The lines in the figure are theoretical and will
be explained below. We note for now that $\eta(0.4)$ is appreciably higher
for the oxidized film than for the unoxidized one and that for the
unoxidized film $\eta(0.4)$ does not saturate, even with a reversed bias of
10V.

Auger spectra of two a-SiH$_x$ films, one freshly etched, and the
other oxidized under identical conditions as the film in Fig. 1, are
shown in Fig. 2. The freshly etched surface (lower line) exhibits a
large Si peak at 96 eV and a small O peak due to some residual surface oxide. The intentionally oxidized surface shows a larger O peak
and a reduced and shifted Si Auger structure indicating an incomplete
oxide of Si. Both spectra show presence of C, presumably due to

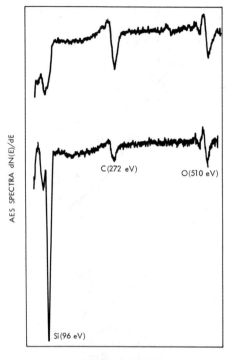

AES SPECTRA dN(E)/dE

C(272 eV)   O(510 eV)

Si(96 eV)

ELECTRON ENERGY E

Fig. 2. Auger electron spectra of a freshly etched (lower line) and a partially oxidized SiH_x surface.

surface contamination. Upon additional oxidation the O peak increased further and the Si transition became characteristic of SiO_2.

We now compare our results with the theoretical model. The photogenerated current was calculated from the charge continuity equation governing drift, diffusion, photogeneration and recombination of charge carriers. The equation was integrated either for a boundary which reflects electrons (corresponding to an insulator impervious to electrons), or one that absorbs electrons (corresponding to an intimate metal semiconductor contact). It was assumed that the potential V has the form $V=V_0 \exp(-x/x_0)$, where V_0 is the built-in potential, x is the distance into the semiconductor from the metal-semiconductor interface and x_0 characterizes the depletion width. The diffusion length for holes, L_p, was assumed to be independent of x. Based on these assumptions $\eta(\lambda)$ was calculated as a function of sample thickness L, optical absorption constant $\alpha(\lambda)$, and of V_0, x_0, and L_p. To fit the experimental data we used for L the measured film thickness of 1.5μm, for V_0 the value of 0.45V derived from the saturated open circuit voltage measured on a solar cell with an intimate $Pd-SiH_x$ contact, and for $\alpha(\lambda)$ the measured values reported in ref. 3. To determine the remaining parameters x_0 and L_p we have plotted in Fig. 3 the calculated values of η as a function of x_0 for the case of strongly absorbing light ($\lambda = 0.4$μm; $\alpha = 5.5 \times 10^5$ cm^{-1}) for both reflecting and absorbing electron boundaries and for the case of weakly absorbing light ($\lambda = 0.65$μm, $\alpha = 1.3 \times 10^4$ cm^{-1}) for an absorbing electron boundary (reflecting boundary gives essentially the same result and was omitted for clarity) and for different values of L_p. The fact that η for strongly absorbing light ($\lambda = 0.4$μm) and an absorbing electron boundary is a strongly varying function of x_0 and is insensitive to L_p, while for weakly absorbing light ($\lambda = 0.65$μm) η is strongly dependent on L_p but only weakly dependent on x_0 provides an unambiguous method for the determination of x_0 and L_p.

The two theoretical curves in Fig. 1 were calculated for $L_p = 0.20$μm and $x_0 = 0.26$μm using absorbing and reflecting boundary conditions, respectively. The agreement is satisfactory except at

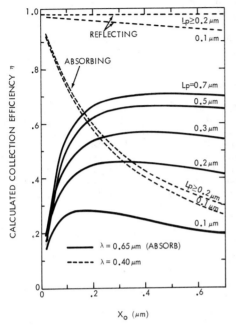

Fig. 3. Calculated collection efficiencies at λ = 0.4μm and at λ = 0.65μm as a function of x_0 with L = 1.5μm, V_0 = 0.45 V, and for different values of L_p.

short wavelengths for the case of the oxidized film, the likely reason being that the semiconductor-insulator boundary is not fully reflecting, as assumed in the calculation. Independent measurements of x_0 by the capacitance technique[5] on a film prepared under similar conditions yielded a value of x_0 = 0.27μm, in excellent agreement with x_0 determined from the collection efficiency. Using the relation $L_p = (kT\mu_p\tau_p/q)^{1/2}$ we compute $\mu_p\tau_p$ = 1.6 x 10^{-8} cm^2/V where μ_p and τ_p are the free-carrier hole mobility and recombination time, respectively. Assuming a value[6] of μ_p = 0.7 cm^2/Vsec we obtain τ_p = 2.3 x 10^{-8} sec. It is interesting to note that a similar value as ours for the $\mu_p\tau_p$ product is reported by Wronski et al.[7] for their best-quality sputtered films, while Moore[8] reports a considerably lower value of $\mu_p\tau_p$ = 3 x 10^{-9} cm^2/V, determined from PEM effect on a DC glow discharge film.

The agreement between the theoretical and experimental collection efficiencies (for the case of the intimate contact) is an independent confirmation of the exponential dependence of the potential on the distance from the interface. The different character of the functional dependence of η on x_0 and L_p for strongly absorbed and weakly absorbed light allows an unambiguous fit of the data and thus provides a method for determining these two important solar cell parameters.

We thank S. Kelemen for the Auger spectroscopy.

REFERENCES

1. D. Gutkowicz-Krusin, et al., Appl. Phys. Lett. 38, 87 (1981).
2. D. Gutkowicz-Krusin, J. Appl. Phys. (to be published).
3. G. D. Cody, B. Abeles, C. R. Wronski, B. Brooks, and W. A. Lanford, J. Non-Cryst. Solids 35-36, 463 (1980).
4. C. R. Wronski, B. Abeles, and G. D. Cody, Solar Cells, 2, 245 (1980).
5. T. Tiedje, C. R. Wronski, B. Abeles, and J. M. Cebulka, Solar Cells, 2, 301 (1980).
6. T. Tiedje, et al., (to be published).
7. C. R. Wronski, T. D. Moustakas, and T. Tiedje (to be published).
8. A. Moore, Appl. Phys. Lett. 37, 327, 1980.

EFFECTS OF GEMINATE RECOMBINATION ON THE PHOTOVOLTAIC EFFICIENCY OF a-Si:H SOLAR CELLS

I. Chen and J. Mort

Xerox Corporation, Webster Research Center,   Webster, N.Y.   14580

ABSTRACT

The photovoltaic characteristics of a-Si:H Schottky barrier cell have been analyzed theoretically taking into account the geminate recombination and the localized state distribution. A comparison of the results with the experimental data in the literature leads to fundamentally different conclusions regarding the limitations in this type of photovoltaic cell. The limitation due to carrier lifetime is unimportant in a cell of typical thickness (~0.5μm), while the geminate recombination can essentially account for observed recombination losses.

A number of measurements[1-3] including xerographic discharge and delayed-collection field measurements have indicated that the quantum efficiency of photogeneration in amorphous Si:H is field-dependent, and may be determined by the Onsager theory of geminate recombination.[4] In this paper we report a theoretical investigation of the effects of geminate recombination on the photovoltaic characteristics of a-Si:H Schottky barrier solar cells.[5]

A typical a-Si:H Schottky barrier cell[6] is shown schematically in the inset of Fig. 1. The semiconductor, usually undoped a-Si:H, of thickness t is bounded in front (x=o) by a high work function metal (e.g. Pt, Pd), and at the rear (x=t) by a heavily doped (n$^+$) a-Si:H layer.

Theoretical calculations of the collection and/or the conversion efficiencies for amorphous silicon solar cells already exist in the literature.[7-10] In this paper a different and more rigorous

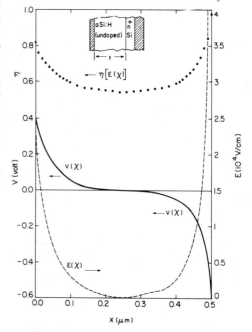

Fig. 1 - The electrostatic potential V(x), and the electric field intensity E(x) in a 0.5μm a-Si:H Schottky barrier cell schematically illustrated in the inset. The dotted curve is the Onsager quantum efficiency with r_o=80A.

approach is taken. The current density, including both the drift and the diffusion com-ponents is calculated by integrating the continuity equations.[11] The unique property of amorphous semiconductors, i.e. the distribution of localized states in the energy gap is explicitly taken into account in solving Poisson's equation for the potential distribution $V(x)$. The results for a cell of thickness $t=0.5\mu m$, is shown in Fig. 1. The boundary value at $x=0$, $V(0)=0.40eV$, is the surface barrier height observed with Pd or Pt contacts.[6] The value at $x=t$, $V(t)=-0.6eV$, is estimated from the work of Spear et al.[12] The corresponding electric field distribution $E(x)$ is also shown (dashed line) in Fig. 1.

The carrier generation rate $G(x)$ with a monochromatic light of intensity F_o is given by

$$G(x) = \alpha F_o \eta [e^{-\alpha x} + f_t e^{-\alpha(2t-x)}]/(1-f_o f_t e^{-2\alpha t}) \qquad (1)$$

where α is the absorption coefficient, f_o and f_t are the fraction of the light internally reflected into the cell at the front and the rear boundaries, respectively and η is the quantum efficiency of photogeneration. If geminate recombination occurs, η is a function of the field E, as determined by the Onsager theory.[4] The values of $\eta(E)$ appropriate to a-Si:H, i.e. the dielectric constant=11.5 and the thermalization length $r_o=10A$ to $90A$ have been calculated by Yip et al.[13] These data combined with $E(x)$ of Fig. 1 yield the quantum efficiency as a function of x, $\eta[E(x)]$. An example with $r_o=80A$ is shown (dotted line) in Fig. 1.

In order to concentrate on the effects of geminate recombination, we shall initially assume in the following discussion that the non-geminate recombination is negligible.

For a given set of geometrical and optical parameters (t,f_o,f_t) the short circuit current $J_{sc}(\lambda)$ can be calculated for monochromatic light with a wavelength λ and an absorption coefficient α. The collection efficiency for this wavelength is then

$$Y[\alpha(\lambda)] = J_{sc}(\lambda)/qF_o \qquad (2)$$

where $\alpha(\lambda)$ is the absorption spectrum[14,15] of the undoped a-Si:H. The total short-circuit current obtained with the solar radiation is the convolution of $Y(\lambda)$ over the solar spectrum $F(\lambda)$,

$$J_{sc} = \int F(\lambda)Y[\alpha(\lambda)]d\lambda \qquad (3)$$

The AMI solar spectrum[16] is used in this calculation. From $\lambda=0.3\mu m$ to $1.02\mu m$, the integrated intensity is 2.06×10^{17} photons/cm^{2}sec and the total power is about 65mW/cm^2 (compared to the total power of ~100 mW/cm^2).

The collection efficiency Y for a $0.5\mu m$ thick cell is shown in Fig. 2 as a function of wavelength, for the cases: (1) the quantum efficiency is both field-independent and unity, designated by $\eta=1$, and (2) the quantum efficiency is determined by geminate recombination according to the Onsager theory, with a thermalization length r_o, designated by $\eta(E,r_o)$ with r_o in A. The results for four values of r_o are plotted. The upper set of five curves are obtained with the idealized condition of $f_o=f_t=1$, i.e. all incident photons are absorbed due to multiple reflection. The lower set of five curves are calculated with $f_o=0$ and $f_t=1$, i.e. the light makes two passes in the undoped aSi:H layer, while no light is transmitted into the n^+ layer. The total J_{sc} calculated for these cases is given in Table I.

When a potential difference V_p between the two boundaries of the cell is induced by exposure to light, the barrier heights at the two boundaries are reduced by a total of V_p. Poisson's equation is solved with new values of the front and the rear barrier heights, and the total current density J calculated , for various values of V_p. The results for the case $f_o=0$ and $f_t=1$ are shown in Fig.3. The intercepts of the curves with the J (vertical) axis are the short-circuit current, and those with the V_p (horizontal) axis give the open-circuit voltage. Table I summarizes these data, and the maximum output power P_{max} and the filling factor FF.

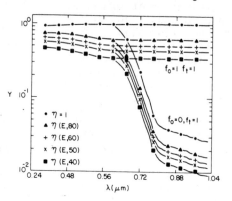

Fig. 2 - The collection efficiency Y for a $0.5\mu m$ a-Si:H cell as a function of wavelength, for two sets of reflection parameter f_o, f_t values and four sets of thermalization lengths r_o.

Since the total solar radiation power is about $100mW/cm^2$, the numbers under the column for P_{max} also give the conversion efficiency in percent. The data shown in Table I are obtained with a specific set of input parameter values. As the latter vary within a reasonable range,

It can be seen from Table I that the short-circuit current and the conversion efficiency are significantly reduced by geminate recombination, while the open-circuit potential and the filling factor are only slightly affected. The results obtained with $f_o=f_t=1$ correspond to an idealized case where all incident photons can be utilized. The set of values with $f_o=0$ and $f_t=1$ represents a more realistic case. However, since the non-geminate recombination has been neglected in these calculations, these values are expected to represent upper limits. It is noteworthy that the results obtained with geminate recombination are very close to the observed values in a-Si:H photovoltaic cells reported by many workers in this field.[6,8,10,17,18] This suggests that if geminate recombination is operative, the loss due to any other recombination process must be relatively insignificant.

This is at variance with current ideas about the limiting factors in a-Si:H solar cells. The general consensus appears to be that the conversion efficiency is limited by carrier recombination of the Shockley-Read-Hall type or a bimolecular bulk process.[6-10] We would like to suggest that there may be some inconsistencies in this viewpoint.

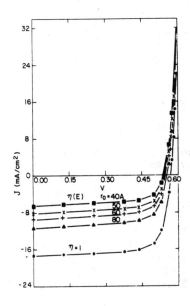

TABLE I. Effects on system parameters of geminate recombination.

η	J_{SC} (mA/cm^2)	V_{OC} (V)	P_{max} (mW/cm^2)	FF
	$f_0 = f_t = 1$			
$n = 1$	32.6	0.588	14.9	0.766
$\eta(E,80)$	20.7	0.573	8.61	0.726
$\eta(E,60)$	17.2	0.568	6.97	0.713
$\eta(E,50)$	14.8	0.564	5.86	0.703
$\eta(E,40)$	11.7	0.555	4.50	0.689
	$f_0 = 0, f_t = 1$			
$\eta = 1$	17.3	0.570	7.39	0.749
$\eta(E,80)$	11.4	0.553	4.31	0.685
$\eta(E,60)$	9.49	0.547	3.54	0.682
$\eta(E,50)$	8.17	0.543	3.01	0.679
$\eta(E,40)$	6.51	0.537	2.36	0.676

Fig. 3 - J-V characteristics for 0.5μm a-Si:H cell, with f_0=0 and f_t=1, and four values of thermalization lengths

In a conventional (crystalline) extrinsic semiconductor, the Shockley-Read-Hall recombination rate is controlled by the minority carrier lifetime. This is a consequence of the equilibrium majority carrier concentration being much larger than any density of photogenerated carriers. Such is not the case in undoped a-Si:H, where the equilibrium majority carrier (electron) density[13] is only ~10^{10}cm^{-3}. For solar intensities of ~10^{17} photons cm^{-2}sec^{-1}, the photogenerated carrier density will be much larger than the equilibrium concentration. The Shockley-Read recombination rate will now be controlled by the *longer* carrier lifetime. This has been confirmed by numerical calculations of the short-circuit currents.[5] In undoped a-Si:H, the electron lifetime (~10^{-5}sec) and diffusion length (~1μm) have been reported to be substantially larger than the corresponding values for holes. However, recent delayed-collection field measurements indicate that the hole diffusion length in undoped a-Si:H can also be as long as ~1μm.[3] We therefore suggest that Shockley-Read-Hall recombination in a-Si:H Schottky solar cells of typical thicknesses ~0.5μm will be unimportant.

The bimolecular recombination introduces non-linearity in J_{sc} with respect to light intensity. Since J_{sc} in a-Si:H solar cells has been observed to be linear in intensity up to (at least) one AM1,[19] we can conclude that the bimolecular process or any process involving intensity dependent lifetime cannot be an important loss mechanism in this type of solar cells. The loss due to geminate recombination, on the other hand, can account for the linearity in intensity as well as the magnitude of the observed value.

References

1.   R. Williams and R.S. Crandall, RCA Review 40, 371 (1979).
2.   J. Mort and S. Grammatica, J. Knights and R. Lujan, Solar Cells 2, 451 (1980).
3.   J. Mort, I. Chen. A. Troup, M. Morgan, J. Knights and R. Lujan, Phys. Rev. Lett. 45, 1348 (1980).
4.   D.M. Pai and R.C. Enck, Phys. Rev. B11, 5163 (1975).
5.   Mathematical details will be presented in a later publication; I. Chen and J. Mort, Appl. Phys. Lett. 37, 952 (1980).
6.   C.R. Wronski, D.E. Carlson and R.E. Daniel, Appl. Phys. Lett. 29, 602 (1976).
7.   B.T. Debney, Solid-State and Electron Devices, 2, 515 (1978).
8.   R. Crandall, Appl. Phys. Lett. 36, 607 (1980).
9.   A. Madan and S.R. Ovshinsky, J. Non-Cryst. Sol. 3536, 171 (1980).
10. D.E. Carlson, The Conf. Records of 14th IEEE Photovoltaic Specialists Conference (1980), p. 291, D.L. Marcel, C.R. Wronski. T. Tiedje, B. Abeles, and G.C. Cody, ibid, p. 1057.
11. A. DeMari, Solid-State Electronics, 11, 33 (1968).
12. W.E. Spear, P.G. LeComber and A.J. Snell, Phil. Mag. B38, 303 (1978). W.E. Spear and P.G. LeComber, Phil. Mag. 33, 935 (1976).
13. K.L. Yip. L.S. Li and I. Chen, J. Chem. Phys. 74, 751 (1981).
14. R.J. Loveland, W.E. Spear and A. Al-Sharbaty, J. Non-Cryst. Sol. 13, 55 (1973/74).
15. D.E. Carlson and C.R. Wronski, Appl. Phys. Lett. 28, 671 (1976).
16. M.P. Tekaekara, "Data on Incident Solar Energy " in *The Energy Crisis and Energy from the Sun*, Institute of Environmental Sciences, (1974).
17. R.C. Crandall, R. Williams and B.E. Tompkins, J. Appl. Phys. 50, 5506 (1979).
18. R.A. Gibson, W.E. Spear, P.G. LeComber and A.J. Snell, J. Non-Crystl. Sol. 35/36, 725 (1980).
19. C.R. Wronski, IEEE Trans. on Electron Devices, ED-24, 351 (1977).

SURFACE CHEMICAL REACTIVITY OF PLASMA-DEPOSITED
AMORPHOUS SILICON

D. E. Aspnes, B. G. Bagley, A. A. Studna, A. C. Adams,
and F. B. Alexander, Jr.
Bell Laboratories, Murray Hill, New Jersey 07974

ABSTRACT

Initial air oxidation rates and limiting oxide thicknesses of
plasma-deposited amorphous silicon (a-Si(H)) films are at least an
order of magnitude less than those of single-crystal silicon.
Spectral changes resulting from either chemically forced or long-
term natural oxidation followed by HF stripping show that oxidation
proceeds by consuming inhomogeneously distributed silicon, thereby
leading to an increased surface roughness and density deficit in
the film.

INTRODUCTION

A knowledge of the surface reactivity of a material is
important for applications involving device fabrication,
particularly with respect to the formation and control of interface
oxides. We report here the results of an investigation of the
growth and chemical removal of air or chemically grown overlayers
on a-Si(H) films. The results are consistent with a columnar
microstructure that is relatively inert but is gradually eroded by
chemical action.

EXPERIMENTAL

Films of a-Si(H) of 7000Å nominal thickness were grown by
plasma deposition onto c-Si substrates at a temperature of 250C.
Reactor conditions of 1 torr pressure, a gas mixture of 1% silane
in argon, and an rf power level of 32 watts were used. The as-
grown surfaces were visually perfect, showing no evidence of light
scattering or visible imperfections.

Pseudo (apparent)-dielectric function spectra $<\varepsilon> = <\varepsilon_1> +$
$i<\varepsilon_2>$ were obtained from 1.5 to 6.0 eV using an automatic spectroscopic ellipsometer described elsewhere.[1] Chemical treatments were
monitored by flowing solutions over the surface of a prealigned
sample, rinsing with the diluent (water or methanol), blow-drying
with filtered N_2, then maintaining the sample in a reduced N_2 flow
to eliminate surface contamination effects, all while taking data
continuously at regular intervals. For these measurements the
ellipsometer was held at 3.5 eV, near the peak in $<\varepsilon_2>$, to minimize
light penetration in the sample and to maximize surface sensitivity.
Effective thicknesses of SiO_2 overlayers were obtained to a
precision of ±0.01Å.

ISSN:0094-243X/81/730307-05$1.50 Copyright 1981 American Institute of Physics

308

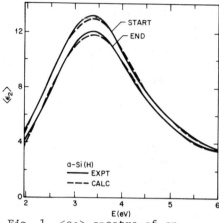

Fig. 1 $<\varepsilon_2>$ spectra of an
a-Si(H) film, as-deposited
(START) and after numerous
oxidation and stripping cycles
(END). Calculated curves are
described in text.

OPTICAL PROPERTIES AND
SAMPLE STRUCTURE

Figure 1 shows $<\varepsilon_2>$ spectra
from 1.95 to 6.0 eV of a typical
film after 1.5h air exposure
followed by HF stripping, and
after a series of forced or
natural oxidations also followed
by HF stripping. The region
below 1.95 eV is dominated by
interference oscillations in the
film. The two spectra are
basically identical to each
other and to that of hydrogen-
free LPCVD a-Si(ref. 2) to within multiplicative constants.
This indicates that the dominant
species contributing to the
polarizability of a-Si(H) in
this spectral range is the
Si-Si bond, and that it is
relatively unaffected by the presence of hydrogen. The magnitude
differences are simply due to differences in the densities of
Si-Si bonds per unit volume. The appearance of interference
oscillations at anomalously high values of $<\varepsilon_2> \sim 4$ together with
the small shifts of the $<\varepsilon_2>$ peaks to lower energies are
characteristic distortions indicating the presence of an overlayer
with a dielectric response between those of bulk and ambient.
This is most likely due to microscopic roughness, because oxides
were chemically stripped before measurement.

Accordingly, we modeled the material as density-deficient
LPCVD a-Si beneath a similar density-deficient overlayer using
standard three-dimensional effective-medium approximation (EMA) and
linear regression analysis techniques.[3] A three-parameter fit
using the void fraction, f_s, of the substrate and thickness, d_o, and
void fraction, f_o, of the overlayer as free variables, resulted
in residuals of 0.56 and 0.46 for the start and end spectra of
Fig. 1, respectively. Because microstructural studies[4] indicated a
columnar microstructure for similar material, we repeated the
calculation for a two-dimensional EMA to more accurately represent
the transverse component of the dielectric tensor of a heterogeneous
material of this microstructure.[5] The residuals calculated in this
model were significantly less, 0.28 and 0.32 respectively. The
improved fit is consistent with a columnar microstructure for these
films.

The free variable values obtained for the as-grown film were
f_s = 0.16±0.01, f_o = 0.32±0.01, and d_o = 100±8Å. After numerous
processing steps these became f_s = 0.19±0.01, f_o = 0.34±0.01, and
d_o = 100±11Å. The uncertainties refer to 90% confidence limits
obtained from linear regression analysis, and do not contain

uncertainties due to systematic errors. The spectra calculated in this model are also shown in Fig. 1 and the fit is seen to be very good. The increase in void fraction 100Å under the surface upon chemical processing is also consistent with a columnar microstructure, because it indicates that oxidation proceeds by unevenly consuming material in a manner that is impossible with a homogeneous sample.

OXIDE REMOVAL

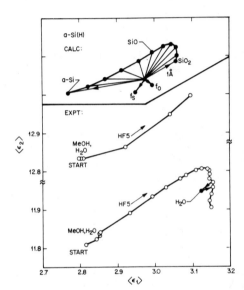

Figure 2 shows the dynamic response of the sample to oxide removal in a solution of 5 vol. % HF in methanol (HF5), both after short (1.5h) atmospheric exposure following deposition, and after many oxidation and stripping cycles. HF5 was used because, unlike water, methanol readily wets the surface and does not leave a residual oxide film (see below). The upper diagram shows the theoretically expected behavior of $<\varepsilon>$ if 1Å of a uniform EMA mixture of $(a-Si)_x (SiO_2)_{1-x}$ is removed from the surface. The points labeled f_s and f_o show the changes expected if the respective void fractions are increased by 0.001. The calculation shows that the initial atmospheric exposure resulted in the accumulation of $\sim$1Å of contamination (detected by its removal in water and methanol), and $\sim$2Å of an insoluble transparent material, probably SiO_2. A c-Si surface exposed to air for a similar period would accumulate a layer at least twice as thick.[6]

Fig. 2 $<\varepsilon>$ trajectories for the as-deposited (upper) and end conditions (lower) shown in Fig. 1. Expected trajectories for several models are shown at the top.

After prolonged air exposure and repeated oxidation-stripping cycles the $<\varepsilon_2>$ value is reduced about 10%, as shown in Fig. 1 and at the bottom of Fig. 2. Yet oxide stripping proceeds identically for the two cases, indicating a common surface chemistry. These two results also provide compelling evidence for an oxidation process that consumes Si-Si bonds well under the surface, as shown by the following argument. The diagram at the top of Fig. 2 shows that $<\varepsilon_2>$ can be lowered while maintaining $<\varepsilon_1>$ fixed only if SiO accumulates or if the void fraction in the surface <u>and</u> bulk regions increases. But 17Å of SiO is needed to reduce $\overline{<\varepsilon_2>}$ by the observed 10%. This should change the surface chemistry, in contrast to our results. We conclude that the more probable mechanism is the uneven removal of bulk material, increasing the density deficit in the outer regions.

A more direct argument can be given by considering the details of the trajectory at the bottom, which shows the results of repeated HF5 treatments alternated with rinses in H_2O. For clarity only one H_2O datum is indicated, although in every case the effect of H_2O was the same. Repeated treatments lead to a saturation followed by a decrease of $<\varepsilon_2>$ which is a small-scale version of the cumulative effect shown in Fig. 2. By referring to the diagram we see that H_2O leaves $\sim 0.3\text{Å}$ of SiO_2 (or similar transparent material) which is removed with HF5. We therefore have direct evidence of the consumption of bulk material in an oxidation-stripping cycle. We emphasize that a <u>cumulative</u> effect as seen in Fig. 2 can occur <u>only</u> if the material is heterogeneous; the removal of material in one dimension as in c-Si, would result always in a return of the trajectory to the same point.

OXIDATION

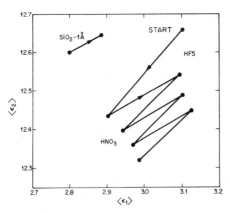

Fig. 3 As Fig. 2, but for forced oxidation with HNO3. The reference increment corresponds to removing 1Å of SiO_2.

Figure 3 shows the results of oxidation forced by chemical means. It is seen that alternate HNO_3 and HF5 treatments result in the growth and removal of several Å of material with a gradual drift downward in the value of $<\varepsilon_2>$. This drift would occur if inhomogeneously distributed a-Si is being consumed (as also occurs with H_2O or natural oxidation). Note that the HF5 line accurately follows the SiO_2 trajectory. The deviations from the SiO_2 line occur during the HNO_3 part of the cycle, where conversion of the bulk material to an oxide is actually taking place.

For this surface-degraded film, Fig. 4 shows similar results, but first with the sample maintained in the dry N_2 ambient for about 1h, then exposed to air. The surprising feature here, in contrast to similar results for c-Si, is the lack of adsorption of atmospheric contaminants or water vapor, and the extremely slow growth of the oxide film. These observations are consistent with the generally inert behavior of a-Si(H) with regard to oxidation or contamination.[7,8]

CONCLUSION

We have presented optical data that are consistent with the model of a columnar microstructure for a-Si(H), with an outer layer that is somewhat less dense than the bulk. The results imply that regions of the heterogeneous material that contribute to the

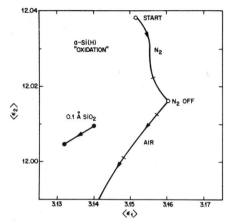

Fig. 4 As Fig. 2, but "oxidation" first in dry N_2, then air. Marks indicate 1h intervals. The reference increment corresponds to growing 0.1Å of SiO_2.

visible-near uv optical parameters are similar in local structure to a-Si. Oxidation studies are interpreted most simply as the consumption of the inhomogeneously distributed a-Si fraction to form SiO_2. The ability to monitor such changes in real time and as a function of energy provides a powerful tool for studying reaction processes and microscopic mechanisms in these materials.

REFERENCES

1. D. E. Aspnes and A. A. Studna, Appl. Opt. 14, 220 (1975); Rev. Sci. Instrum. 49, 291 (1978).
2. B. G. Bagley, D. E. Aspnes, and A. C. Adams, Bull. Amer. Phys. Soc. 25, 12 (1980).
3. D. E. Aspnes, J. B. Theeten, and F. Hottier, Phys. Rev. B20, 3292 (1979).
4. J. C. Knights, J. Non-Crystalline Solids 35 & 36, 159 (1980).
5. The normal component can be ignored to a good approximation because the dominant contribution to an ellipsometrically measured <ε> spectrum comes from the component along the intersection of the surface and plane of incidence (D. E. Aspnes, J. Opt. Soc. Am. 70, 1275 (1980)).
6. D. E. Aspnes and A. A. Studna (to be published).
7. D. E. Aspnes, B. G. Bagley, A. A. Studna, C. J. Mogab, and F. B. Alexander, Jr., Bull. Amer. Phys. Soc. 22, 1263 (1977).
8. H. Fritzsche and C. C. Tsai, Solar Energy Materials 1, 471 (1979).

312

EFFECT OF THERMAL ANNEALING ON THE STRUCTURAL AND ELECTRICAL PROPERTIES OF THE Pd-a-Si:H INTERFACE

C. C. Tsai, R. J. Nemanich, and M. J. Thompson*
Xerox Palo Alto Research Center, Palo Alto, CA 94304

ABSTRACT

The interface between Pd and hydrogenated amorphous Si is probed by interference enhanced Raman spectroscopy and Schottky electrical measurements. With the growth of crystalline Pd_2Si, which is accelerated at elevated temperatures, the Schottky barrier improves by lowering both the ideality factor and reverse-biased saturation current. After low temperature annealing at 180-230°C, Schottky diodes become almost ideal with an ideality factor of 1.05 and a barrier height of 0.97eV. Auger depth profile reveals that the annealed interface becomes essentially oxygen free. In contrast, no silicides form on aged Si, and the Schottky diodes remain nonideal after annealing.

INTRODUCTION

The metal-semiconductor interface plays an important role in many semiconductor devices. It is fascinating that few atomic layers at the interface can dominate the performance of the entire semiconductor device through the formation of various types of contacts. From studies of metals on crystalline Si (c-Si) it has been established that silicides form at the interface and the composition and structure of these compounds are dependent on the thermal history of the sample.[1] We have chosen the interface between Pd and hydrogenated amorphous Si (a-Si:H) for our study for two reasons. First, there has been considerable interest in making Schottky barrriers on a-Si:H using both Pt and Pd for large area device applications including solar cells. Secondly, Pd-silicides are of the easiest, most stable silicides to form on c-Si. By simultaneously investigating the structural and electrical properties of the Pd-a-Si:H interface as a function of thermal annealing, we hope to improve our understanding of the physics of the metal-a-Si:H interface.

The structure of interfaces are probed using interference enhanced Raman scattering (IERS).[2,3] Through optical interference effects this technique permits observation of spectral features due to thin film structures that are < 2nm in thickness. The electrical properties of interfaces are determined by measuring the current density versus voltage characteristics of Schottky barriers. In addition, Auger electron spectroscopy gives the compositional depth profile of the interface. Emphasis is made on the effect of the native oxide on a-Si:H, since impurities at interfaces are known to inhibit silicide growth on c-Si.[1]

*On sabbatical leave from the Department of Electronics, Univ. of Sheffield, Sheffield, England.

EXPERIMENTAL

The IERS method[2] employs a multilayer sample configuration-a very thin (2-6nm) layer of Pd is thermally evaporated onto a 10nm thin film of a-Si:H, which then lies on top of a 40nm transparent SiO_2 spacer and an Al reflector. Thicknesses of the layers are adjusted according to a computer calculation so that most incident laser radiation is absorbed by Pd and a-Si:H, and the electrical field intensity is strongest near the Pd-a-Si:H interface. Using this technique backscatter Raman spectra can be obtained from very thin films with intensities enhanced 10-1000 times over that from the corresponding bulk samples.[2] Backscatter Raman experiments were carried out with a 514.5nm Ar^+ laser operating at a relatively low power level of ~ 40mW to minimize sample heating.

Schottky diodes were fabricated by thermally evaporating 4-10nm thick, 1mm-diameter Pd pads onto a 0.2-2μm thick layer of undoped a-Si:H, which lies on top of a 50nm thick n^+ a-Si:H film. Ni, Mo, or Cr bottom electrodes were sputtered onto the quartz substrates prior to the plasma deposition of the n^+ layer. A large sample-to-source distance minimized sample heating during the Pd deposition.

The a-Si:H films were deposited at the anode at a temperature of 230°C in a diode system[4] where a pure SiH_4 plasma was excited with 1-2W of rf power. This is a well characterized material known to contain ~8 at.% hydrogen and very few defects. Before the Pd deposition all a-Si:H films suffered an exposure to air and were therefore etched in a 10% HF solution to remove some surface oxide prior to the Pd evaporation. All annealing studies and thin film depositions (except a-Si:H) were made in diffusion pump vacuums.

RESULTS AND DISCUSSION

As has been described previously,[3] rather similar Pd-silicides form on thin a-Si:H films as compared to those on bulk c-Si both in terms of crystal structures and formation temperatures. Shown in Fig. 1 are the Raman spectra which indicate the interface structures and reaction products of Pd on a-Si:H. Curve (a) represents the as-deposited sample measured within hours after the Pd deposition. While spectral features dominated by the broad peak at ~ 480cm^{-1} are due to the amorphous Si network vibrations, several sharp lines appeared from ~90 to 210cm^{-1} which are attributed to a crystalline silicide phase with a composition near Pd_2Si. The Pd network, however, has no Raman active modes. The power of IERS is demonstrated by the fact that silicide features were clearly evident immediately after deposition, and it was estimated that < 2nm Pd was consumed to form Pd_2Si. The silicide growth continues at a slow rate at room temperature, and accelerates at elevated temperatures. Curve (b), obtained after 15 minute annealing at 150°C, indicates further growth of the Pd_2Si lines relative to the a-Si features. Subsequent annealing at 230°C introduced new spectral features (curve(c)). After

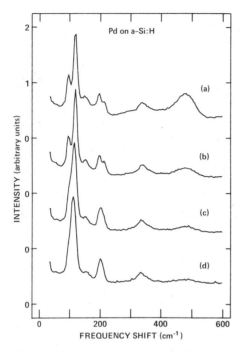

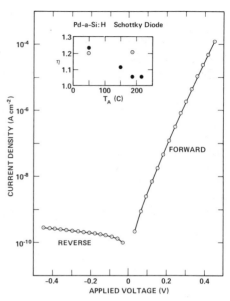

Fig. 1. Raman spectra of Pd on a-Si:H-(a) as deposited; (b), (c), and (d) after 15 minute annealing at 150, 230, and 300°C, respectively.

Fig: 2. J-V characteristics of as-deposited Pd Schottky diodes on fresh or etched a-Si:H. The insert shows the dependence of the ideality factor on the annealing temperature for Pd on fresh or etched a-Si:H (closed circles), and on aged a-Si:H (open circles).

300°C annealing the spectrum became dominated by these new features (curve (d)), which have been attributed to another crystalline silicide phase with a composition also near Pd_2Si.

Now let us discuss the corresponding electrical measurements. The current density (J) of a practical Schottky diode at a given temperature T depends on the applied voltage (V) according to the equation

$$J = J_0 \exp[(qV/\eta kT) - 1] \qquad (1)$$

where J_0 is the saturation current density and $\eta (\geq 1)$ the diode ideality factor. An ideal Schottky diode has $\eta = 1$. Assuming the thermionic emission theory applies, the barrier height can be obtained from the T-dependence of J_0. A more detailed discussion on Pd-a-Si:H Schottky diodes is given elsewhere.[5]

The J-V characteristics of the as-deposited Schottky diodes which are shwon in Fig. 2, exhibit a high rectification ratio with an initial ideality factor of 1.23. The diode is not stable at room temperature. Following the growth of the Pd$_2$Si phase at the interface, both η and the reverse-biased saturation current decrease. Thermal annealing, which accelerates the silicide growth, also speeds up changes in the diode characteristics. A 15-minute annealing at 150°C causes a significant drop of η to 1.11, while a similar change can be achieved by aging at room temperature for several weeks. Meanwhile the Pd pads often changed color from a metallic appearance to brown, which is also an indication of silicide formation. Additional annealing at 180°C, which corresponds to further consumption of Si and Pd to form silicides, makes nearly ideal diodes with $\eta \sim 1.05$. Moreover, their T-dependence of the J-V characteristics measured between 190 to 380 K follows the thermionic emmision theory and yields a barrier height of 0.97eV. The Schottky barriers now become very stable at room temperature. Additional annealing at 230°C converts most of the first Pd$_2$Si structure into the second phase. Nevertheless, the diode characteristics remain almost ideal. The annealing behavior of η is shown by the closed circles in the insert in Fig. 2. This almost ideal diode behavior has been consistently and reproducibly obtained through thermal annealing in the range of 180-230°C.

It is unlikely that heat treatments below the deposition temperature of a-Si:H would vary the material significantly enough to account for such drastic changes in the electrical properties of samples. Rather we believe the improved Schottky barrriers are a direct result of the silicide growth. With the progressive growth of silicides, the interface is moving deeper into the bulk of a-Si:H.

Since all a-Si:H films suffered some air exposure prior to the Pd evaporation, Auger spectroscopy was employed to investigate where the oxide resides. The compositional depth profile of an aged a-Si:H film without the Pd top electrode indicates that oxidation of a-Si:H causes a ~ 0.5nm thin oxide to form in 6 weeks and is confined to the surface. To examine the effect of annealing on the oxide distribution, a compositional depth profile was obtained from a 300°C annealed diode

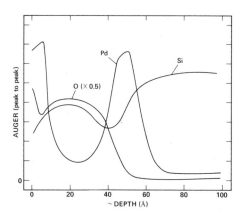

Fig. 3. Auger depth profile of a Pd-a-Si:H diode annealed to 300°C for 15 minutes.

which consisted of a 6nm Pd film on an unetched fresh a-Si:H film, which is shown in Fig. 3. Most dramatic is the fact that the oxygen level dropped below the detection limit before reaching the silicide-a-Si:H interface. And oxides originally present at the interface were relocated above the silicide layer. Although Si usually is the dominant diffusive species in silicide growth on c-Si, the Auger result suggests that Pd diffusion through the oxide is responsible for the initial silicide formation in the present case.

While removal of native oxides on c-Si is essential to ensure uniform silicide growth on c-Si, but no difference in the annealing behaviors was found on a-Si:H whether the a-Si:H was freshly prepared ($<$ 1 hour air exposure) or aged and then etched. However, completely different results were obtained when we repeat the Pd deposition on a-Si:H samples that were stored for several months. No evidence of silicide formation was observed even after annealing to 400°C. The J-V characteristics also indicated nonideal Schottky diodes with η remained high as shown by the open circles in the insert in Fig. 2. Since aged a-Si:H films are not expected to have significantly thicker oxides that the "fresh" ones,[6] these results suggest that the oxide coverage becomes more uniform in the aged samples. Thus the aged samples lack weak points in the oxide layer which facilitate the silicide formation.

We believe that two effects account for the almost ideal Schottky behavior after vacuum thermal annealing. One is the removal of oxides from the interface region. The other is that the interface moves deeper into the bulk of a-Si:H. Consequently a more "bulk"-like a-Si:H material, which presumably has fewer defects and impurities than the surface, is involved in the formation of the Schottky barrier. The silicide growth, however, is responsible for both effects.

The authors are indebted to R. I. Johnson, and R. A. Lujan for their assitance in sample preparation.

REFERENCES

1. For a review see G. Ottaviani, J. Vac. Sci. Technol. 16, 1112 (1979).
2. G. A. N. Connell, R. J. Nemanich, and C. C. Tsai, Appl. Phys. Lett. 36, 31, (1980); R. J. Nemanich, C. C. Tsai, and G. A. N. Connell, Phys. Rev. Lett. 44, 273 (1980); C. C. Tsai and R. J. Nemanich, J. Non-Cryst. Solids, 35 & 36, 1203 (1980).
3. C. C. Tsai, R. J. Nemanich, and T. W. Sigmon, J. Phys. Soc. Japan 49, Suppl. A, 1265 (1980); R. J. Nemanich, C. C. Tsai, M. J. Thompson, and T. W. Sigmon (to be published).
4. J. C. Knights, Proc. of Conf. on Structure and Exitations in Amorphous Solids, ed. by G. Lucovsky, and F. L. Galeener (AIP, NY, 1976), p. 296.
5. M. J. Thompson, N. M. Johnson, R. J. Nemanich, and C. C. Tsai (to be published).
6. H. Fritzsche, and C. C. Tsai, Solar Energy Materials 1, 471 (1979).

DIFFUSION LENGTH OF HOLES IN a-Si:H BY THE SURFACE PHOTOVOLTAGE METHOD*

J. Dresner, D. J. Szostak, and B. Goldstein
RCA Laboratories
Princeton, NJ 08540

The diffusion length L for holes in undoped a-Si:H films has been measured by using a variation of the Surface Photovoltage Method[1] where the sample was illuminated with unmodulated light and the surface photovoltage ΔV was measured with a vibrating Kelvin probe. The measurements were performed in high vacuum ($\sim 5 \times 10^{-9}$ Torr); this made it possible to remove the surface oxide by argon ion sputtering and thus vary the nature of the surface barrier. The composition of the surface was monitored by Auger Electron Spectroscopy. The samples were prepared by decomposition of SiH_4 in a DC glow discharge at substrate temperatures of $T_s = 330^{\circ}C$ and $T_s = 240^{\circ}C$.

Values of L in the range 0.33μ to 0.45μ were found for samples prepared at both substrate temperatures. After prolonged illumination (60 hours of ~1 Watt/cm^2) a reduction to L = 0.17μ was observed. The original value of L was restored after annealing at 200°C. We have also found that in a sample made at $T_s = 330^{\circ}C$, L had a constant value of 0.4μ over a range of illumination from 7×10^{13} to 5×10^{16} photons/cm^{2}sec. Since one expects illumination to decrease the width of the surface depletion layer, this results suggests that our measurement of L is not influenced by the surface charge field.

1) A.M. Goodman, J. Appl. Phys. 32, 2550 (1961)

*This research was supported by Solar Energy Institute under Contract No. XJ-9-8254 and by RCA Laboratories, Princeton, NJ 08540

PROBLEMS REGARDING THE CONDUCTANCE IN a-Si:H FILMS*

H. Fritzsche and M. Tanielian
University of Chicago, Chicago, IL 60637

ABSTRACT

The doping dependence of the effect of adsorbed water on the conductance of plasma-deposited a-Si:H films is explained by assuming that adsorbed water donates about 5×10^{10} electrons/cm^2 and produces an accumulation layer in n-type samples and a depletion layer in p-type samples. The anomalously large conductivity prefactor σ_0 in intrinsic films and the decrease of σ_0 with decreasing conductivity activation energy are discussed in terms of homogeneous and heterogeneous models for electronic conduction.

INTRODUCTION

It is remarkable that, after years of active research into the properties of plasma-deposited amorphous silicon, we are still unable to account for the simplest material characterization: the electrical conductance. First, the distinction between bulk and surface conductance is difficult to achieve; small amounts of adsorbates, oxide layers, and even the substrate affect measurements with coplanar electrodes.[1] We shall discuss these problems in the first section. However, even when the conductivity is measured under conditions which reduce space charge effects, its value and temperature dependence cannot be successfully interpreted with the conventional model for amorphous semiconductors. This model predicts for conductivity due to extended state transport above a mobility edge:

$$\sigma = \sigma_0 \exp(-E_a/kT) \qquad (1)$$

where σ_0 is about 600 ohm^{-1}cm^{-1}. There are two surprising problems with this model: (i) when E_a is between 0.9 and 1.0 eV, the prefactor σ_0 reaches values of order 10^6 ohm^{-1}cm^{-1}, and (ii) σ_0 decreases with decreasing E_a according to the empirical Meyer-Neldel rule, when E_a is changed either by doping,[1-4] different preparations,[2] or light-induced changes in defect concentration.[5] We shall discuss the high σ_0 values and the relation between σ_0 and E_a in terms of various models proposed to explain the observed values. We suggest the possibility that compositional and structural heterogeneities affect the transport properties in these films.

SURFACE AND BULK CONDUCTANCE: THE EFFECT OF ADSORBED WATER

After an a-Si:H film is heat-dried at 160° in vacuum and darkness, its conductance at T=300K is strongly affected by various adsorbates or insulating overlayers which act as electron donors or acceptors.[6] Figure 1 shows the effect of water adsorption on the conductance at 300K as a function of E_a of the samples in the heat-dried state A. The films were deposited at a rate of 1.5 Å/s on Corning 7059 substrates held at 500 < T_s<550K in a (9:1) Ar to SiH$_4$ plasma mixture. PH$_3$ or B$_2$H$_6$ were used as dopant gases. The ordinate of Figure 1 shows the maximum conductance G$_B$ measured after initiation of a flow of nitrogen containing 20% relative humidity relative

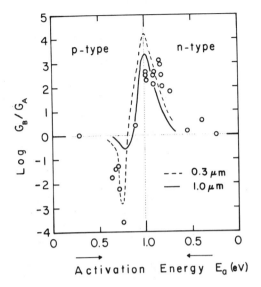

Fig. 1. Effect of adsorbed water on conductance as a function of doping. Curves are the result of simple model calculations.

to G_A of the heat-dried state. The increase in G observed for n-type and near intrinsic samples is interpreted as resulting from an electron accumulation layer produced by the adsorbed water. Since the space charge conductance dominates the bulk conductance, the effect is quite insensitive to thickness except for highly doped samples in which G_B/G_A is small because the Fermi level E_F lies in a region of high density of states $N(E)$. For p-type samples the decrease in G is the result of a hole depletion region. It is important to note that decreases in G by 2 or 3 orders of magnitude require that the depletion region must extend through most of the sample thickness.

Very large changes are, therefore, observed only for 0.3-0.4 μm thick samples.

The curves marked 0.3 μm and 1.0 μm are the results of model calculations for two film thicknesses in which water donates a charge Q to the bulk, creating a space charge layer. The bulk density of states $N(E)$ is based on the capacitance measurements of Tiedje et al.[7] and B = 0.08 eV

$$N(E) = N_0 \cosh (E/B) \qquad (2)$$

where $N_0 = 2 \times 10^{15}$ eV^{-1} cm^{-3}, and the best fit charge donated to the film $Q = 5 \times 10^{10}$ el/cm^2. Given the simplicity of the calculation, we feel the agreement between experiment and theory in Figure 1 supports this model for the effect of adsorption on the conductance. An improved fit with the data is expected when the change of $N(E)$ with doping, the distribution of surface states, and the initial surface band bending of the heat-dried state A can be taken into account.

THE RELATION BETWEEN σ_0 AND E_a

The prefactor σ_0 of Eq. (1) increases with E_a and reaches values exceeding 10^6 ohm^{-1} cm^{-1}. Figure 2 shows this trend as well as the scatter of the results from the Dundee group,[2] from RCA,[4] and from our group. In judging the relation between σ_0 and E_a, only samples of the same laboratory should be compared because of systematic differences in the preparation conditions between laboratories. Our data include both n- and p-type samples but only those which obey Eq. (1) between 300 and 480K. We do not observe the decrease in the slope of the $\ln\sigma$ vs. 1/T curve to a lower E_a above T=420K, as re-

320

ported by Spear et al.[2] We sometimes observe a decrease in slope below 350K. This occurs also in several samples of the Marburg group.[3] This extra, low-T conductance is quite surface sensitive, and we, therefore, identify it with some form of surface conductance.

Assuming conduction in extended states, one expects

$$\sigma = eN_c \, \mu\exp(-\Delta E/kT) \qquad (3)$$

where $\Delta E = E_c - E_F$ for electrons. With reasonable values for the mobility $\mu = 5 \ cm^2/Vs$, for the effective density of states $N_c = 2.5 \times 10^{19} \ cm^{-3}$ at E_c, the prefactor in Eq. (3) is 20 $ohm^{-1} \ cm^{-1}$. Using this value, we calculated ΔE at T=300K from Eq. (3). The right-hand scale of Fig. 2 shows $E_a - \Delta E$; this is the unaccounted part of the activation energy. Only about 0.07 eV of this difference can be due to the inward shift of the band states with temperature. In the following we discuss two models for the anomalously large values of σ_o (or of $E_a - \Delta E$) and its dependence on E_a: (i) Spear et al.'s suggestion[2] of a T-dependence of the mobility edge and (ii) conduction in heterogeneous materials.

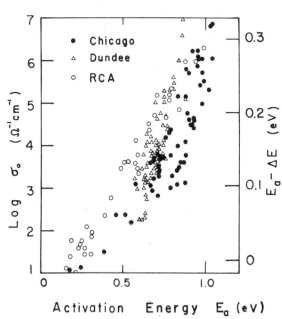

Fig. 2. Dependence of σ_o on E_a. Chicago data include both n- and p-type samples. Sample marked * had visible microstructure.

Spear et al.[2] suggested that an increasing number of the weakly localized tail states below the T=0 mobility edge become extended as T is increased. This leads to a downward shift of E_c which is linear with T above 200K. According to Spear et al. the temperature coefficient is larger the higher E_c lies (at T=0) above E_A, the edge of the tail states. This separation in turn is expected to be largest for samples having high disorder and large random potentials. These are then the samples with large E_a and σ_o values.

Several experimental results may be used to test this hypothesis. One expects that the disorder is enhanced by (a) light-induced creation of defects,[5] (b) doping, (c) compensating double doping,[8] and (d) annealing which leads to effusion of hydrogen. Process (a) indeed increases E_a and σ_o in qualitative agreement with the model. Doping, however, causes a rapid decrease in these values, as shown in Figure 2, and compensation as well as hydrogen effusion do not yield unusually large σ_0 values. Moreover, drift mobility experiments suggest that the conduction band tail is much narrower[9] than the valence band tail,[10] yet n-type and p-type samples are essentially indistinguishable in Figure 2.

We agree with Spear et al.[2] that the T-dependence of E_c and E_v should not be ignored. However, we do not find the suggested correlation of the magnitude of this dependence with disorder. In our samples we also do not find the bending over of the conductivity curves to a lower E_a above T=430K where in Spear et al.'s model the mobility edge essentially approaches the end of the tail states.

Even though all avenues of explaining the anomalous behavior of the conductivity have not been fully explored within homogeneous conduction models, one should consider the possibility that the conduction properties are strongly influenced by structural and compositional heterogeneities. Morphologies on the 100-1000 Å scale have been observed in many samples[11,12] with grains or columns containing only a few at. % hydrogen separated by intergrain regions enriched with mono- and polyhydrides of silicon. Moreover, gettered oxygen as well as other impurities and atoms from dopant gases probably enhance the heterogeneities. Some dopant gases, such as B_2H_6, were found to influence strongly the film morphology.[12] Even though no microstructure could be observed by scanning electron microscopy in the majority of samples used in Figure 1, structural and compositional heterogeneities might be present but difficult to detect because of contrast and resolution limitation.

Two models for heterogeneity will be considered. Thus, heterogeneities may arise from fluctuations in the random distribution of hydrogen and of doping atoms or from granular models in which grains of higher conductivity are surrounded by thin high resistive regions. The former situation can be treated by percolation theory whereas in the latter case the conduction is impeded by the barriers of the intergrain regions.

Fluctuation models have been discussed by Brodsky[13] and by Overhof and Beyer.[14] Using only long-range Coulomb potential fluctuations, the latter authors were able to explain the $E\mu=0.005-0.15$ eV difference between the activation energies of the conductivity and the thermopower S(T) observed in a-Si:H doped with P or Li. They obtained[3]

$$\ell n \sigma(T) - (e/k)S(T) = C - E\mu /kT .   \qquad (4)$$

They also found an increase in C with $E\mu$ by about 10^3. Although this relationship between C and $E\mu$ agrees quite well with the experimental values obtained from Eq. (4), it does not yield the increase of σ_0 with E_a shown in Figure 2 because $E\mu$, and hence C, tends to decrease with increasing E_a. However, their model for N(E) leads to a temperature shift of $E_F(T)$ which produces a decrease of σ_0 from 10^4 ohm^{-1} cm^{-1} at $E_a = 0.8$ eV to 10^2 ohm^{-1} cm^{-1} at $E_a = 0.4$ eV when one assumes $\mu = 25$ cm^2/Vs and a constant value $E\mu = 0.1$ eV. The higher σ_0 values for larger E_a remain unexplained.

Granular models are often used to describe the transport properties of polycrystalline semiconductors. They predict,[15] in essential agreement with experiments, that the Hall coefficient R measures the carrier concentration within the grains whereas the conductivity has an additional activation energy ϕ which corresponds to an effective barrier height. This naturally leads to an activated Hall mobility $R\sigma\propto\exp(-\phi/kT)$. Similarly, the thermopower S, which is determined by an open-circuit voltage measurement, is expected to correspond closely to S of the grains near the contacts. This leads to an activation energy difference between $\ln\sigma$ and S of $E\mu = \phi$. One is reminded of the warning by Bube[16] that similarities between crystalline and amorphous semiconductors may have entirely different origins. However, the magnitudes of $E\mu$ and of the Hall mobility activation energy[17] in a-Si:H are nearly the same. Furthermore, a substantial increase of σ_0 with E_a is most frequently found in heterogeneous, nonstoichiometric semiconducting alloys[18] and in materials which consist of observable grains surrounded by resistive barriers.

The conductivity prefactor of a granular amorphous material has not yet been calculated. It will be enhanced, however, by the temperature dependence of the effective barrier height and by the fact that the applied field is no longer uniform over the sample length but concentrated at the resistive barriers which add up to a small fraction of this length.

We end with the following question and problem. Does σ_0 also decrease when the separation E_c-E_F (or E_F-E_v) is lowered by charging the material without changing in any way N(E)? If that is so, then the conventional analysis of the field effect[19] is incorrect and greatly overestimates the deduced density of states.

*Supported in part by the NSF-MRL program at The University of Chicago and by NSF Grant DMR8009225.

1. H. Fritzsche, Solar Energy Materials 3, 447 (1980).
2. W. E. Spear, D. Allan, P. LeComber, and A. Ghaith, J. Non-Cryst. Solids 35/36, 357 (1980).
3. W. Beyer and H. Overhof, Solid State Commun. 31, 1 (1979).
4. D. E. Carlson and C. R. Wronski, Topics in Applied Physics, Vol. 36, ed. M. H. Brodsky (Springer, New York, 1979), p. 287.
5. D. L. Staebler and C. R. Wronski, J. Appl. Phys. 51, 3262 (1980).
6. M. Tanielian, et al., J. Non-Cryst. Solids 35/36, 575 (1980).
7. T. Tiedje, et al., Solar Cells 2, (1980).
8. R. A. Street, D. K. Biegelsen, and J. C. Knights, to be published.
9. T. Tiedje, et al., Appl. Phys. Lett. 36, 695 (1980).
10. A. R. Moore, Appl. Phys. Lett. 31, 762 (1977).
11. J. Knights, J. Non-Cryst. Solids 35/36, 159 (1980).
12. E. A. Schiff, et al., Appl. Phys. Lett. 38, 92 (1981).
13. M. H. Brodsky, Solid State Commun. 36, 55 (1980).
14. H. Overhof and W. Beyer, to be published.
15. G. H. Blount, et al., J. Appl. Phys. 41, 2190 (1970); M. G. Mathew and K. S. Mendelson, J. Appl. Phys. 45, 4370 (1974).
16. R. H. Bube, J. Appl. Phys. 47, 2223 (1976).
17. T. Dresner, Appl. Phys. Lett. 37, 742 (1980).
18. G. Busch, Helv. Phys. Acta 19, 189 (1946).
19. Nancy B. Goodman and H. Fritzsche, Phil. Mag. B42, 149 (1980).

A Study of Amorphous Si:H:F Alloys Using
MIS Tunnel Junctions**

I. Balberg* and D. E. Carlson
RCA Laboratories, Princeton, NJ, 08540, U.S.A.

ABSTRACT

The effect of fluorine inclusion on the amorphous silicon-hydrogen alloys is studied by the measurements of G-V and C-V characteristics of MIS devices where S is such an alloy. It is found that fluorine is either eliminating deep gap states or adding new donor states, but there is no evidence for elimination of states closer than 0.2 eV to the band edges. The inclusion of fluorine does not significantly change the resistivity or the activation energy (10^2 Ωcm and $\sim$0.2 eV) of amorphous films heavily doped with phosphorus. The very low values for the resistivity and the activation energy ($\stackrel{<}{\sim} 10^{-1}$ Ωcm and 0.02 eV) reported for silicon-hydrogen-fluorine alloys are associated with the crystallization of these alloys.

INTRODUCTION

Recently Madan et al[1] have reported reasonably efficient solar cells ($\eta \sim$ 6.3%) using glow discharge decomposition of H_2 and SiF_4. Comparison of this material with a-Si:H shows that it has the same photoconductivity but a significantly improved doping efficiency. In particular, conductivities as high as 10^1 $(\Omega$ cm$)^{-1}$ and activation energies as low as 0.02 Ev were reported for phosphorus or arsenic doped films. These observations were attributed to the reduction of the density of states near and above mid-gap.[2]

In order to evaluate the role of the fluorine on the density of states and the doping efficiency, we have carried out a systematic study of the G-V and C-V characteristics of MIS (metal-insulator-semiconductor) structures where S was an amorphous silicon-hydrogen-fluorine alloy (a-Si:H:F).

EXPERIMENTAL CONDITIONS

The MIS junction used for the present study has the same structure as the four terminal devices described in earlier studies[3].

*Present address: The Racah Institute of Physics, The Hebrew University, Jersualem, Israel.
**Research reported herein was supported by Solar Energy Research Institute, under Contract No. XJ-9-8254, and by RCA Laboratories, Princeton, NJ, 08540, U.S.A.

ISSN:0094-243X/81/730323-06$1.50 Copyright 1981 American Institute of Physics

The amorphous material was deposited in one of four glow discharge systems; a dc proximity system, an ac (60Hz) system, an rf (13.56 MHz) system and an rf magnetron-diode glow-discharge system. The flow rates and pressures of the discharge atmosphere (mixtures of SiH_4 and SiF_4) were the same as in our previous work [3]. The effect of the substrate temperature, T_s, on the material was studied for the temperature interval $330 \geq T_s \geq 200°C$. The doping levels, to be quoted below, are given by the ratio of the dopant gas, (PH_3 or SiF_4), to the silane in the gas mixtures.

The measurement technique which has been described in detail previously [3] is based on a modulation of the applied dc bias by a small test signal and the detection of the ac current through the MIS device. The in-phase current is proportional to the conductance of the device, G, while the out-of-phase current is proportional to ωC where ω is the test signal frequency and C is the capacitance of the device. In the present study all measurements were taken using a test signal amplitude of 1 mV and a frequency of $2\pi \times 10^3$ rad/sec.

EXPERIMENTAL RESULTS

The composition of several films were determined by means of both secondary ion mass spectroscopy (SIMS) and electron probe microanalysis. For a dc discharge in 10% SiF_4, 90% SiH_4, the film consisted of ~89 at.% silicon, ~10 at.% hydrogen, ~0.43 at.% fluorine and ~0.8 at.% oxygen. Films made in pure SiH_4 (Liquid Carbonic, CCD grade) discharges under similar operating conditions usually contained ~10 - 12 at.% hydrogen and ~0.1 - 0.5 at.% oxygen. (For all films, the nitrogen and carbon content was always less than 0.1 at.%). The phosphorus content of doped films was found to be generally 2 to 3.5 times larger than that present in the gas phase. Electron diffraction measurements taken on films used in the present study did not reveal any evidence for crystallinity.

Fig. 1 shows the variation of resisitivity with substrate temperature for a series of films made in a dc discharge system. The effect of adding SiF_4 is to reduce the resistivity by a factor of less than two in sharp contrast to the large effects reported by Madan et al [2]. The most conductive material produced in the present study had a resistivity of 75 Ω-cm and an activation energy of 0.17 eV ($PH_3/SiH_4 = 10^{-2}$ and $SiF_4/SiH_4 = 10^{-1}$).

Before considering the role of the fluorine in the amorphous alloy, consider the behavior of the non-fluorinated material. The "conductance well" observed for undoped or lightly doped a-Si:H is

associated with tunneling of electrons from the metal into the semiconductor conduction band for a negative bias, and from the semiconductor valence band to the metal for a positive bias[3]. In cases
where the semiconductor is very resistive, the voltages V_c and V_v at
which the conductance rises sharply are proportional to $E_c - E_F$ for
V_c (<0) and $E_F - E_v$ for V (>0). Thus, the ratio:

$$V_c/V_v = (E_c - E_F)/(E_F - E_v) \tag{1}$$

is a good measure of the location of the Fermi level [3]. When the
material becomes more n-type or more conducting, the ratio V_c/V_v,
will become larger than $(E_c - E_F)/(E_F - E_v)$[4,5].

In Fig. 2 we show the effect of phosphorus doping on the G-V
and C-V characteristics of a-Si:H. In undoped a-Si:H the conductance
well is nearly symmetric and contains no peak while the capacitance
is constant and equals the geometrical capacitance. At intermediate
doping levels ($PH_3/SiH_4 \stackrel{\sim}{\sim} 10^{-3}$), the G-V characteristic is rounded
and there is a peak in the conductance which depends on the test sig-
nal frequency (see Fig. 2(a)). These results can be interpreted by
assuming [4,5] that the doped a-Si:H behaves as a crystalline semiconductor which has a peak in the density of surface states at the
energy level $E = E_c - 0.45$ eV. With increasing doping levels the
conductance peak disappears while the capacitance peak appears to
move towards larger negative voltages as shown in Fig. 2(b). A step-
like structure is observed in the conductance due to tunneling into
states which are located below the midgap. The density of these
states is known to be enhanced by phosphorus doping[3].

The apparent sharp decrease of the capacitance at voltages for
which the conductance rises sharply is due to the phase variation in
the lock-in detector. The increase of the capacitance from positive
to negative voltages may be a combination of the capacitance peak
shift (to be expected with the rise of E_F) and a capacitance increase
associated with sensing states below midgap. The narrowing of the
conductance well is associated with the increasing conductivity of the
semiconductor which causes an increase in the voltage drop across the
oxide for a given applied bias. The narrowing of the well and the
shift in the Fermi level towards higher energies thus moves the
peak in the G-V and the C-V characteristics out of the well.

In Fig. 2(c) we see the effect of a further increase in the
doping as the conductance well narrows due to the increasing conductivity of the semiconductor. The structure in the G-V characteristic is masked by the sharp rise of the metal-to-bands tunneling
conductance. The capacitance has now an additional increase for an
applied positive bias due to the ionized donors (as is the case in
MOS devices) and/or to the sensing of the states above the midgap
which can be achieved in the highly conducting materials [5] (having
a shorter time constant for the generation-recombination process).

The results shown in Fig. 2 are similar to those obtained with other deposition methods.

The effect of fluorine on a material which is intermediately doped ($PH_3/SiH_4 \sim 10^{-3}$) is demonstrated in Fig. 3 ($SiF_4/SiH_4 = 10$). The effect of fluorine is to lower the resistivity and to eliminate the peak in both the G-V and C-V characteristics. Comparison of this figure to Fig. 2 indicates that the effect of the fluorine is the same as increasing the doping from about $PH_3/SiH_4 \sim 10^{-3}$ to about $PH_3/SiH_4 = 10^{-2}$. Similar results were obtained with other glow discharge methods.

In Fig. 4 we show the effect of an order of magnitude increase in the fluorine content on a highly doped ($PH_3/SiH_4 \sim 10^{-2}$) material. The behavior shown in Fig. 4(a) is similar to the behavior shown in Fig. 2(b), and the behavior shown in Fig. 4(b) is similar to that shown in Fig. 2(c). These results confirm that the effect of fluorine is similar to the effect of increasing the doping level. Also there are no drastic changes in the resistivity or the characteristics which may indicate changes in the density of states close to the band edges. Comparison of Figs. 3 and 4 indicates that the doping efficiency does not improve significantly when SiF_4/SiH_4 exceeds 10^{-1}.

The relative position of the Fermi level in the fluorinated material has been determined to be ~ 0.2 eV below E_c from the I-V characteristics [3].

DISCUSSION

In the present study the inclusion of fluorine may be either adding new donor states or may be removing defect states near midgap. The first effect may be explained by the fact that fluorine has donor levels in crystalline silicon which are located at $E_c - 0.21$ eV and $E_c - 0.66$ eV [6,7]. The first level may act then as a donor level as long as it is above E_F. However, neither this effect nor the elimination of deep centers can explain an E_F which is closer to E_c than about 0.2 eV. The explanation for the high conductivity and low activation energy observed by Madan et al. [2] has to be based on a mechanism of elimination of states close to the band edges. Since these states are usually tail states due to the disordered nature of the amorphous material, they can be eliminated by crystallization. Such effects have been observed in materials prepared by glow discharge [8]. This study showed that at high rf power deposition or at low deposition rates the Si:H alloy crystallizes yielding a phosphorus-doped material with conductivity of about 10 $(\Omega cm)^{-1}$ and an activation energy of 0.02 eV. The fact that the crystallization is enhanced by the dopants may explain the discrepancy between Madan et al's density of states and their resistivity and activation energy results. The field effect measurements were carried out on a material which was not heavily doped while the low resistivity and activation energy are associated with heavily doped material, where crystallization is more likely.

The electrical and structural properties of the films used in the present study may have been influenced by the large concentration of oxygen ($\sim$0.8 at.%). However, by increasing the power density in a dc discharge we have recently succeeded in making high conductivity films ($\sim$10 Ω^{-1} cm^{-1}), and electron diffraction measurements confirm the films are microcrystalline.

Hence the effect of crystallization can explain the low resistivity and the low activation energy found in some Si:H and Si:H:F alloys. The effect of fluorine in the amorphous Si:H:F alloys is to either eliminate deep defect-states in the gap or add new donor levels, and thus improve the doping efficiency as long as the Fermi level is below the band tail states ($E_c - E_F \gtrsim 0.2$ eV).

REFERENCES

1.   A. Madan, J. McGill, W. Czubatyj, J. Yang and S. R. Ovshinsky, Appl. Phys. Lett.

2.   A. Madan, S. R. Ovshinsky and E. Benn, J. Phil. Mag. 40, 259 (1979).

3.   I. Balberg, Phys. Rev. B, October (1980).

4.   I. Balberg and D. E. Carlson, Phys. Rev. Letters 43, 58 (1979).

5.   I. Balberg, J. Electronic Materials, 9, 797 (1980).

6.   P. Su, A. Sher, Y. H. Tsuo and J. A. Moriarty, Appl. Phys. Letters 36, 991 (1980).

7.   A. Goetzberger, E. Klausmann and M. J. Schulz, CRC Critical Reviews in Solid State Sciences 6, 1 (1976).

8.   A. Matsuda, S. Yamasaki, K. Nakagawa, H. Okushi, K. Tanaka, S. Iizima, M. Matsumura and H. Yamamoto, Japan J. Appl. Phys. 19, L305 (1980).

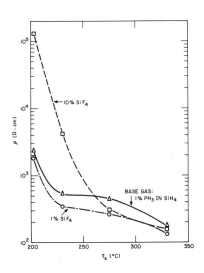

Fig. 1.   Resistivity as a function of substrate temperature for a series of phosphorus-doped films made in a dc glow discharge system.

328

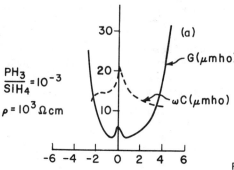

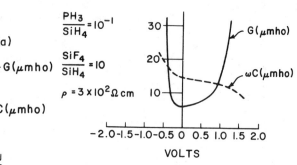

Fig. 3. The G-V and C-V characteristics obtained for a MIS device where S is intermediately doped a-Si:H ($PH_3/SiF_4 = 10^{-3}$) with a high ($\gtrsim$ 2 at.%) fluorine content ($SiF_4/SiH_4 = 10$). The amorphous material was deposited in an rf magnetron-diode glow-discharge system.

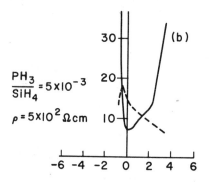

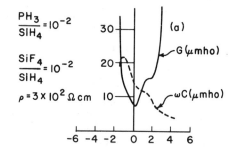

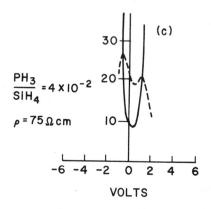

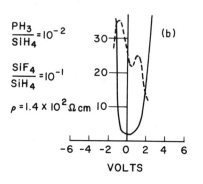

Fig. 2. The effect of increasing phosphorus doping level from 10^{-3} (a) through 5×10^{-3} (b) to 4×10^{-2} (c) on the G-V and C-V characteristics of a MIS device, where S is n-type a-Si:H. The amorphous material was deposited in an ac glow discharge system.

Fig. 4. The effect of increasing fluorine content from ~0.05 at.% (a) to ~0.5 at.% (b) on the G-V and C-V characteristics of a MIS device where S is highly doped n-type a-Si:H. The amorphous material was deposited in a dc glow discharge system.

THICKNESS DEPENDENCE OF THE RESISTIVITY OF AMORPHOUS HYDROGENATED SILICON ON VARIOUS SUBSTRATES*

Gordon O. Johnson,** J. A. McMillan and E. M. Peterson
Solid State Science Division
Argonne National Laboratory, Argonne, IL 60439

ABSTRACT

The Staebler-Wronski effect has been studied in glow-discharge a-Si(H) by making thickness vs. resistivity measurements for films produced under varying deposition conditions and on different substrates. For films grown on sapphire, the resistivity in both the photo-induced and annealed states remains constant with film thickness except for an increase in resistivity for films less than .2 μm thick. The results on all the films are consistent with both the photo-induced and annealed states exhibiting bulk resistivity. Films grown on microscope slides behave similarly to films grown on sapphire for applied fields of less than 10 V/cm but for larger fields exhibit a switching effect. This switching, unlike the switching observed in amorphous chalcogenide semiconductors is characterized by long rise and decay times, from several minutes at 150 °C to hours at room temperature.

INTRODUCTION

In 1977, Staebler and Wronski[1] made the first observation of photo-induced changes in the dark conductivity of amorphous silicon. Since that time, several explanations for the observed effects have been suggested[1-4] but no consensus as to the origin of the effect has been reached.

Solomon et al.[3] deduced, using the field effect technique, that the high resistivity, photo-induced state was a bulk state characterized by a flat band condition at the film surfaces while the low resistivity, annealed state was characterized by interfacial charges which produced band bending at the interfaces. This band bending could give rise to either a higher or lower resistivity layer as compared to the bulk. For the annealed state it was proposed that the bands were bent upward resulting in a highly conducting layer with a lower activation energy. This view seems to be supported by Malhiot et al.,[5] who reported that their samples exhibited a thickness independent resistance in the annealed state.

On the other hand, Ast and Brodsky[6,7] measured the conductivity of phosphorous doped samples, concluding that the resistivity was thickness independent, except for a high resistivity layer about .2 μm thick.

---

*Work supported by the U.S. Department of Energy.
**Permanent address: Walla Walla College, College Place, WA 99324.

Likewise, Staebler and Wronski,[4] and Jansse et al.[8] concluded
that the annealed state was a bulk state on the basis of their measurements of the forward bias characteristics of Schottky diodes made
from a-Si(H) films. Tanielian et al.[9] also believe that their experiments with various absorbates indicate that the photo-induced and
annealed states are bulk states.

An examination of the conductivity vs. temperature curves for
a-Si films prepared by the various groups that have studied the
Staebler-Wronski effect indicates that preparation conditions[10] and
perhaps the substrate chosen may influence the magnitude of the
change between the photo-induced and annealed states very strongly.
For this reason we decided to study thickness vs. resistivity curves
for sets of a-Si grown under different deposition conditions, and also
using different substrates.

EXPERIMENTAL DETAILS

All of the films used were prepared by the RF decomposition of
silane in a conventional diode deposition apparatus which gives essentially zero bias on the electrode holding the substrate. The RF
frequency was 7 mHz. The substrates used were either quartz, sapphire, or Clay Adams #3015 microscope slides. The planar electrodes
for electrical measurements were electron beam evaporated niobium and
were placed on the substrate before depositing the films. The electrodes were spaced at either .5 or 1 mm and almost always produced
ohmic contacts. The resistivity measurements were all carried out at
a pressure $< 10^{-5}$ Torr. A typical experiment consisted of heating
the sample at 150 °C for several hours to degas, and then illuminating at room temperature for from 2 to 24 hours. All resistivity measurements were made while heating or cooling at the uniform rate of
ca. 1 °/min. to avoid effects produced by rapid temperature changes.[11]

RESULTS AND DISCUSSION

The electrical resistivity and activation energy in both the
photo-induced and annealed states are shown in Figs. 1 and 2 vs.
thickness for sets of films grown under different deposition conditions. The resistivity is constant for films thicker than .2 μm for
both the photo-induced and annealed states. For thinner films there
is an increase in resistivity, especially for the thinnest films which
are about .05 μm thick. The activation energy of the films of Fig. 1
does not appear to increase as the films get thinner. For the films
of Fig. 2 there seems to be an increase in activation energy for films
thinner than .2 μm. The increase in resistivity and activation energy
for the annealed state of Fig. 2 is similar to that observed by Ast
and Brodsky[6] for P-doped films except that the changes in our films
start at a thickness of about .2 μm instead of .5 μm. The changes
which occur in the resistivity and activation energy are very similar
for the photo-induced and annealed states indicating that the high resistivity of the thin films is not caused by the annealing process and
is independent of the Staebler-Wronski effect. It seems likely, that
the increase in resistivity is connected with a decrease in hydrogen

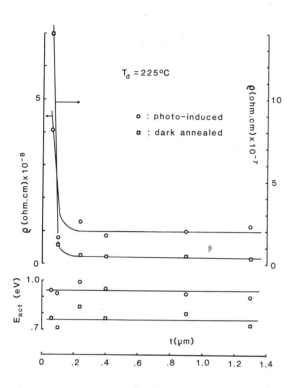

$T_d = 225°C$

o : photo-induced

□ : dark annealed

Fig. 1. Resistivity and
activation energy for
a-Si(H) films prepared
from 10% SiH_4-Argon
mixtures at 225 °C,
power = 1 watt,
pressure = .08 Torr and
electrode spacing = 7.3
cm.

Fig. 2. Resistivity and
activation energy for
a-Si(H) films prepared
from 10% SiH_4-Argon mixtures at 335 °C,
power = .8 W,
pressure = .13 Torr and
electrode spacing = 4.8
cm.

content observed at both
the free surface and the
substrate-film interface.

Neither of these sets
of films reproduced the
results of Malhiot et al.[5]
who found that the resis-
tance of films deposited
on microscope slides did
not change with thickness.
In an effort to reproduce
their results, we depos-
ited films on glass and
sapphire substrates at
the same time. The films
deposited on sapphire are
shown in Fig. 2. The
temperature dependence of
the resistance of one of
these films is shown in
Fig. 3. Notice that there
is only about a factor of
10 between the resistance
of the photo-induced and

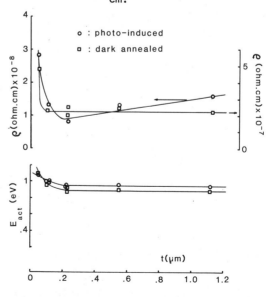

o : photo-induced

□ : dark annealed

annealed states. The resistance of the corresponding film deposited on microscope slide glass is shown in Fig. 4. There is now a 4 decade difference in the resistance of the photo-induced and annealed

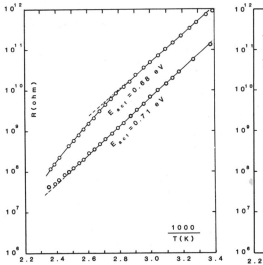

Fig. 3. Resistance of the photo-induced and annealed states for a 1.13 μm a-Si(H) film deposited on sapphire.

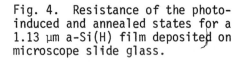

Fig. 4. Resistance of the photo-induced and annealed states for a 1.13 μm a-Si(H) film deposited on microscope slide glass.

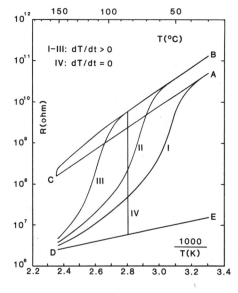

Fig. 5. Switching effect of the a-Si(H) glass system.

state at room temperature and the activation energy of the annealed state is now only .16 eV instead of .75 eV. The resistance of all

the other films deposited on microscope slide glass has a similar
temperature dependence. The resistance of the glass substrate alone
is also shown in Fig. 4. The differences in resistance between the
films of Fig. 3 and 4 are not due to differences in the Staebler-
Wronski effect between the films but are instead due to a peculiar
switching effect found in films deposited on microscope slide glass.
A schematic diagram of this switching behavior is shown in Fig. 5.
With applied fields of about 100 V/cm and following our usual heating and annealing schedule, path II is followed from the photo-
induced state B to the fully annealed state D. If the applied field
is only 50 V/cm, the start of annealing is delayed and path III is
followed from B to D. For very small applied fields (10 V/cm) the
film never anneals to D. Instead, path BCA is followed. This path
looks very much like a normal Staebler-Wronski cycle. If the film is
heated and annealed with no applied field and a field of 100 V/cm is
then applied, the resistance of the film changes from C to D. Path I
from A to D is for a 300 V/cm field starting from point A. If the
film is heated with no applied field to T $\cong$ 80 $^\circ$C and then a field of
200 V/cm is applied while the temperature remains constant, path IV
will be taken over a period of several hours. If a field of 1000 V/cm
is applied at point A and the temperature kept constant, the resistance will at first not change at all. However, after about 10 minutes, the resistance will begin to change towards lower values. The
change, however, is very gradual and even after 6 hours the resistance
is still changing. If the film is taken to E with 100 V/cm field
and then the field is reversed, the resistance will gradually move
irreversibly to point A. In order to return to E with the 100 V/cm
field, the film must be taken through a heating and annealing cycle.

We also compared the resistivities of films deposited on sapphire and quartz at the same time, but there were never any differences between the two.

REFERENCES

1. D. L. Staebler and C. R. Wronski, Appl. Phys. Letters 31, 292
    (1977).
2. S. R. Elliott, Phil. Mag. B39, 349 (1979).
3. I. Solomon, T. Dietl and D. Kaplan, Le Journal de Physique 39,
    1241 (1978).
4. D. L. Staebler and C. R. Wronski, J. Appl. Phys. 51, 3262 (1980).
5. C. Malhiot, J. F. Currie, S. Sapieha, M. R. Weetheimer and A.
    Yelon, J. Non-Crystalline Solids 35 and 36, 207 (1980).
6. D. G. Ast and M. H. Brodsky, J. Non-Crystalline Solids 35 and
    36, 611 (1980).
7. D. G. Ast and M. H. Brodsky, Phil. Mag. B41, 273 (1980).
8. D. Jousse, R. Basset, S. Delionebus and B. Bourdon, Appl. Phys.
    Letters 37, 208 (1980).
9. M. Tanielian, H. Fritzsch, C. C. Tasi, and E. Symbalisty, Appl.
    Phys. Letters 33, 353 (1978).
10. D. I. Jones, A. A. Gibson, P. G. LeComber and W. E. Spear,
    Solar Energy Mats. 2, 93 (1979).
11. D. G. Ast and M. H. Brodsky, Inst. Phys. Conf. Ser. 43, 1159
    (1979).

334

INTERFERENCE FRINGE ANALYSIS OF a-Si:H SCHOTTKY BARRIER CELLS

David L. Staebler

RCA Laboratories*   Laboratories RCA Ltd.
Princeton, NJ 08540   and   Zurich, Switzerland

ABSTRACT

The photoresponse of a-Si:H Schottky barrier cells has interference fringes at long wavelengths. It is shown that the modulation strength of the fringes can vary with applied voltage. Measurements were made on Pt Schottky barrier cells produced by glow
discharge at RCA Laboratories, Princeton, and in cells produced by
low pressure CVD at Laboratories RCA Ltd., Zurich. The results are
compared to a computer model calculation. The variation in fringes
are found to be due to changes in the width of the carrier collection region. In the cells tested, primary photocurrent for sub-
bandgap excitation is due to carriers generated in or very close
to the Pt-layer.

INTRODUCTION

The absorption coefficient of amorphous silicon is low at
optical wavelengths longer than 800 nm. As a result, Pt Schottky
barrier cells can have strong interference fringes, both in reflectivity and photocurrent, because of optical resonance between the
Pt layer and the reflecting substrate. This paper shows how such
fringes can be used to analyze the photocurrent for sub-bandgap
light. A theoretical analysis is presented first. Experimental
results follow.

THEORY

Figure 1 shows the structure used in this analysis. It consists of a reflecting substrate, a layer of undoped a-Si:H about
500 to 700 nm thick, an a 5-nm-thick Pt-layer. (The thin n-layer
normally used to make good contact to the substrate is ignored in
this analysis for simplicity.) The region marked W is the collection width, the region in which there is sufficient built-in
electric field to collect all optically generated holes. When the
cell is illuminated with monochromatic light, multiple reflections
within the a-Si:H sets up the standing wave pattern shown in
Figure 1. This pattern causes fringes in the collection efficiency
spectrum. As is shown below, the strength of the fringes depends
on W.

* Present Address.

ISSN:0094-243X/81/730334-05$1.50 Copyright 1981 American Institute of Physics

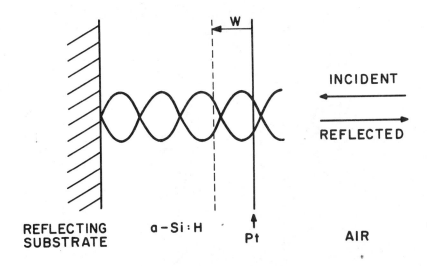

Fig. 1. Pt-Schottky-barrier cell structure used in this study, showing the optical standing waves caused by the interference of incident and reflected light.

The collection efficiency was calculated with a computer program, assuming a 5-nm-thick Pt-layer and a 675-nm-thick a-Si:H layer. The a-Si:H optical absorption was taken from the data of Crandall [1] for undoped material. The optical constants for the substrate were taken from those for pure Fe, and should not be too different from those for stainless steel. I also assumed that each photon absorbed in W produces a free hole and electron that are collected at opposite sides (the hole at the Pt, the electron at the stainless steel), and that photons absorbed outside of W do not generate any primary photocurrent.

Figure 2 shows the calculated results. The top curves are the collection efficiencies (charges collected per incident photon) for different values of W. The bottom curve shows the reflectivity of the entire cell. It is subtracted from unity to show the correlation with the efficiency fringes. The data show clearly that the strength of the efficiency fringes depends on W. In particular, the fringes become prominent when W approaches 25 nm. In a simplified view, this happens because W is less than the distance between nodes in the optical standing wave (Figure 1). If W is much larger, it contains many nodes, and the fringes are weaker.

336

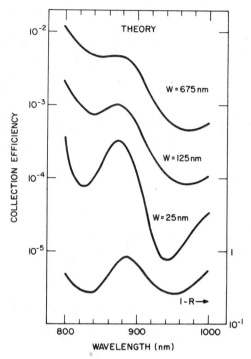

Fig. 2. Calculated values of collection efficiency and reflectivity for the structure shown in Fig. 1.

EXPERIMENT

Figure 3 shows experimental results for a Pt-Schottky-barrier
cell on stainless steel. The a-Si:H was produced in a dc glow discharge at a substrate temperature of ~330°C. The cell thickness
was ~600 nm. W was more than 400 nm, as determined from the collection efficiency spectrum in visible light [2]. Nevertheless,
the zero bias curve in Figure 3 is consistent with a W less than
125 nm (see Figure 2). Note particularly the shape of the experimental fringe minimum at λ = 920 nm. It is similar to the theoretical curve for W = 25 nm.

The top curve in Figure 3 shows the photoconductivity spectrum
measured with a forward bias beyond flat band. This current comes
from electrons generated throughout the entire thickness of the
a-Si:H layer [1]. Indeed, the fringes are weak, consistent with
the top curve of Figure 2, where W is equal to the full thickness
of the cell.

Results for a cell made by LPCVD and post hydrogenation [3]
are given in Figure 4. The fringes are prominent. For λ > 900 nm,
they don't depend on bias; the curves just shift up and down. For
λ ~ 800 nm, the reverse bias increases the collection efficiency,
but decreases the fringe modulation.

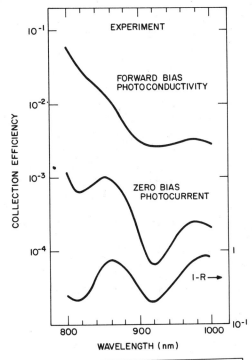

Fig. 3. Measured values for an a-Si:H cell. The zero bias curve shows the spectrum for primary photo-current, while the top curve is that for photoconductivity.

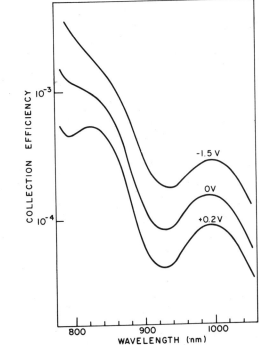

Fig. 4. Collection efficiency for a LPCVD cell, measured at a reverse bias of 1 volt, zero bias, and a forward bias of 0.2 volt.

DISCUSSION

Both cells have strong fringes in the primary photocurrent for $\lambda > 900$ nm, similar to that calculated for W = 25 nm. There are two possible reasons why the apparent W is only 25 nm. One is that W decreases to this value for sub-bandgap light. The other is that the current is dominated by internal photoemission of electrons from the Pt [4]. This current should also have strong interference fringes [5]. Indeed, I verified this with another computer analysis. The fringing should be similar to that calculated for W = 25 nm. In addition, the photoemission current should vary with applied bias as shown in Figure 4. A reverse bias should decrease the energy threshold for photoemission, and thus increase the current [5]. At 800 nm, current due to collection of holes from the a-Si:H begins to dominate, as shown by the decrease in fringes.

The magnitude of the measured collection efficiency is much more than the value predicted for W = 25 nm (Figure 2). This favors the internal photoemission model for $\lambda > 900$ nm. Crandall [1] has seen sub-bandgap photocurrent due to collection of holes via gap state transport, with weak fringes in undoped samples. In the cells studied here, this current may be obscured by the larger current due to internal photoemission.

The author acknowledges A. Bell for help in the calculations, H. Keiss for the use of his experimental equipment, and R. Keller for technical assistance. The cells were provided by J. Dresner and A. Widmer. This research was supported by Solar Energy Research Institute, under Contract No. XJ-9-8254, and by RCA Laboratories, Princeton, NJ, and Laboratories RCA Ltd., Zurich, Switzerland.

REFERENCES

1. R. S. Crandall, Solar Cells 2, 319 (1980).
2. C. R. Wronski, IEEE Transactions on Electron Devices ED24, 351 (1977).
3. D. L. Staebler and A. Widmer, presented at March Meeting of the German Physical Society, Freudenstadt, W. Germany, 1980.
4. C. R. Wronski, B. Abeles, G. D. Cody and T. Tiedje, Appl. Phys. Lett. 37, 96 (1980).
5. R. Williams, Semiconductors and Semimetals, Vol. 6, p. 97 (Academic Press, New York, 1970).

Author Index